*Each page of this book has
stolen hours from our family life.
We hope that our Wives Layla and Brunella
will appreciate this repairing dedication.*

Springer

Milano
Berlin
Heidelberg
New York
Barcelona
Hong Kong
London
Paris
Singapore
Tokyo

Luigi Allegra • Francesco Blasi (Eds)

Chlamydia pneumoniae
The Lung and the Heart

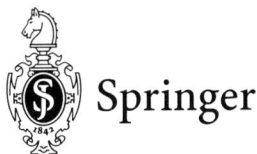 Springer

LUIGI ALLEGRA
FRANCESCO BLASI
Institute of Respiratory Diseases
University of Milan
IRCCS Ospedale Maggiore
Milan, Italy

The Editors and Authors wish to thank ABBOTT S.p.A. for the support
and help in the realization of this volume

© Springer-Verlag Italia, Milano 1999

ISBN 88-470-0047-5

Library of Congress Cataloging-in-Publication data: applied for

Cover design: Simona Colombo
Typesetting: Photo Life (Milan)
Printing and binding: Staroffset (Cernusco sul Naviglio, Milan)

Printed in Italy

SPIN: 10704070

Table of Contents

List of Contributors

Luigi Allegra
Institute of Respiratory Diseases,
University of Milan,
IRCCS Ospedale Maggiore,
Via F. Sforza 35, 20122 Milan, Italy

Cristina Arosio
Institute of Respiratory Diseases,
University of Milan,
IRCCS Ospedale Maggiore,
Via F. Sforza 35, 20122 Milan, Italy

Gian Luca Biscione
Department of Respiratory Medicine,
University of Naples "Federico II",
Monaldi Hospital, 80100 Naples, Italy

Peter Black
Department of Medicine,
University of Auckland,
Private Bag 92019, Auckland,
New Zealand

Francesco Blasi
Institute of Respiratory Diseases,
University of Milan,
IRCCS Ospedale Maggiore,
Via F. Sforza 35, 20122 Milan, Italy

Jens Boman
Department of Clinical Virology,
University of Umeå, 901 85 Umeå,
Sweden

Lee Ann Campbell
Department of Pathobiology,
University of Washington,
Seattle,WA 98195, USA

Roberto Cosentini
Emergency Medicine Department,
IRCCS Ospedale Maggiore,
Via F. Sforza 35, 20122 Milan, Italy

Laura Fagetti
Institute of Respiratory Diseases,
University of Milan,
IRCCS Ospedale Maggiore,
Via F. Sforza 35, 20122 Milan, Italy

Charlotte A. Gaydos
Department of Medicine,
Division of Infectious Diseases,
The Johns Hopkins University,
Baltimore, MD 21205-2196, USA

Giuliana Gialdroni Grassi
Chair of Chemotherapy,
University of Pavia, Via Taramelli 5,
27100 Pavia, Italy

J.Thomas Grayston
Department of Epidemiology,
University of Washington,
Seattle, WA 98195, USA

Sandeep Gupta
Department of Cardiological Sciences,
St. George's Hospital Medical School,
Cranmer Terrace, London SW17 0RE, UK

Enrique Gurfinkel
Department of Internal Medicine,
Coronary Care Unit, Favaloro Foundation,
Avenida Belgrano 1746,
1093 Buenos Aires, Argentina

David L. Hahn
Family Practice Department,
Dean Medical Center, Arcand Park Clinic,
3434 East Washington Ave.,
Madison, WI 53704, USA

Margaret R. Hammerschlag
Department of Pediatrics,
State University of New York Health
Science Center at Brooklyn,
Brooklyn, NY 11203-2098, USA

Sebastian L. Johnston
University Medicine (810),
University of Southampton,
Southampton General Hospital,
Tremona Road,
Southampton SO16 6YD, UK

Juan Carlos Kaski
Coronary Artery Disease Research Group,
Department of Cardiological Sciences,
St. George's Hospital Medical School,
Cranmer Terrace, London SW17 0RE, UK

Cho-chou Kuo
Department of Pathobiology,
University of Washington,
Seattle,WA 98195, USA

Maija Leinonen
National Public Health Institute,
Department in Oulu, P.O.Box 310,
90101 Oulu, Finland

Joachim Lorenz
Department of Pulmonary and Intensive
Care Medicine and Infectious Diseases,
District Hospital Lüdenscheid,
Paulmannshöherstrasse 14,
58515 Lüdenscheid, Germany

Michael S. Niederman
Pulmonary & Critical Care Medicine,
Winthrop-University Hospital,
222 Station Plaza North, Suite 400,
Mineola, NY 11501, USA,
and SUNY at Stony Brook

Rosanna W. Peeling
Laboratory Centre for Disease Control,
Health Canada, 1015 Arlington Street,
Winnipeg, Manitoba, Canada R3E 3R2

Pekka Saikku
Chlamydia Laboratory, National Public
Health Institute, Department in Oulu,
P.O.Box 310, 90101 Oulu, Finland

David A. Smith
Coronary Artery Disease Research Group,
Department of Cardiological Sciences,
St. George's Hospital Medical School,
Cranmer Terrace, London SW17 0RE, UK

Paolo Tarsia
Institute of Respiratory Diseases,
University of Milan,
IRCCS Ospedale Maggiore,
Via F. Sforza 35, 20122 Milan, Italy

San-pin Wang
Department of Pathobiology,
University of Washington,
Seattle, WA 98195, USA

History of *Chlamydia pneumoniae* (TWAR)

J.T. Grayston, S.-P. Wang

Isolation of TW-183

The history of the TWAR organism, now called *Chlamydia pneumoniae,* began in Taiwan in 1965. A field trial was under way testing an inactivated yolk sac-grown trachoma vaccine [1]. The trial was carried out in children, the endpoint being reduction in the incidence of clinical trachoma. At that time there was no adequate method to measure antibody response, and the organisms could be isolated only in the yolk sac of the embryonated egg. The children were followed by means of periodic isolation attempts from conjunctival swabs. A swab collected on 20 November 1965 from a child with the clinical diagnosis of trachoma dubium was frozen until 15 February 1966 and then inoculated in the yolk sac of embryonated eggs. This isolation attempt was the 2715th in our laboratories at the U.S. Medical Research Unit, No. 2, in Taipei. Dr. Russell Alexander was in charge of the laboratory at the time of these isolation attempts. In the first passage all eggs survived for 13 days and no elementary bodies were demonstrated on Macchiavello's stain of yolk sac smears. A second blind passage was routinely made, and in the yolk sac of these eggs, typical elementary bodies of *Chlamydia* were demonstrated. The isolate was named TW-183, because it was the 183rd isolate in the laboratory. It was assumed that the isolate was a *Chlamydia trachomatis* strain.

Characterization of TW-183

New isolates were immunotyped in the mouse toxicity prevention test. This was a laborious test that depended on the fact that high-titer *C. trachomatis* yolk sac suspensions killed mice within 18 h after intravenous injection. This toxic death could be prevented by prior immunization of the mice with a sub-lethal dose of a homologous strain [2]. Cross-challenge experiments had by that time demonstrated six separate immunotypes of *C. trachomatis* (now serovars A–F) [3]. In order to define a new immunotype we required three isolates that cross-protected with each other but not with any of the known immunotypes.

In typing tests, TW-183 repeatedly failed to produce toxic death in mice, even with a 40% yolk sac suspension. When it was used as an immunizing strain, it failed to protect against any of the established immunotypes. We assumed it was an as yet unidentified immunotype and waited to find other new isolates with which it would cross-protect.

A suspension of TW-183 was heat-inactivated and employed as antigen in the complement fixation (CF) test for *Chlamydia* with known positive sera. It reacted similarly to established *Chlamydia* CF antigen. This method is a classic way to demonstrate that a new isolate belongs to the *Chlamydia* genus.

TW-183 was tested by intracerebral inoculation of suckling mice. No symptoms or death were produced, suggesting that it was unlikely to be a lymphogranuloma venereum (LGV) organism. It was tested for its ability to cause follicular conjunctivitis in monkeys. Despite two separate challenges to the right eye of three monkeys, no follicular conjunctivitis resulted; only mild inflammatory changes could be seen. These findings were unlike those with any *C. trachomatis* isolate previously tested.

During 1968 and 1969, the micro-immunofluorescence (MIF) serologic test for *Chlamydia* was developed [4]. One of its first uses was to replace the mouse toxicity prevention test for immunotyping isolates of *C. trachomatis*. By 1972 we had typed 400 isolates from around the world and classified them into 15 serovars. TW-183 remained untypeable.

TW-183 Is Not *Chlamydia trachomatis*

In 1970 cell culture for *Chlamydia* became available. A fourth egg passage of TW-183 was inoculated to HeLa 229 cell culture. The inclusions observed were iodine stain-negative. When stained with Giemsa the inclusions were densely packed, did not indent or displace the nucleus, and lacked vacuolar structures. This morphology is characteristic of *C. psittaci* and not *C. trachomatis*.

Antibody Against TW-183

TW-183 as antigen in the MIF test appeared similar qualitatively in the immunofluorescent reaction with homologous antisera to that seen with the established *C. trachomatis* serovars. TW-183 was used as antigen in the MIF test to explore the presence of antibody in several different groups of human sera. Since the isolate was originally from the eye of a child, it was tested against a group of sera from 32 families observed for the incidence and prevalence of trachoma [5]. The sera from 191 family members were tested against 11 *C. trachomatis* serovars and TW-183. Most of the antibody found against *C. trachomatis* was serovar C or B. Antibody against TW-183 was frequently found in these families in both children and adults, but it was not related to the presence or absence of eye disease. Table 1 shows the prevalence of antibody against TW-183 and all *C. trachomatis* types by age group. Antibody was common against TW-183 (68%) and against *C. trachomatis* (58%), but there was no evidence of a relation

Table 1. *Chlamydia* MIF antibody in families from rural Taiwan studied for trachoma

Age in years	No. tested	% with antibody	
		TW-183	*C. trachomatis*[a]
0–4	20	15	15
5–9	61	51	49
10–14	43	81	53
15–29	11	64	82
30–39	27	81	81
40–49	12	83	92
50+	17	94	76

[a] Antibody against any of 11 *C. trachomatis* immunotypes

between the two. These MIF tests used an IgMAG conjugate. Conjugates for individual immunoglobulin fractions were not yet available. The higher percentage of antibody in adult males than in females, which has been extensively demonstrated 20 years later, was seen here. The highest titer TW-183 antibody was found in 10- to 14-year-olds. Two had antibody titers of ≥ 512, which suggested recent infection.

Sera from other studies in Taiwan were explored for the presence of antibody against TW-183, in order to gain insight into the importance of this organism. A very high prevalence of antibody was found in an aboriginal population, and a high prevalence in Taiwan Chinese.

One hundred women with cervicitis at the National Taiwan University Hospital clinic were tested with 11 *C. trachomatis* serovars and TW-183. Any *C. trachomatis* serovars antibody was found in 38%, while 61% had antibody against TW-183. This was early evidence that infection with TW-183-like organisms is more common than *C. trachomatis* infection, even in persons with a clinical disease often caused by *C. trachomatis*. There was also a high prevalence of TW-183 antibody found in young adult Chinese bar girls (66%) and American airmen (71%) on Taiwan.

In retrospect, these findings fit in very well with what is now the well-known seroepidemiology of *C. pneumoniae*. At the time, the results were surprising. Such a high frequency of *Chlamydia* antibody in apparently normal populations had no precedent. We did conclude that the untypeable TW-183 was probably not a cause of eye disease but was a very common infection. Although the serological findings were perplexing they did prepare us to understand the significance of the later findings with TW-183 and pneumonia.

IOL-204/207

Another interesting development in the history of TWAR in the 1970s was a publication from England which included a sentence stating that an isolate called IOL-207 from a conjunctival scraping from a child with trachoma in Iran was similar immunologically to TW-183 [6]. No data showing this relationship was published then or subsequently. Unfortunately, the early history of IOL-207 is confused and uncertain. Professor Barrie R. Jones of the Institute of Ophthalmology, University of London, came to our laboratory in early 1970 to be instructed in the technique of the MIF test. At that time we began an exchange with Professor Jones of a number of eye and genital tract *Chlamydia* isolates we were attempting to fit in to the immunotyping scheme. For example, Professor Jones's laboratory had a new isolate that fit in with isolates that we had obtained that became the new serovar G.

Among the untypeable strains that we provided to Professor Jones was TW-183. In the exchange of untypeable strains we received an isolate, labeled IOL-207, said to be from the eye of a child in Iran. We were subsequently advised in May of 1970 that an error had been made in the designations of isolates, and the one that we received should have read IOL-204, an isolate from the vagina of a woman in England, who had a *Chlamydia* punctate keratitis. We found that the now relabeled isolate, IOL-204, produced iodine-negative inclusions in cell culture. We informed Professor Jones of this fact because of the potential danger to personnel of a pathogenic *C. psittaci* strain. In a June 1971 letter, Professor Jones stated that they had confirmed that this strain produced iodine-negative inclusions. Then, in a July 1971 letter, he explained in some detail about the isolation of IOL-204 from the fourth passage of eggs, and how it had been confused with the vaginal isolate. He stated that "there is no doubt that IOL-204 came from eggs inoculated with scrapings from an eye in Iran". Dr. Jones raised the possibility of some cross-contamination during the four yolk sac passages before the isolate was found.

Subsequently, the Jones group published several serologic studies with this isolate now called IOL-207 as antigen [7, 8]. It was described as atypical *Chlamydia* with characteristics of both *C. trachomatis* and *C. psittaci*. Its inclusions were iodine-negative but it was susceptible to sulfadiazine and caused follicular conjunctivitis in baboons. Except for iodine staining, these are characteristics of *C. trachomatis* isolates not TW-183.

TW-183 Is Associated with Pneumonia

During the 1970s there was increased interest in the possible role of *C. trachomatis* in respiratory infections. This culminated in the demonstration by Dr. Marc Beem at the University of Chicago that pneumonia with a prominent croup-like cough in infants under the age of 6 months could be caused by *C. trachomatis* [9]. Also during the 1970s both our laboratory and that of Dr. Julie Schachter at the University of California in San Francisco were finding some serologic evidence suggesting that *C. trachomatis* might be causing pneumonia and other respiratory infections in adults. The MIF antibody responses in persons with respiratory infections were not the clear-cut antibody rises with good definition commonly seen with acute *Chlamydia* infection.

After the discovery that the TWAR agents caused respiratory infections, re-testing of these sera with TWAR antigen at the same time as *C. trachomatis* antigens made it clear that the antibody titer rises were against TWAR.

The most important step in the elucidation of the role of TW-183 in human respiratory disease came from Dr. Pekka Saikku's fellowship studies in our laboratories. Dr. Saikku came to Seattle in January of 1978 to study the *Chlamydia* MIF test. He brought several groups of sera from Finland from respiratory infection outbreaks in which *Chlamydia* CF antibody was present. After learning the MIF technique he planned to test these sera with the many *C. trachomatis* immunotypes available in our laboratory.

The sera from one outbreak was of particular interest, because it seemed unlikely that *C. psittaci* was the cause of the CF-positive outbreak. This was because of the very mild nature of the pneumonitis and the absence of any bird vectors in this area in winter. The outbreaks were discovered only on routine tuberculosis chest X-ray screening of mostly teenagers and young adults.

When Dr. Saikku tested sera from this outbreak, he was unable to find evidence of significant antibody against any of the *C. trachomatis* serovars. We then suggested that he try TW-183 as antigen, since it remained an untypeable strain to which there was considerable antibody in populations. Significant antibody titer rises and abundant IgM antibody against TW-183 in these sera provided evidence that *Chlamydia* organisms related to TW-183 were the probable cause of the outbreak of pneumonitis [10]. Table 2 shows some of these antibody responses.

Table 2. Results of tests for antibody to *Chlamydia* for seven young men with pneumonitis from whom paired serum specimens were available

Patient no. (age, years)	Days after onset that serum was obtained	Antibody titers[a] MIF test with TW-183		
		IgM	IgG	CF
1 (18)	19	128	512	128
	40	32	512	32
2 (17)	19	256	128	64
	41	32	256	32
3 (16)	30	256	1024	1024
	46	0	2048	102
4 (15)	19	256	512	64
	50	16	512	32
5 (18)	25	128	256	128
	45	128	512	128
6 (18)	19	256	128	32
	36	32	128	16
7 (18)	23	512	1024	128
	34	256	1024	128

None of the patients had antibody to eight individual or pooled elementary body antigens of *C. trachomatis* or to strain 6BC
[a] Reciprocal of final serum dilution

TWAR Causes Acute Respiratory Infections

Because of our continuing interest in pneumonia and acute respiratory infections more severe than the common cold, we had instituted a surveillance of these illnesses in the drop-in medical clinic at the University of Washington's student health service. Following the serologic findings of Dr. Saikku's sera, we began to study the serum pairs and the throat swabs for *Chlamydia* organisms. We inoculated the throat swabs into the yolk sac of embryonated eggs in addition to cell culture. We were fortunate that the throat swab from the 39th student tested had a number of *Chlamydia* inclusions in the first pass in cell culture that could be identified by indirect immunofluorescence. The isolate was successfully propagated in HeLa 229 cell culture and became isolate AR-39 [11].

We began to refer to the group represented by these new isolates as TW-183/AR-39-like organisms. In manuscripts or grant applications the repeated use of the phrase "TW-183/AR-39-like organisms" was fatiguing to the typist and she used the abbreviation TWAR, and when the manuscript was typed the word processor substituted TW-183/AR-39-like organisms for TWAR. We adapted the abbreviation TWAR as the name for the group represented by these isolates.

Additional isolates immunologically similar to the TWAR organisms were made in the student health service study. Some were made directly in cell culture, but often they were isolated only in the yolk sac of the embryonated egg.

The University Student ARD Study completed investigation of 386 patients in a 2.5-year period. From these subjects eight TWAR isolates had been made from 13 patients showing serologic evidence of infection. In our publication of the findings we suggested that the TWAR strains were most likely a new human *C. psittaci* strain transmitted from human to human without a bird or animal reservoir. They had been responsible for 12% of the pneumonia illnesses and 5% of the bronchitis over the 2.5-year period [11].

We made use of two epidemic situations to provide conclusive evidence that the association of the TWAR organisms with acute respiratory disease was etiologic. One was in Finnish military conscripts, the other in University of Washington students [12, 13]. A high proportion of the pneumonia illnesses during the outbreaks were associated with TWAR organisms, both by isolation and serology. With similar laboratory studies available on control groups during the epidemic periods, it was possible to conclude that the TWAR organisms caused the pneumonia illnesses.

Epidemiology of TWAR Infection

To extend our knowledge of the epidemiology and the clinical diseases caused by this group of organisms, we studied by MIF serology serum banks from a variety of epidemiologic studies of respiratory infections. Most important were sera made available from studies in the Seattle area by John Fox and by Hjordis Foy, and from throughout Denmark by Carl Mordhorst. The frequency of infection with the TWAR organisms was documented through age-specific population prevalence and incidence antibody studies [14, 15]. We also gained knowledge of the periodicity of TWAR infection [16], its geographical spread [16], and its incubation period [17].

The etiologic, epidemiologic, and clinical data were summarized by the end of the 1980s and presented a reasonably complete outline of the role of the TWAR organisms in respiratory infections [18].

TWAR Becomes *Chlamydia pneumoniae*

Also at the end of the 1980s there were two new important milestones in the history of TWAR organisms. After 1985, in addition to the studies just described, important advances in our understanding of the organisms were coming from laboratory studies. Ted Kuo demonstrated on electron micrography that the elementary bodies of TWAR organisms differed from those of *C. trachomatis* and *C. psittaci*. They were pear-shaped with a periplasmic space and a loose outer membrane [19]. At the same time, Lee Ann Campbell and her students showed that while the TWAR isolates were closely related with one another, they were less than 10% related by DNA homology with *C. trachomatis* and *C. psittaci* organisms [20]. These two findings, along with the immunological separateness of the TWAR organisms from known *C. psittaci* and *C. trachomatis* strains, led to the acceptance of the TWAR organisms as a new species of the genus *Chlamydia* named *Chlamydia pneumoniae* after the clinical syndrome most frequently associated with infection [21].

While infections of the respiratory tract remain the primary infection caused by *C. pneumoniae*, the organism has been associated with several important chronic diseases. The evidence for an association with atherosclerosis and coronary heart disease is the most fully developed, but data suggesting that the organism may be associated with other chronic diseases have also appeared. Information on *C. pneumoniae* and atherosclerosis and other chronic illnesses is presented elsewhere in this book.

This history has taken TWAR to the point of speciation of the organism as *C. pneumoniae*, at which time considerable information was available on its epidemiology, clinical picture, and microbiology. This rapid expansion of knowledge about *C. pneumoniae* in the space of a few years makes one wonder what the future will bring to the understanding of this important pathogen.

References

1. Woolridge RL, Grayston JT, Chang IH, Cheng KH, Yang CY, Neave C (1967) Field trial of a monovalent and of a bivalent mineral oil adjuvant trachoma vaccine in Taiwan school children. Am J Ophthalmol 63:619-624
2. Wang S-P, Grayston JT (1963) Classification of trachoma virus strains by protection of mice from toxic death. J Immunol 90:849-856

3. Alexander ER, Wang S-P, Grayston JT (1967) Further classification of TRIC agents from ocular trachoma and other sources by the mouse toxicity prevention test. Am J Ophthalmol 63:443-452

4. Wang S-P, Grayston JT (1970) Immunologic relationship between genital TRIC, lymphogranuloma venereum, and related organisms in a new microtiter indirect immunofluorescence test. Am J Ophthalmol 70:367-374

5. Grayston JT, Gale JL, Yeh LJ, Yang CY (1972) Pathogenesis and immunology of trachoma. Trans Assoc Am Physicians 85:203-211

6. Dwyer RS, Treharne JD, Jones BR, Herring J (1972) Chlamydial infection. Results of micro-immunoflurescence tests for the detection of type-specific antibody in certain chlamydial infections. Br J Vener Dis 48:452-459

7. Darougar S, Forsey T, Brewerton DA, Rogers LL (1980) Prevalence of antichlamydial antibody in London blood donors. Br J Vener Dis 56:404-407

8. Burney P, Forsey T, Darougar S, Sittampalam Y, Booth P, Chamberlain R (1984) The epidemiology of chlamydial infections in childhood: a serological investigation. Int J Epidemiol 13:491-495

9. Beem MO, Saxon EM (1977) Respiratory-tract colonization and a distinctive pneumonia syndrome in infants infected with *Chlamydia trachomatis*. N Engl J Med 296:303-310

10. Saikku P, Wang S-P, Kleemola M, Brander E, Rusanen E, Grayston JT (1985) An epidemic of mild pneumonia due to an unusual strain of *Chlamydia psittaci*. J Infect Dis 151:832-839

11. Grayston JT, Kuo C-C, Wang S-P, Altman J (1986) A new *Chlamydia psittaci* strain, TWAR, isolated in acute respiratory tract infections. N Engl J Med 315:161-168

12. Ekman MR, Grayston JT, Visakorpi R, Kleemola M, Kuo C-C, Saikku P (1993) An epidemic of infections due to *Chlamydia pneumoniae* in military conscripts. Clin Infect Dis 17:420-425

13. Grayston JT, Aldous MB, Wang S-P, Kuo C-C, Campbell LA, Easton A, Altman J (1993) Evidence that *Chlamydia pneumoniae* causes pneumonia and bronchitis. J Infect Dis 168:1231-1235

14. Wang S-P, Grayston JT (1990) Population prevalence antibody to *Chlamydia pneumoniae*, strain TWAR. In: Bowie WR, Caldwell HD, Jones RP et al (eds) Chlamydial infections. Cambridge University Press, Cambridge, UK, pp 402-405

15. Aldous MB, Grayston JT, Wang S-P, Foy HM (1992) Seroepidemiology of *Chlamydia pneumoniae* TWAR infection in Seattle families, 1966-1979. J Infect Dis 166:646-649

16. Mordhorst CH, Wang S-P, Myhra W, Grayston JT (1990) *Chlamydia pneumoniae*, strain TWAR, infections in Denmark 1975-1987. In: Bowie WR, Caldwell HD, Jones RP et al (eds) Chlamydial infections. Cambridge University Press, Cambridge, UK, pp 418-421

17. Mordhorst CH, Wang S-P, Grayston JT (1994) Transmission of *Chlamydia pneumoniae* (TWAR). In: Orfila J, Byrne GL, Chernesky MA et al (eds) Chlamydial infections. Esculapio, Bologna, pp 488-491

18. Grayston JT, Campbell LA, Kuo C-C, Mordhorst CH, Saikku P, Thom DH, Wang S-P (1990) A new respiratory tract pathogen: *Chlamydia pneumoniae* strain TWAR. J Infect Dis 161:618-625

19. Chi EY, Kuo C-C, and Grayston JT (1987) Unique ultrastructure in the elementary body of *Chlamydia* sp. strain TWAR. J Bacteriol 169:3757-3763

20. Cox RL, Kuo C-C, Grayston JT, Campbell LA (1988) Deoxyribonucleic acid relatedness of *Chlamydia* sp. strain TWAR to *Chlamydia trachomatis* and *Chlamydia psittaci*. Int J Syst Bacteriol 38:265-268

21. Grayston JT, Kuo C-C, Campbell LA, Wang S-P (1989) *Chlamydia pneumoniae* sp. nov. for *Chlamydia* sp. strain TWAR. Int J Syst Bacteriol 39:88-90

Chlamydia pneumoniae: Culture Methods

C.-C. Kuo

Evolution of Chlamydial Culture Methods

After T'ang et al. in Peking first successfully cultivated trachoma organisms in chick embryo in 1957, egg culture became a standard method of isolation and growth of *Chlamydia trachomatis* [1]. The researchers' success was owed to the use of streptomycin, but not penicillin, for control of contamination. Since egg culture is not only cumbersome for cultivation but also for purification of organisms from yolk sacs, finding a sensitive cell culture method was vigorously pursued. In 1965, Gordon and Quan described a method for isolation of trachoma agents in McCoy cell culture using a flat-bottomed culture vial [2]. To enhance the sensitivity, McCoy cells were irradiated with γ-radiation and centrifugation was applied during the absorption period after specimens were inoculated to culture vials. The procedure was simplified by Ripa and Mårdh, who replaced γ-radiation with the use of cyclo-heximide [3]. In their method non-irradiated McCoy cells were used. To enhance the sensitivity of McCoy cells to *C. trachomatis* growth, cycloheximide was added to culture medium for cultivating infected cells. Cycloheximide inhibits host cell protein synthesis but does not affect chlamydial metabolism; thus, it reduces the competition for nutrients between host cells and parasites and enhances the growth of chlamydial organisms. This cell culture method was quickly adapted, and replaced egg culture for isolation and growth of *C. trachomatis*. Other modified methods have appeared and been used, such as the use of DEAE-dextran-treated HeLa 229 cells [4]. However, the crucial factors are centrifugation and cycloheximide. The use of 96-well microtiter plates for isolation of *C. trachomatis* was first introduced by McComb and Puzniak in 1974 [5] and later popularized by Yoder et al. in 1981 for handling large volumes of clinical specimens [6].

The first *C. pneumoniae* isolate, TW-183, was obtained in embryonated egg yolk sac in 1965 from the eye of a child in Taiwan during a trachoma vaccine study [7]. In our initial attempt to isolate *C. pneumoniae* from the respiratory tract, we used both egg and HeLa 229 cell cultures [7]. It was found that egg culture was less sensitive than HeLa cell culture for isolation of *C. pneumoniae*. Essentially, the cell culture method for *C. trachomatis* was adapted for *C. pneumoniae*. HL [8, 9] and Hep-2 [10, 11] cells were found to be more sensitive than HeLa cells and have become the cell lines of choice for isolating and growing *C. pneumoniae*.

Egg Culture

Seven-day old embryonated chick eggs are used for yolk sac inoculation [7]. Inoculated eggs are incubated at 35 °C. Yolk sac membranes are harvested either when the eggs are killed by the growth of chlamydiae or, if the eggs survive, on day 12 or 13 before hatching. Smears are then made from the yolk sac membrane on microscopic slides, and stained with basic fuchsin (Macchiavello's stain) or fluorescent antibody (FA) for detection of elementary bodies (EBs). Macchiavello's stain is less sensitive than direct FA stain using *C. pneumoniae*-specific monoclonal antibody in detection of *C. pneumoniae* EBs [7].

Cell Culture

HeLa 229 Cells

The first respiratory *C. pneumoniae* isolate, AR-39, was obtained from a university student with pharyngitis in Seattle, Washington, USA in 1983 by HeLa 229 cell culture [7]. We originally used HeLa 229 cells for isolation of *C. pneumoniae*, because it was the cell line we were using at that time – and are still using – for isolation and growth of *C. trachomatis* in our laboratory [12]. Although HeLa 229 cells are sensitive for isolation of *C. pneumoniae*, serial passages of *C. pneumoniae* isolates in HeLa cells were often unsuccessful. Of 25 *C. pneumoniae* strains isolated in HeLa cells, only three were adapted directly to grow in bottle culture after 15–17 passages in vial culture [7]. Cell culture adaptation succeeded with another five strains by inoculation of egg passage 1 or 2 into HeLa cells. However, two egg isolates still failed to pass in HeLa cells.

HL Cells

A human line, HL cells, was originally described by Cavallaro and Monto [13] to be sensitive for isolation and propagation of respiratory syncytial virus. Cles and Stamm found that HL cells were sensitive for laboratory propagation of *C. pneumoniae* strain TW-183 [8]. We further showed that the isolation and propagation of wild *C. pneumoniae* strains were dramatically better than we had observed in HeLa 229 cells [9]. We therefore switched from HeLa 229 to HL cells for routine isolation and propagation of *C. pneumoniae* in 1989.

A kinetic study of growth of *C. pneumoniae* in HL cells showed that *C. pneumoniae* organisms undergo multiple developmental cycles in continuous cultures of HL cells [9]. This phenomenon has not been observed with the trachoma biovar of *C. trachomatis* in HeLa, McCoy, and L cells [14], or in HL cells [9]. The infectivity assays of growth of *C. pneumoniae* in HL cells showed a maturation cycle of 3 days. However, the increases were 100 times greater from day 0 to day 3 than from day 3 to day 6, because the inoculum was centrifuged onto new cell monolayers on day 0 but not on day 3. The difference may be accounted for by the centrifugation effect and more homogeneous infection of the whole monolayer. Therefore, we recommend passage of cell cultures every 3 days.

Studies by Cles and Stamm [8] and Kuo and Grayston [9] suggest that one cell culture system cannot be recommended for the isolation and growth of both *C. pneumoniae* and *C. trachomatis.* While HL cells appeared to be as sensitive as HeLa cells for ocular strains of *C. trachomatis,* they were 100–1000 times less sensitive for genital strains when HeLa cell-adapted strains were used for comparison [9].

Hep-2 Cells

Another cell line commonly used for isolation and growth of *C. pneumoniae* is Hep-2 [10, 11]. Its sensitivity is similar to that of HL cells.

Other Cells

Other cells commonly used in chlamydial cultures, including McCoy, L-929, and BHK-21 [7, 8], have been tested for their sensitivity to *C. pneumoniae.* None of these cells showed any advantage over HeLa 229 or HL cells for growth of *C. pneumoniae.*

Technical Considerations (Table 1)

Enhancement and Optimal Conditions for Cell Culture

Several treatments that have been used to enhance the growth of *C. trachomatis* have been applied to enhance the growth of *C. pneumoniae* [9]. These are: pretreatment of cell monolayers with 25–30 µg/ml of DEAE-dextran before inocula-

Table 1. Optimal cell culture conditions

Cell lines	HL, Hep-2
Enhancement	Centrifugation of inoculum Incorporation of cycloheximide to culture medium for incubation of infected cells: concentrations depend on cell lines Incubation at 35 °C
Detection of inclusions	Direct FA, genus- or *C. pneumoniae*-specific monoclonal antibody
Serial passages	Pass every 3 days Slow expansion Transfer from vial to flask cultures

tion, centrifugation of inoculum, and incorporation of a host cell metabolic inhibitor such as cycloheximide. Pretreatment with DEAE-dextran enhances the growth of *C. pneumoniae* in HeLa cells about two times, but not in HL cells [7–9]. Centrifugation ($900 \times g$ for 60 min) is the most effective enhancement method among the three treatments. The infectivity of *C. pneumoniae* is enhanced 1000 times in HeLa 229 cells and 100 times in HL cells [7, 9]. Cycloheximide treatment enhances the infectivity of *C. pneumoniae* three times in HeLa cells and 15 times in HL cells at the optimal concentrations of 0.9 and 0.6 μg/ml, respectively [7, 9].

As with growing the trachoma biovar of *C. trachomatis*, the optimal temperature of incubation of *C. pneumoniae* is 35 °C. The burst size is three times greater at 35 °C than at 37 °C [9]. The optimal time of harvesting is 3 days for both HeLa 229 cells [7] and HL cells [9].

Detection of Inclusions in Cell Culture

Detection of inclusions is best done by FA stain. For initial screening a fluorescein-conjugated genus-specific monoclonal antibody is usually used to cover all three species of *Chlamydia*. Differentiation of the species can be done by using a monoclonal antibody specific to either *C. pneumoniae* or *C. trachomatis* [7]. The preparations of direct FA conjugate for these three antibodies are available commercially. *C. psittaci* species-specific monoclonal antibody is not available. Acetone, but not methanol, should be used for fixation of cover slips for FA staining if *C. pneumoniae* species-specific monoclonal antibodies are used for inclusion stain, because methanol treatment destroys the reactivity of *C. pneumoniae*-specific antigens with antibodies against *C. pneumoniae* [15]. This precaution also applied to the micro-IF serologic test for assaying *C. pneumoniae* specific antibodies in serum. Iodine stain, which is used for staining *C. trachomatis* inclusions, will not stain *C. pneumoniae* inclusions because they contain no glycogen [7]. *C. pneumoniae* inclusions are difficult to detect with May-Grünwald Giemsa stain, which is often used for staining *C. trachomatis* inclusions and for morphological observation of chlamydial cell cultures in general.

Number of Passages Required for Isolation

It has been a common practice to do at least two passages in isolation of chlamydiae from clinical samples. In our experience with isolation of *C. pneumoniae* from pharyngeal swabs with HeLa 229 or HL cells, 90% (36/40 isolates) of positives were obtained in the first passage and the remaining 10% in the second passage when two passages were done. The number of organisms detected in pharyngeal swab specimens in acute respiratory tract infection were small; 83% of specimens contained less than 10 inclusion-forming units in 0.1 ml of inoculum from a swab sample eluted in 1 ml of SPG transport medium. Additional number of passages have been advocated by some investigators. In the study of isolation of *C. pneumoniae* from coronary atheromatous tissues, Maass et al. did ten passages [16]. They were able to obtain 11 isolates from 70 specimens using Hep-2 cells in multi-well culture plates. The isolates were identified by FA stain in the second to fifth passages. Factors to be considered in multiple passages are increased labor costs for a small increment of additional positives, and the chance of cross contamination with open-vessel culture using multi-well plates instead of sealed-culture vials.

Sensitivity of Cell Culture Isolation

Sensitivity of cell culture for diagnosis of acute *C. pneumoniae* respiratory infection is reasonable, at about 60%. In our studies of serologically confirmed acute respiratory infection, including pneumonia, bronchitis, and pharyngitis, the isolation rates from throat swabs were 24/49 (59%) in students at the University of Washington, Seattle [17], and 25/43 (58%) in a military epidemic of *C. pneumoniae* in Kajaani, Finland [18]. These isolation rates are as good as isolation of *C. trachomatis* from the conjunctiva in trachoma, from the urethra in male urethritis, and from the cervix in female cervicitis. However, isolation from the chronic stage is much more difficult. Culture is often negative even from tissues, while PCR may be positive. The reasons for the difficulty in isolation in chronic stages are (1) that the infection in the chronic stage involves deeper tissues, such as lung interstitial macrophages, arterial wall macrophages, and smooth muscle cells; (2) the titers are low due to poor growth in these cells and to immune suppression of multiplication and maturation of the organism; and (3) these sites are not readily accessible by routine sample collection methods.

Sampling Sites

What is the best site for taking clinical samples for laboratory diagnosis of acute respiratory infection by culture? Boman et al. [19] compared samples collected simultaneously from nasopharynx, throat, and sputum and found rates of 80% (12/15) from nasopharynx, 63% (12/19) from throat, and 64% (14/22) from sputum.

Serial Passages in Cell Culture

The key to success in serial passages, to raise the titer from the first isolation in vial culture to growth in bottle culture for large-scale production of organisms, is "slow expansion". Pass cultures every 3 days in the same number of vials (usually three vials per isolate; stain one vial for assaying titers and pass the remaining two vials to new cultures) until more than 50% of cells are infected before increasing the number of vials. Transfer 20–30 vials of highly infected cells into a small size bottle. No centrifugation is necessary for bottle or flask cultures. Then, continue passages in a small bottle to raise titer before going to large bottles. Split to more bottles after the titers have increased by checking the titer periodically by titrating harvests at passage. To ensure good infection, cultures should be inoculated with greater than 1 multiplicity of infection (MOI). A culture bottle or flask of 112 cm^2 surface area with 100% infection should yield greater than 1×10^8 IFUs/ml per flask after purification.

Handling and Storage of Specimens

C. pneumoniae organisms are sensitive to temperature and freezing process [20]. Like other chlamydial organisms, *C. pneumoniae* organisms are best stored in buffers containing sucrose and glutamic acid, such as SPG (sucrose, 75 g; KH$_2$PO$_4$, 0.52 g; Na$_2$HPO$_4$, 1.22 g; glutamic acid, 0.72 g; H$_2$O to 1 l; pH 7.4–7.6) and 2SP (sucrose, 68.47 g; KH$_2$PO$_4$, 0.6 g; K$_2$HPO$_4$, 2.83 g; H$_2$O to 1 l; pH 7.4–7.6). Addition of 10% fetal calf serum to the transport medium has been shown to further enhance the stability [21].

Exposure of *C. pneumoniae* organisms at room temperature for 1 day inactivates 99% of the infectivity [20]. Storage of *C. pneumoniae* organisms in SPG at refrigerator temperature (4 °C) for 1 day inactivates 30% of the infectivity. Slow freezing is better than quick freezing. The infectivity is reduced by only 23% when specimens are kept in the refrigerator for 0.5–4 h before freezing at –75 °C, in comparison with 61% inactivation when specimens are frozen directly at –75 °C. Therefore, if isolation can be done within 24 h after specimen collection, it is better to store specimens in a refrigerator without freezing. If isolation cannot be done within 24 h, the specimens should be stored in a deep freezer. No difference is observed when specimens are thawed slowly or quickly after freezing at -75 °C.

References

1. T'ang F, Chang H, Huang Y, Wang K (1951) Studies on the etiology of trachoma with special reference to isolation of the virus in chick embryo. Chin Med J 75:429-447
2. Gordon FB, Quan AL (1965) Isolation of the trachoma agent in cell culture. Proc Soc Exp Biol Med 118:354-359
3. Ripa KT, Mårdh PA (1977) Cultivation of *Chlamydia trachomatis* in cycloheximide-treated McCoy cells. J Clin Microbiol 6:328-331
4. Kuo C-C, Wang S-P, Wentworth B, Grayston JT (1972) Primary isolation of TRIC organisms in HeLa 229 cells treated with DEAE-dextran. J Infect Dis 125:665-668
5. McComb DE, Puzniak CI (1974) Micro cell culture method for isolation of *Chlamydia trachomatis*. Appl Microbiol 28:727-729
6. Yoder BL, Stamm WE, Koester CM, Alexander ER (1981) Microtest procedure for isolation of *Chlamydia trachomatis*. J Clin Microbiol 13:1036-1039
7. Kuo C-C, Chen H-H, Wang S-P, Grayston JT (1986) Identification of a new group of *Chlamydia psittaci* strains called TWAR. J Clin Microbiol 24:1034-1037
8. Cles LD, Stamm WE (1990) Use of HL cells for improved isolation and passage of *Chlamydia pneumoniae*. J Clin Microbiol 28:938-940
9. Kuo C-C, Grayston JT (1990) A sensitive cell line, HL cells, for isolation and propagation of *Chlamydia pneumoniae* strain TWAR. J Infect Dis 162:755-758
10. Wong KH, Skelton SK, Chan YK (1992) Efficient culture of *Chlamydia pneumoniae* with cell lines derived from the human respiratory tract. J Clin Microbiol 30:1625-1630
11. Roblin PM, Dumornay W, Hammerschlag MR (1992) Use of Hep-2 cells for improved isolation and passage of *Chlamydia pneumoniae*. J Clin Microbiol 30:1968-1971

12. Kuo C-C, Wang S-P, Grayston JT (1977) Growth of trachoma organisms in HeLa 229 cell culture. In: Hobson D, Holmes KK (eds) Nongonococcal urethritis and related infections. American Society for Microbiology, Washington DC, pp 328-336

13. Cavallaro JJ, Monto AS (1972) HL cells, a sensitive line for the isolation and propagation of respiratory syncytial virus. Proc Soc Exp Biol Med 140:507-510

14. Moulder JW, Hatch TP, Kuo C-C, Schachter J, Storz J (1984) *Chlamydia* Jones, Rake and Sterns. In: Krieg NR (ed) Bergey's manual of systematic bacteriology, vol 1. Williams & Wilkins, Baltimore, pp 729-735

15. Wang S-P, Grayston JT (1991) *Chlamydia pneumoniae* elementary body antigenic reactivity with fluorescent antibody is destroyed by methanol. J Clin Microbiol 29:1539-1541

16. Maass M, Bartels C, Engel PM, Mamat U, Sievers HH (1998) Endovascular presence of viable *Chlamydia pneumoniae* is a common phenomenon in coronary artery disease. J Am Coll Cardiol 31:827-832

17. Grayston JT, Kuo C-C, Wang S-P, Altman J (1986) A new *Chlamydia psittaci* strain TWAR, isolated in acute respiratory tract infection. N Engl J Med 315:161-168

18. Ekman M-R, Grayston JT, Visakorpi R, Kleemola M, Kuo C-C, Saikku P (1993) An epidemic of infections due to *Chlamydia pneumoniae* in military conscripts. Clin Infect Dis 17:420-425

19. Boman J, Allard A, Persson K, Lundborg M, Juto P, Wadell G (1997) Rapid diagnosis of respiratory *Chlamydia pneumoniae* infection by nested touchdown polymerase chain reaction compared with culture and antigen detection by EIA. J Infect Dis 175:1523-1526

20. Kuo C-C, Grayston JT (1988) Factors affecting viability and growth in HeLa 229 cells of *Chlamydia* sp. strain TWAR. J Clin Microbiol 26:812-815

21. Maass M, Dalhoff K (1995) Transport and storage conditions for cultural recovery of *Chlamydia pneumoniae.* J Clin Microbiol 33:1793-1796

Serology for *Chlamydia pneumoniae* (TWAR)

S.-P. Wang

Introduction

As many other medical sciences, serology for *Chlamydia pneumoniae* (TWAR) has been improved according to our demand to cope with the progress of the knowledge on the organisms.

The time-honored serological method for *Chlamydia* is the complement fixation (CF) test [1], which has served for serodiagnosis of *C. psittaci* (CPs) infections, mainly due to transmission from naturally infected psittacine birds and LGV infections. These chlamydial infections have systemic rather than local involvement in man. Likewise, the CF test has also been useful for serodiagnosis of primary TWAR infection. CF reaction is based on antibody reaction with common genus LPS (lipopolysaccharide) antigen which is shared by all chlamydiae. The CF test does not distinguish between different *Chlamydia* species. We now know that TWAR infection is much more common; many persons diagnosed as having psittacosis based on the CF test, without good evidence of avian transmission, in reality had TWAR infection.

When the other oculogenital infection of *C. trachomatis* (CT) became the major problem of human infections, the CF method was found not to be very useful, due to its lack of sensitivity and specificity. In our search for a more effective serological method, the micro-immunofluorescence (micro-IF or MIF) technique was developed [2, 3]. First of all, the MIF test was developed for the purpose of serotyping for CT organisms to substitute a tedious, in vivo mouse toxicity prevention test [4]. It worked nicely and efficiently to classify the species of CT into 18 serovars [5–9]. It also depicted an untypeable strain, TW-183, which was originally considered to be a CT strain, because it was isolated from the eye during the trachoma studies. Later this untypeable strain led to the discovery of a new species, *C. pneumoniae* (TWAR) [10].

Historically, an epidemic of respiratory tract infection occurred in Finland [11] and was suspected to be due to some sort of *Chlamydia*, because the patients were serologically reactive with LGV antigen in the CF test. However, it was unlikely to be due to an avian transmission or to oculogenital spreading. The patients' sera did not react to one of our common isolates (strain Ps-1) of *C. psittaci*, or to any CT serovar in the MIF test. A MIF test with TW-183 was finally attempted and suggested an association of TW-183 as the cause of the epidemic. TW-183 was still considered to be a variety of CPs strain at that time, because, unlike the CT organism, it produced glycogen-negative inclusions in cell culture [12].

Encouraged by the findings, investigators [13] initiated studies of re-isolation of the organisms from respiratory tract illness and extensive uses of MIF for serodiagnosis and seroepidemiology. Most of our current knowledge in regard to TWAR infection is derived from studies with TWAR MIF serology. It includes: (1) an association of TWAR with acute respiratory tract infection [13]; (2) the occurrence of TWAR epidemics [14, 15]; (3) the description of antibody prevalence in populations [16, 17]; (4) the spread of infections by studies of serum banks [18]; (5) confirmation of the finding of the association of TWAR and coronary heart diseases [19–21]; (6) the similarity of test results using a variety of TWAR strains derived from around the world [22].

Certainly, the development of other serological tests, such as ELISA, is being attempted by other investigators. This chapter will focus the discussion on MIF serology for TWAR infection. Standardization of the test has been attempted to determine the extent of inter-laboratory variation in the use of MIF assay for serodiagnosis of TWAR infections [23].

MIF for TWAR Serology

Some Features of TWAR MIF

In the MIF system, where *Chlamydia* elementary bodies are used as test antigen, cross-reactions do occur among the serovars of the same species, such as C and A, E and D, and F and G serovars of CT species. However, cross-reactions among different species, namely between CT serovar and TWAR organisms, or CPs and TWAR organisms, have not been seen. Only a single serovar has so far been recognized in TWAR organisms. This increases specificity of MIF with TWAR organisms.

Another interesting feature of MIF serology in primary TWAR infection is that IgM antibody tends to be more persistent, and more slowly replaced by IgG antibody, than in CT infection. This makes IgM antibody response unique and an important marker for serodiagnosis of acute infection.

MIF Test Procedures

Antigen Preparation

The antigen used in the MIF test is whole elementary bodies of TWAR organisms. We have used HeLa 229 cells and the more sensitive HL cell line for growth of the organism. Cell cultures highly infected with TWAR are homogenized, and the bacterial suspensions are purified by Rinografin centrifugation and treated with formalin in a final concentration of 0.02%. Although formalin kills the organisms, it does not alter the quality of surface antigen for the test. The formalinized and concentrated bacterial suspension (approximately 10^9 organisms/ml) can be stored at 4 °C for many years. An equal amount (0.1 ml) of 2%–3% formalinized normal yolk sac suspension (NYS) is added, and the mixture is sonicated for a few seconds prior to placement on the microscope slide to ensure homogeneity of the suspension. The NYS is added to enhance adhesion of the organisms to the slide and to facilitate location of antigen spots under the microscope. Test antigens should produce strong typical fluorescence with TWAR monoclonal antibody and have a density appropriate for observation of evenly distributed elementary bodies under the fluorescent microscope (FA scope).

Test Procedures

Glass microscope slides should be chemically clean to prevent loss of the antigens from the slide during washing procedures. Dip pen points (e.g., Hunt Fine Pens #104, Hunt Manufacturing, Statesville, N.C., USA) are employed for placement of antigens on the slides. A template (Fig. 1) with prior marking is placed under a clean slide to guide placement. The template has a central 15 mm × 15 mm area with 16 dots arranged 5 mm apart from each other. In conjunction with an accurately marked microscope stage (Fig. 2) viewing of each dot is made easy.

A dot of test antigen is placed with a pen point over each of 16 spots before the test slide is removed from the template. If more than one *Chlamydia* antigen is used, antigen dots may be placed within a 2-mm area using the first antigen dot as guide. A clean pen point is used for each antigen. Thus 16 single TWAR antigen dots or 16 groups of different *Chlamydia* antigen dots can be placed on one slide. The slides are air-dried before being fixed in pure acetone for 15 min at room temperature. Serial twofold serum dilutions (1:8 to 1:1024) are made in a microtiter using a micropipette with tip and applied to the slide with a bacteriological loop. A loop of the highest dilution of serum is overlaid on the TWAR antigen dot or group of anti-

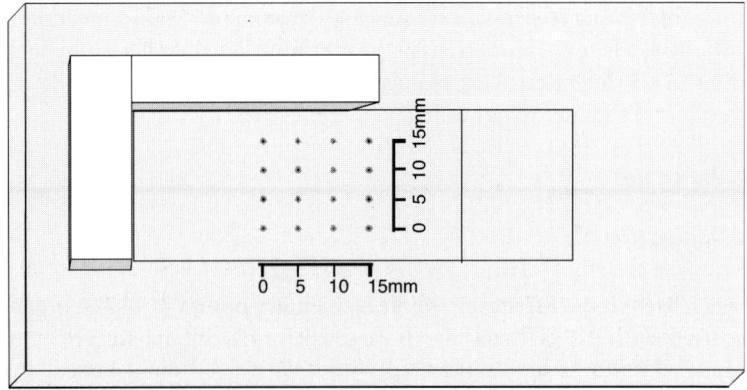

Fig. 1. Template for antigen placement on a slide

gen dots. The loop is blotted on a clean paper towel and lower dilution overlaid on the next antigen group. The application continues serially to the lower dilution. As many as 16 loops of serum can be placed on one slide. The slides are then placed in a moist chamber (or simply in a covered plate with a wet paper towel underneath) and incubated at 37 °C for 30 min. After incubation, the slides are rinsed gently by dips and drains for each slide using a forceps in four changes of 0.01 M phosphate-buffered saline and three changes of distilled water. The slides are placed on their sides and air-dried at room temperature. A fluorescent conjugate of anti-human immunoglobulin is then applied on the slides with a bacteriological loop. They are incubated at 37 °C for 30 min and the process of dip-and-drain washing and drying is repeated as before. A cover slip is mounted with mounting fluid over the antigen spots on top of the slide. The slides are usually read immediately, but can be kept at refrigerator temperature for a few days without losing fluorescence.

Fluorescein Conjugates

Anti-IgM, -IgG, or -IgA labeled with fluorescein isothiocyanate and, as counter-stain, rhodamin-conjugated bovine albumin (RBA) or Evans blue, are obtained from commercial sources. Proper dilution of fluorescein conjugate is determined by testing dilutions of 1:30 to 1:50 with a high-titer positive serum to find the dilution with maximum fluorescence. Conjugate is distributed in small quantities (0.2-ml aliquots) and kept frozen at −20 °C. Upon use, approximately 1/15 volume of RBA, or Evans blue to a concentration of 0.05%, is added to the thawed conju-gate dilution. The mixture of counterstain and conjugate is kept at 4 °C until con-sumed. Either counterstain may be used.

Microscopic Examination

An FA scope, such as Zeiss Axioskop with epifluorescence, works well for the MIF method. A mercury vapor HBO 50 W/AC L1 lamp provides the light source. Binoc-ular observation is made using $10 \times$ ocular lenses and $10 \times$ (Neofluar $10 \times / 0.30$) and $40 \times$ (Plan Neofluar $40 \times / 0.75$) objective lens. A low-power $10 \times$ objective lens is used to locate antigenic spots, and a high-power $40 \times$ lens (without oil immer-sion) is used to observe immunofluorescence. Alignment scales placed on the microscope's stage and used in association with the horizontal and vertical cen-tering greatly assist in viewing the antigen dots (Fig. 2).

The labels will have scale marks matching the dot placement on the slide, markings at 0, 5 mm, 10 mm, and 15 mm. The vertical alignment label is placed on the stage, on top of the existing indicator marks, and the horizontal alignment label is placed on the slide holder mechanism. Exact placement of the labels is not crucial but correct positioning of the travel pointers is. Use a reference slide and low magnification to align a dot. Place the vertical and horizontal travel pointers to match accordingly. Figure 2 demonstrates this being done for a dot offset 5 mm from both the vertical and horizontal axis. You may now use the travel pointers and scale marks to align the microscope with any of the 16 dots.

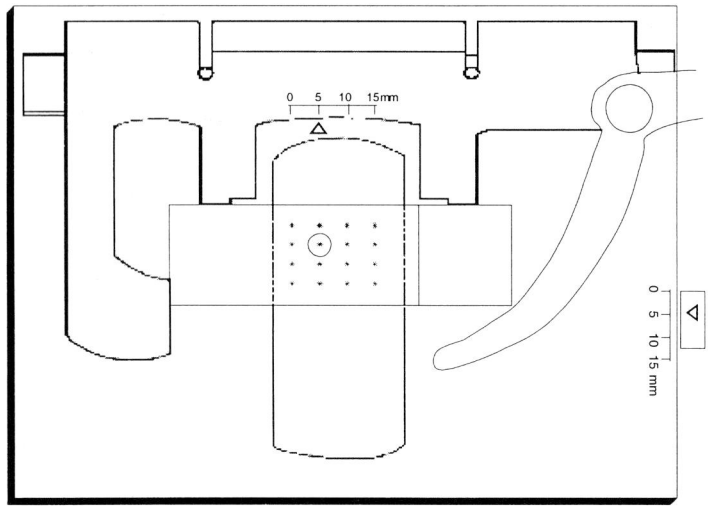

Fig. 2. FA scope stage with row and column markers

Serological Test

It is advised to do a pilot screening of each serum to test a single dilution of 1:8 with anti-IgM, anti-IgG, and, if desired, anti-IgA fluorescein conjugates. Positive sera at 1:8 dilution are then titrated only with the positive immunoglobulin. The screening is useful not only to eliminate unnecessary titration but also as extra confirmation of positive serological results. Each patient should have at least two serum specimens obtained several weeks apart. Paired sera, if available, from each patient should be tested concurrently to assist in determination of significant titer change.

Removal of Rheumatoid Factor from Human Serum

It is known that some patients may have the rheumatoid factor (RF), anti-IgM IgG (autoimmune antibody to self immunoglobulin, particularly to IgM), which can cause a false-positive reaction [24]. Any positive IgM antibody should be considered for such a possibility. The test is the Gullsorb test. To 10 μl of undiluted serum in a microfuge tube, 40 μl of rabbit anti-human IgG and 30 μl of PBS are added, making a 1:8 dilution of human serum. A microfuge tube of serum dilution without rabbit anti-human IgG is the control. Both microfuge tubes are incubated at 37 °C for 60 min and then centrifuged at 20 000 g for 5 min. The treated and non-treated (control) supernates are titrated for IgM antibody for TWAR in the MIF test. When the treated serum yields the same or higher titer as the control, the IgM antibody is considered true, while a complete loss or a decreased titer in the treated serum indicates a false IgM reaction.

Endpoint Determination

Only fluorescence associated with evenly distributed elementary bodies is considered positive. Fluorescence associated with unevenly distributed particles, particularly without clear elementary body morphology, is not positive. True antibody reactions should gradually lose fluorescence intensity with increasing serum dilution. The false reactions tend to show a sudden decrease of fluorescence in higher serum dilutions. The endpoint (titer) is defined by the reciprocal of the highest antibody dilution which yields an unequivocal recognition of individual elementary body particles under high-power (10×40) magnification. Reactions of higher dilution should be studied until questionable and negative reactions are seen. The serum dilution with the unequivocally positive reaction is taken as an endpoint. Because this determination is qualitative and may be difficult due to the slow fall-off in intensity of fluorescence, paired sera should always be tested together to assist in the determination of antibody titer change.

Prezone Phenomenon

Although it is rare at low dilutions of serum, an excess of antibody may obstruct positive immunofluorescence. In these rare cases, lower dilutions of serum (including 1:8) may falsely appear to be negative. A reaction exhibiting a strong green background, or any question about the reaction, should be confirmed by titration.

Interpretation of Results

The MIF test uses both IgM and IgG antibodies to interpret results. The best serological evidence of acute TWAR infection is a fourfold rise in antibody titer in paired sera. In addition, a titer of 1:16 or greater in the IgM fraction, or 1:512 or greater in the IgG fraction is considered presumptive evidence of current or recent infection.

The patterns of antibody response to acute TWAR infection have been identified: one is associated with primary infection, the other with reinfection. In primary infection, a prompt CF antibody response is seen. TWAR IgM antibody appears later, about 3 weeks after onset of illness. Antibody in IgG may not appear until 6–8 weeks after onset. In reinfection, CF and IgM antibody may not appear or may appear only at low titers. The IgG antibody titer rises quickly, often in 1–2 weeks, and may reach a titer of 512 or more.

Understanding these patterns is important in interpreting serological studies of TWAR infections. In a first infection, if the second serum is obtained less than 3 weeks after onset, the antibody response can be missed. In reinfections, the absence of CF and IgM antibody can make it difficult to distinguish between acute infection and persistent antibody from past infection. Follow-up serologies on patients with an acute antibody response reveal that, while IgM usually begins to fall within 2 months and usually disappears 4–6 months after an acute infection,

IgG persists and may be detected for over 3 years after acute infection in some patients. For the serological diagnosis of TWAR infection, paired serum specimens should be obtained whenever possible. The presence of a high titer of antibody alone provides a much less precise serological diagnosis than a fourfold rise in titer from paired sera. This is especially true for elderly patients, who may have persistently high IgG titers.

Sensitivity of the MIF Test

From the beginning of TWAR studies, MIF serology has consistently been the most sensitive method for diagnosing acute infection. Isolation, and to a lesser extent PCR, has been dependent on careful handling of laboratory specimens. Even under the best circumstances, demonstration of organism has been less successful than serology in identifying acute infection.

We examined throat swabs from several groups of patients for the presence of TWAR by cell culture and PCR and tested several serum specimens from them by MIF. We found excellent correlation between positive serology by MIF and detection of the organism. The organism was demonstrated by isolation and/or PCR in 62%–75% of persons positive by serological tests, but not in patients who did not have serologic evidence of infection [25].

References

1. Meyer KF, Eddie B (1956) Psittacosis. In: Lennett EH, Schmidt NJ (eds) Diagnostic procedures for virus and rickettsial diseases (2nd edn). American Public Health Association, New York, pp 399-430
2. Wang S-P, Grayston JT (1970) Immunological relationship between genital TRIC, lymphogranuloma venereum, and related organisms in a new microtiter indirect immunofluorescence test. Am J Ophthalmol 70:367-374
3. Wang S-P (1971) A micro-immunofluorescence method. Study of antibody response to TRIC organisms in mice. In: Nichols RL (ed) Trachoma and related disorders caused by chlamydial agents. Excerpta Medica, Amsterdam, pp 273-218
4. Wang S-P, Grayston JT (1963) Classification of trachoma virus strains by protection of mice from toxic death. J Immunol 90:849-856
5. Wang S-P, Grayston JT (1971) Classification of TRIC and related strains with microimmunofluorescence. In: Nichols RL (ed) Trachoma and related disorders caused by chlamydial agents. Excerpta Medica, Amsterdam, pp 305-321
6. Wang S-P, Grayston JT, Gale JL (1973) Three new immunologic types of trachoma-inclusion conjunctivitis organisms. J Immunol 110:873-879
7. Kuo C-C, Wang S-P, Grayston JT, Alexander ER (1974) TRIC type K, a new immunological type of *Chlamydia trachomatis*. J Immunol 113:591-596
8. Wang S-P, Grayston JT (1975) *Chlamydia trachomatis* immunotype J. J Immunol 115:1711-1716
9. Wang S-P, Grayston JT (1991) Three new serovars of *Chlamydia trachomatis*, Da, Ia, and L2a. J Infect Dis 163:403-405
10. Grayston JT, Kuo C-C, Campbell LA, Wang S-P (1989) *Chlamydia pneumoniae* sp. nov. for *Chlamydia* sp. strain TWAR. Int J Syst Bacteriol 39:88-90

11. Saikku P, Wang S-P, Kleemola M, Braner E, Rusanen E, Grayston JT (1985) An epidemic of mild pneumonia due to unusual *Chlamydia psittaci*. J Infect Dis 151:882-839

12. Kuo C-C, Chen H-H, Wang S-P, Grayston JT (1986) Characterization of TWAR strains, a new group of *Chlamydia psittaci*. In: Oriel D, Ridgway G, Schachter J, Taylor-Robinson D, Ward M (eds) *Chlamydia* infections. Cambridge University Press, Cambridge, UK, pp 321-324

13. Grayston JT, Kuo C-C, Wang S-P, Altman J (1986) A new *Chlamydia psittaci* strain TWAR isolated in acute respiratory tract infections. N Engl J Med 315:161-168

14. Mordhorst CH, Wang S-P, Grayston JT (1986) Epidemic "ornithosis" and TWAR infections in Denmark 1976-85. In: Oriel D, Ridgway G, Schachter J, Taylor-Robinson D, Ward W (eds) *Chlamydia* infections. Cambridge University Press, Cambridge,UK, pp 325-328

15. Kleemola M, Saikku P, Wang S-P, Visakorpi R, Grayston JT (1988) Pneumonia epidemic in military trainees in Finland caused by TWAR, a new chlamydia organism. J Infect Dis 157:230-236

16. Wang S-P, Grayston JT (1990) Population prevalence antibody to *Chlamydia pneumoniae* strain TWAR. In: Bowie WR, Caldwell HD, Jones RP, Mårdh PA, Ridgway GL, Schachter J, Stamm WE, Ward ME (eds) Chlamydial infections 1990. Cambridge University Press, Cambridge, UK, pp 402-405

17. Kuo C-C, Jackson LA, Campbell LA, Grayston JT (1995) *Chlamydia pneumoniae* (TWAR). Clin Microbiol Rev 8:451-461

18. Aldous MB, Grayston JT, Wang S-P, Foy HM (1992) Seroepidemiology of *Chlamydia pneumoniae*, TWAR infections in Seattle families 1966-1979. J Infect Dis 166:646-649

19. Thom DH, Wang S-P, Grayston JT, Siscovick DS, Stewart DK, Kronmal RA, Weiss NS (1991) *Chlamydia pneumoniae* strain TWAR antibody and angiographically demonstrated coronary heart disease. Arterioscler Thromb 11:547-551

20. Thom DH, Grayston JT, Siscovick DS, Wang S-P, Weiss NS, Daling JR (1992) Association of prior infection with *Chlamydia pneumoniae* and angiographically demonstrated coronary artery disease. JAMA 268:68-72

21. Melnick SL, Shahar E, Folsom AR, Grayston JR, Sorlie RD, Wang S-P, Szklo M (1993) Past infection by *Chlamydia pneumoniae* strain TWAR and asymptomatic carotid atherosclerosis. Am J Med 95:499-504

22. Wang S-P, Grayston JT (1994) The similarity of *Chlamydia pneumoniae* (TWAR) isolate as antigen in the microimmunofluorescence (MIF) test. In: Orfila J, Byrne GI, Chernsky MA, Grayston JT, Jones RP, Ridgway GL, Saikku P, Schachter J, Stamm WE, Stephens RS (eds) *Chlamydia* infections 1994. Esculapio, Bologna, pp 181-184

23. Peeling RW, Wang S-P, Grayston JT, Blasi F, Boman J, Clad A, Freidank H, Gaydos CA, Gnarpe J, Hagiwara T, Jones RB, Orfila J, Persson K, Puolakkainen M, Saikku P, Schachter J (1998) *Chlamydia* serology: inter-laboratory variation in micro-immunofluorescence results. In: Stephens RS, Byrne GI, Christiansen G, Clarke IN, Grayston JT, Rank RG, Ridgway GL, Saikku P, Schachter J, Stamm WE (eds) Chlamydial infections. Proceedings of the 9th International Symposium on Human Chlamydial Infection, Napa, CA, 21-28 June, 1998, ISBN 0-9664383-0-2, pp 159-162

24. Verkooyen RP, Hazenberg MA, van Haaren GH, van den Bosch JM, Snijder RJ, van Helden HP, Verbrugh HA (1992) Age-related interference with *Chlamydia pneumoniae*: micro-immunofluorescence serology due to circulating rheumatoid factor. J Clin Microbiol 30:1289-1290

25. Wang S-P, Grayston JT (1998) *Chlamydia pneumoniae* (TWAR) micro-immunofluorescence antibody studies: 1998 update. In: Stephens RS, Byrne GI, Christiansen G, Clarke IN, Grayston JT, Rank RG, Ridgway GL, Saikku P, Schachter J, Stamm WE (eds) Chlamydial infections. Proceedings of the 9th International Symposium on Human Chlamydial Infection, Napa, CA, 21-28 June, 1998, ISBN 0-9664383-0-2, pp 155-158

Chlamydia pneumoniae: Molecular Biology Methods

J. BOMAN, C.A. GAYDOS

Introduction

Chlamydia pneumoniae is an obligate intracellular bacterium which is difficult to diagnose by conventional means. Concerning serology, several problems are involved such as non-standardization of reagents and the technical complexity of the assay. Culture of the organism in tissue culture is the current gold standard to demonstrate that a patient is infected by viable *C. pneumoniae*, but the use of culture for detection of *C. pneumoniae* is problematic because of low sensitivity. Since *C. pneumoniae* can cause severe clinical disease, correct diagnosis and therapy are important. Faster, more sensitive and less laborious methods are therefore required. The ability of the polymerase chain reaction (PCR) technique to rapidly amplify small amounts of specific nucleic acid has made this technique an important diagnostic tool with potential to offer clinical laboratories a convenient means to detect *C. pneumoniae* rapidly and reliably. Although significant improvements have been made in developing molecular methods for the detection of *C. pneumoniae*, several problems remain. For example, a variety of different PCR-based assays have been developed, and one important issue is comparison of methods and standardization of the protocols. Nevertheless, increased use of automation and the introduction of commercial diagnostic kits will improve standardization and availability. Furthermore, use of new molecular techniques, such as quantitative PCR and sequence analysis, will promote research applications and improve the effectiveness for diagnosis of *C. pneumoniae*.

Methodological Aspects

Given the limitation of traditional diagnostic methods, nucleic acid amplification (NAA) techniques will improve our ability to detect *C. pneumoniae* accurately and in good time. Routine implementation of NAA techniques, however, requires consideration of several methodological issues, including the selection of appropriate gene targets for amplification, choice of appropriate primers, specimen collection, nucleic acid preparation, detection and attenuation of inhibitors of the amplification reaction, detection of amplification products and control of contamination and non-specific reactions [1–3]. Because of the complex interactions of the PCR components, no single PCR protocol will be applicable for all situations. Consequently, each new PCR application is likely to require new optimization procedures. Suboptimal reaction conditions may arise for a number of reasons, including inappropriate primers, improper time and temperature conditions, variable polymerase quality, temperature inconsistencies across the block of the thermal cycler and incorrect Mg^{2+} concentrations [4]. Stringent annealing temperatures during the first cycles will help to increase specificity, and touchdown PCR [5] with decreasing annealing temperatures may increase specificity [6, 7]. Nested PCR with amplification in two steps utilizing two different primer pairs may also greatly increase both the sensitivity and the specificity of the PCR procedure [7, 8].

Recently, Verkooyen et al. reported that diagnosis of a *C. pneumoniae* infection is still difficult and the choice of a gold standard remains problematic [9]. The lack of a consensus standard makes it difficult to evaluate new methods, and a stringent gold standard should be used for evaluation of diagnostic tests. The fact that *C. pneumoniae* may be carried in the respiratory tract for prolonged periods [10] makes it even more difficult to compare different diagnostic tests, especially detection methods, with serologic methods. As PCR can detect the presence of *C. pneumoniae* DNA from non-infectious reticulate bodies as well as from non-viable elementary bodies, PCR tests in general are expected to be more sensitive than culture methods. Detection of cDNA by reverse-transcription PCR of messenger RNA may be a useful complement to cell culture in assessing whether the *C. pneumoniae* infection is active/productive [11].

Guidelines have been developed to minimize the risk of false-positive results due to contamination. It is important to pay attention to these recommendations, including meticulous laboratory techniques, strict physical separation of work areas and containment devices, inactivation protocols and environmental decontamination [12, 13]. The use of strongly positive controls should be avoided and several well-characterized negative controls and multiple reagent controls should be included with each amplification [14]. The positive controls should consist of low and very low DNA levels for *C. pneumoniae*. The negative controls should include all PCR components except target DNA and follow the whole procedure from extraction of the nucleic acid to detection of amplification product. Confirmation of all positive findings by reanalysis is recommended to minimize the risk of false positives due to sporadic contamination events [13, 15].

False-negative results may be due to inhibitors, volume sampling error, human error, inadequate extraction of nucleic acid, equipment failure, reagent problems such as inappropriate magnesium concentration and primer synthesis, low sensitivity of the detection system or poor specimen quality [12]. False negatives can often be detected by use of good-quality control procedures, and positive controls that amplify weakly but consistently should be selected [14]. Complicated DNA extraction methods for removal of PCR inhibitors may be used in research laboratories, but create work-flow problems in diagnostic laboratories. In order to identify inhibitors of the PCR, the negative samples can be spiked with small amounts of target DNA [16] or one may include a competitive hybrid internal control for each sample that is co-amplified in the reaction with the same primers as used for the real target [17]. Inhibitory samples can then be reanalyzed after dilution of the processed sample, storage at 4 °C, freeze-thawing, heating, or by sample treatment with an alternative extraction protocol [17]. Dilution of samples is a simple method that may improve amplification by reduction of inhibitors, but the sensitivity may be reduced as a result of dilution of target DNA. The use of a nested PCR minimizes the problem with PCR inhibitors substantially [8].

In theory, using a larger volume of the sample in the amplification reaction may increase the sensitivity but this strategy may be hampered by an unacceptable increase in the level of PCR inhibitors in a subset of the samples [1, 18]. Amplification of human genes such as the β-globin gene can be valuable for confirming the presence of human DNA in the sample [15], but is not recommended as a test of inhibition since the number of copies of this gene in each sample may be much higher than the number of copies of the C. pneumoniae target gene.

Some DNA polymerases are more suitable than others for specific tasks; it is therefore worth comparing enzymes from different suppliers. Some enzymes may be less susceptible than others to specific inhibitors [4].

The specimen collection depend on the type of clinical condition. Suitable specimens for detection of C. pneumoniae include sputum [6, 7], bronchoalveolar lavage (BAL) [19], swabs of nasopharynx and throat [7, 8], gargled-water [20], and tissues from biopsy or autopsy [21]. C. pneumoniae DNA may also be detected in blood specimens [15, 22, 23] but the tecniques require further evaluation. A recent study comparing different respiratory sampling sites [7] appears to show that sputum samples are superior to nasopharyngeal and throat swabs in terms of the diagnostic yield. Nasopharyngeal and throat samples are of value in patients who cannot produce a sputum sample [7]. However, not all protocols seem to be useful for detection of C. pneumoniae in sputum [9].

For collection of nasopharyngeal specimens, a Dacron fiber-tipped swab with a plastic shaft is preferred over a calcium alginate fiber-tipped swab with an aluminium shaft, since the latter may contain PCR inhibitors [24].

Chlamydia transport media intended primarily for cell culture may not be optimal for collection and transport of samples that should be analyzed by a NAA test [25]. When only PCR is to be performed, simpler collection buffers that do not contain PCR inhibitors should be used [2]. Black et al. [8] found that transport media commonly used for chlamydial swab specimens may be inhibitory in the PCR. Therefore, both sampling devices and transport media should be checked for the presence of PCR inhibitors. After collection, the samples should be transported to the laboratory as soon as possible and kept at 4 °C or frozen at –70 °C.

For routine diagnostic purposes, a simple method for processing clinical samples is desirable. The precise technique used for extraction of nucleic acid depends on the type and amount of starting material [26]. Few studies have been published comparing different processing methods on clinical specimens containing C. pneumoniae organisms. Gnarpe and Eriksson compared the Amplicor sputum sample preparation kit (Roche Diagnostics) with proteinase K treatment on throat samples and found that the sensitivity of the *C. pneumoniae* PCR was increased by treatment involving more complete lysis of the cells [27]. Daugharty et al. [28] evaluated seven procedures for extracting chlamydial DNA from buffy coats spiked with *Chlamydia* elementary bodies. They found that the QIAamp kit (Qiagen) was the extraction method of choice due to its simplicity, rapidity and sensitivity. Maass and Dalhoff [29] assessed the presence of PCR inhibitors in 75 BAL specimens after treatment by three common sample preparation methods. PCR inhibitors were present in 31% of the samples processed by heat treatment and in 12% of the samples for which single-step proteinase K digestion was used. However, PCR inhibitors were efficiently attenuated after digestion with a complex cetyltrimethylammonium bromide (CTAB) purification method followed by phenol-chloroform extraction. Wilson et al. [30] compared four methods for DNA extraction from dilutions of cultured *Chlamydia*: a guanidine isothiocyanate/silica method, an extraction method using Chelex, boiling samples followed by high-speed centrifugation, and proteinase K treatment. The proteinase K digestion-based method was more sensitive than the guanidine isothiocyanate/silica-based method. Further, the Chelex-based method was less sensitive than the guanidine isothiocyanate/silica-based method, and boiling of the elementary bodies did not appear to release *C. pneumoniae* DNA for PCR.

If a swab is used for collection, the tube should be vortexed with glass beads before removal of the swab from the transport medium. Sputum samples and other viscous samples should be treated with a mucolysing agent (e.g. *N*-acetylcysteine), then washed and concentrated before DNA extraction [7, 31]. Nonetheless, further studies need to be done before general recommendations for specimen collection and preparation can be made with confidence.

It is important to choose a gene sequence that is conserved within the species to avoid failure of the PCR due to mismatches between the target gene and the primers. Moreover, the sequence should differ significantly from other gene sequences including sequences of other *Chlamydia* species in order to avoid false-positive results due to amplification of non-*C. pneumoniae* sequences.

Several different targets, primers and reaction protocols have been described for the detection of *C. pneumoniae* DNA. The PCR protocol described by Tong and Sillis [6] using a nested touchdown PCR with a target within the major outer membrane protein (MOMP)-coding gene has proved to be both sensitive and specific when compared with other diagnostic methods including cell culture and MIF serology [6, 7]. The outer primers amplify a 333-bp product from both *C. pneumoniae* and *C. psittaci*, but do not amplify DNA from *C. trachomatis*. One of the internal primers is specific for *C. pneumoniae*; therefore, only the first-stage product from *C. pneumoniae* can be amplified in the nested PCR, yielding a 207-bp product. 16S rRNA genes [32] have also been widely used as the target, and a combined PCR-enzyme immunoassay (PCR-EIA) method developed by Gaydos et al. has proven specific and fairly sensitive for detection of *C. pneumoniae* in respiratory specimens, although its sensitivity may be improved [33–35]. The method combines the sensitivity and specificity of PCR with a convenient and objective detection system based on EIA technique after hybridization with an RNA probe.

Black et al. [8] used a nested primer strategy for direct species-specific detection of the 16S rRNA gene of *C. pneumoniae*. The test was applied to 58 swab specimens and was found to be as sensitive as culture or serology for detection of *C. pneumoniae* infection. Black and colleagues also concluded that single-step PCR may be unreliable for direct testing of clinical specimens unless a nested PCR is performed, sensitive PCR product detection methods are used, or steps are taken to eliminate inhibitors in the transport medium or in the specimen itself. The satisfactory performance of nested PCR has recently been confirmed [10].

Wilson et al. [30] have designed a "one-tube nested PCR" using two primer pairs with different melting points (T_m) in one reaction mixture for amplification of a *C. pneumoniae*-specific region of the 16S rRNA gene. Jantos et al. [16] have described a simplified PCR-EIA test based on the 16S rRNA primers described by Gaydos et al. [32]. Biotin-labelled *C. pneumoniae* PCR products hybridize to a digoxigenin-labeled probe. The complex is then captured in streptavidin-coated microtiter plates and detected using anti-digoxigenin peroxidase conjugate and a colorimetric substrate. This PCR-EIA test was found to be much more sensitive than visualization of PCR products on agarose gel and as sensitive as Southern blot hybridization. A commonly used PCR system for detection of *C. pneumoniae* DNA was developed by Campbell et al., derived from a cloned 474-bp *Pst*I *C. pneumoniae*-specific fragment [36]. A modification of this PCR test was performed by Khan and Potter [37] who designed a fourth primer and developed a nested PCR with the internal primers generating a product of 204 bp.

If a one-step-based PCR method is used, detection of the PCR product by a specific probe-based hybridization assay is recommended for increased sensitivity and specificity [38]. Microplate-based colorometric methods with enzyme immunoassays (PCR-EIA) may give comparable results to Southern or dot blot hybridization and offer some advantages in terms of simplicity and speed [2, 16, 30, 33]. For detection of products generated by nested PCR, agarose gel electrophoresis followed by ethidium bromide staining seems to be a reliable detection method [7, 8]. Development of quantitative methods for detection of *C. pneumoniae*-specific nucleic acid has begun but the advanced instrumentation is expensive. Direct quantitative real-time DNA and RNA detection is now possible by using specifically designed automated equipment, such as the Perkin Elmer Applied Biosystem 7700 DNA sequence detector [26].

Beside PCR, several alternative amplification techniques have been developed. These techniques may all be useful alternatives for detection of *C. pneumoniae*, but no study has yet been published describing the application of any of these methods for this purpose. Moreover, no commercial amplification test is currently available for detection of *C. pneumoniae*.

Diagnostic Aspects

Several clinical studies using PCR for the detection of *C. pneumoniae* have been published [7–9, 33, 39]. Although the performance of many PCR methods seems very good, some of these are cumbersome and time-consuming and not easily adapted or practical for routine laboratories. In addition, the risk of contamination is greatly increased by testing of large numbers of specimens [38]. More studies need to be conducted that determine the sensitivity and specificity of PCR by testing a large number of clinical specimens from symptomatic and asymptomatic individuals [40]. The samples should be tested in parallel using culture and one or several alternative amplification methods (e.g., PCR targeting alternative gene sequences). Serology should also be performed to distinguish a carrier state from acute infection [7, 33].

Introduction of highly sensitive NAA techniques such as PCR may increase our ability to identify carriers of *C. pneumoniae*. As a consequence, the interpretation of results may occasionally be problematic when there is not a corresponding serologic response. In symptomatic patients, detection of a persistent and perhaps harmless *C. pneumoniae* co-infection may obscure the true etiology. Therefore, a single PCR result must always be viewed with caution and interpreted in the context of the patient's symptomatology and together with other diagnostic procedures and clinical findings. Continuous education of clinicians, in proper use and interpretation of the amplification-generated results, and in the limitations of the tests, is of great importance.

C. pneumoniae has emerged as a common and important respiratory pathogen and appropriate therapy can be offered early in the disease course provided that a rapid and reliable diagnostic test is available. During an outbreak of *C. pneumoniae* among University of Washington students, Grayston and colleagues found that PCR is a promising technique for quickly demonstrating the organism in clinical specimens [39].

Dalhoff and Maass [19] used a PCR method based on published primers [36] and showed that *C. pneumoniae* may be frequently detected by PCR in samples from the lower respiratory tract of hospitalized patients with pneumonia, but is uncommon in immunocompetent non-pneumonia patients, confirming that the PCR results obtained on BAL samples are of clinical relevance in immunocompetent patients. Also, Gaydos et al. [34] demonstrated a prevalence of 11% by PCR in BAL of immunocompromised patients with pneumonia. This finding was confirmed by Dalhoff and Maass [19], who detected *C. pneumoniae* in 13% of BAL samples collected from 47 HIV-infected persons who were evaluated because of opportunistic lung disease or for staging of pulmonary involvement in systemic diseases. In the upper respiratory tract, *C. pneumoniae* may be detected also in healthy subjects [41].

The PCR technique is commonly used, alone or in combination with other methods, for the detection of *C. pneumoniae* in the cardiovascular system. *C. pneumoniae* DNA has been detected in atherosclerotic plaques in several studies [21, 42, 43] but the frequency of positive results varies from 0% to 100% [44–47]. This variation may be explained by the use of different populations as well as different PCR techniques.

Conclusions

The application of NAA technology to *Chlamydia* research and routine diagnostics opens up new possibilities for direct detection of *C. pneumoniae*. With further improvements, this principle will certainly provide diagnostic laboratories with powerful and rapid means for direct identification of *C. pneumoniae* in a variety of clinical specimens. Until simplification and standardization of the NAA-based techniques have been achieved and/or commercial kits have been developed, these new techniques should be implemented with caution, and attention should be paid to strict quality control procedures to obtain reliable results.

References

1. Ieven M, Goossens H (1997) Relevance of nucleic acid amplification techniques for diagnosis of respiratory tract infections in the clinical laboratory. Clin Microbiol Rev 10:242-256
2. Palmer HM (1994) The chlamydiales and mycoplasmatales. In: Ehrlich GD, Greenberg SJ (eds) PCR-based diagnostics in infectious diseases. Blackwell, Boston, pp 493-510
3. Martin GP, Timmers E (1997) PCR and its modifications for the detection of infectious diseases. In: Lee HH, Morse SA, Olsvik O (eds) Nucleic acid amplification technologies: application to disease diagnosis. BioTechniques, Eaton, Cambridge, Mass, pp 79-99
4. Wilson IG (1997) Inhibition and facilitation of nucleic acid amplification. Appl Environ Microbiol 63:3741-3751
5. Don RH, Cox PT, Wainwright BJ, Baker K, Mattick JS (1991) "Touchdown" PCR to circumvent spurious priming during gene amplification. Nucleic Acids Res 19:4008
6. Tong CYW, Sillis M (1993) Detection of *Chlamydia pneumoniae* and *Chlamydia psittaci* in sputum samples by PCR. J Clin Pathol 46:313-317
7. Boman J, Allard A, Persson K, Lundborg M, Juto P, Wadell G (1997) Rapid diagnosis of respiratory *Chlamydia pneumoniae* infection by nested touchdown polymerase chain reaction compared with culture and antigen detection by EIA. J Infect Dis 75:1523-1526
8. Black CM, Fields PI, Messmer TO, Berdal BP (1994) Detection of *Chlamydia pneumoniae* in clinical specimens by polymerase chain reaction using nested primers. Eur J Clin Microbiol Infect Dis 13:752-756
9. Verkooyen RP, Willemse D, Casteren SC, Joulandan SA, Snijder RJ, van den Bosch JM, van Helden HP, Peeters MF, Verbrugh HA (1998) Evaluation of PCR, culture, and serology for diagnosis of *Chlamydia pneumoniae* respiratory infections. J Clin Microbiol 36:2301-2307
10. Hammerschlag MR, Chirgwin K, Roblin PM, Gelling M, Dumornay W, Mandel L, Smith P, Schachter J (1998) Persistent infection with *Chlamydia pneumoniae* following acute respiratory illness. Clin Infect Dis 14:178-182
11. Khan MA, Potter CW, Sharrard RM (1996) A reverse transcriptase-PCR based assay for in-vitro antibiotic susceptibility testing of *Chlamydia pneumoniae*. J Antimicrob Chemother 37:677-685
12. Whelen AC, Persing DH (1996) The role of nucleic acid amplification and detection in the clinical microbiology laboratory. Annu Rev Microbiol 50:349-373
13. Kwok S, Higuchi R (1989) Avoiding false positives with PCR. Nature 339:237-238
14. Kwok S (1990) Procedures to minimize PCR-product carry-over. In: Innis MA,

Gelfand DH, Sninsky JJ, White TJ (eds) PCR protocols – A guide to methods and applications. Academic Press, San Diego, pp 142-145

15. Boman J, Soderberg S, Forsberg J, Birgander LS, Allard A, Persson K, Jidell E, Kumlin U, Juto P, Waldenstrom A, Wadell G (1998) High prevalence of *Chlamydia pneumoniae* DNA in peripheral blood mononuclear cells in patients with cardiovascular disease and in middle-aged blood donors. J Infect Dis 178:274-277

16. Jantos CA, Roggendorf R, Wuppermann FN, Hegemann JH (1998) Rapid detection of *Chlamydia pneumoniae* by PCR-enzyme immunoassay. J Clin Microbiol 36:1890-1894

17. Pham DG, Madico GE, Quinn TC, Enzler MJ, Smith TF, Gaydos CA (1998) Use of lambda phage DNA as a hybrid internal control in a PCR-enzyme immunoassay to detect *Chlamydia pneumoniae*. J Clin Microbiol 36:1919-1922

18. Andersen AB, Thybo S, Godfrey-Faussett P, Stoker NG (1993) Polymerase chain reaction for detection of *Mycobacterium tuberculosis* in sputum. Eur J Clin Microbiol Infect Dis 12:922-927

19. Dalhoff K, Maass M (1996) *Chlamydia pneumoniae* pneumonia in hospitalized patients. Clinical characteristics and diagnostic value of polymerase chain reaction detection in BAL. Chest 110:351-356

20. Pruckl PM, Aspock C, Makristathis A, Rotter ML, Wank H, Willinger B, Hirschl AM (1995) Polymerase chain reaction for detection of *Chlamydia pneumoniae* in gargled-water specimens of children. Eur J Clin Microbiol Infect Dis 14:141-144

21. Kuo C-C, Shor A, Campbell LA, Fukushi H, Patton DL, Grayston JT (1993) Demonstration of *Chlamydia pneumoniae* in atherosclerotic lesions of coronary arteries. J Infect Dis 167:841-849

22. Naidu BR, Ngeow Y-F, Pang T (1997) MOMP-based PCR reveals presence of *Chlamydia pneumoniae* DNA in respiratory and serum samples of patients with acute *C. pneumoniae*-associated infections. J Microbiol Methods 28:1-9

23. Naidu BR, Ngeow Y-F, Kannan P, Jeyamalar R, Khir A, Khoo KL, Pang T (1997) Evidence of *Chlamydia pneumoniae* infection obtained by the polymerase chain reaction (PCR) in patients with acute myocardial infarction and coronary heart disease. J Infect 35:199-200

24. Wadowsky RM, Laus S, Libert T, States SJ, Ehrlich GD (1994) Inhibition of PCR-based assay for *Bordetella pertussis* by using calcium alginate fiber and aluminium shaft components of a nasopharyngeal swab. J Clin Microbiol 32:1054-1057

25. Black CM, Tharpe JA, Russell H (1992) Distinguishing *Chlamydia* species by restriction analysis of the major outer membrane protein gene. Mol Cell Probes 6:395-400

26. O'Leary JJ, Engels K, Dada MA (1997) The polymerase chain reaction in pathology. J Clin Pathol 50:805-810

27. Gnarpe J, Eriksson K (1995) Sample preparation for *Chlamydia pneumoniae* PCR. APMIS 103:307-308

28. Daugharty H, Skelton SK, Messmer T (1998) Chlamydia DNA extraction for use in PCR: stability and sensitivity in detection. J Clin Lab Anal 12:47-53

29. Maass M, Dalhoff K (1994) Comparison of sample preparation methods for detection of *Chlamydia pneumoniae* in bronchoalveolar lavage fluid by PCR. J Clin Microbiol 32:2616-2619

30. Wilson PA, Phipps J, Samuel D, Saunders NA (1996) Development of a simplified polymerase chain reaction-enzyme immunoassay for the detection of *Chlamydia pneumoniae*. J Appl Bacteriol 80:431-438

31. Sillis M, White P, Caul EO, Paul ID, Treharne JD (1992) The differentiation of *Chlamy-*

dia species by antigen detection in sputum specimens from patients with community-acquired acute respiratory infections. J Infect 25[Suppl 1]:77-86

32. Gaydos CA, Quinn TC, Eiden JJ (1992) Identification of *Chlamydia pneumoniae* by
    DNA amplification of the 16S rRNA gene. J Clin Microbiol 30:796-800
33. Gaydos CA, Roblin PM, Hammerschlag MR, Hyman CL, Eiden JJ, Schachter J, Quinn
    TC (1994) Diagnostic utility of PCR-enzyme immunoassay, culture, and serology for
    detection of *Chlamydia pneumoniae* in symptomatic and asymptomatic patients. J
    Clin Microbiol 32:903-905
34. Gaydos CA, Fowler CL, Gill VJ, Eiden JJ, Quinn TC (1993) Detection of *Chlamydia
    pneumoniae* by polymerase chain reaction-enzyme immunoassay in an immunocom-
    promised population. Clin Infect Dis 17:718-723
35. Gaydos CA, Eiden JJ, Oldach D, Mundy LM, Auwaerter P, Warner ML, Vance E, Burton
    AA, Quinn TC (1994) Diagnosis of *Chlamydia pneumoniae* infection in patients with
    community-acquired pneumonia by polymerase chain reaction enzyme immunoas-
    say. Clin Infect Dis 19:157-160
36. Campbell LA, Perez Melgosa M, Hamilton DJ, Kuo C-C, Grayston JT (1992) Detection
    of *Chlamydia pneumoniae* by polymerase chain reaction. J Clin Microbiol 30:434-439
37. Khan MA, Potter CW (1996) The nPCR detection of *Chlamydia pneumoniae* and
    Chlamydia trachomatis in children hospitalized for bronchiolitis. J Infect 33:173-175
38. Schmidt BL (1997) PCR in laboratory diagnosis of human *Borrelia burgdorferi* infec-
    tion. Clin Microbiol Rev 10:185-201
39. Grayston JT, Aldous MB, Easton A, Wang SP, Kuo C-C, Campbell LA, Altman J (1993)
    Evidence that *Chlamydia pneumoniae* causes pneumonia and bronchitis. J Infect Dis
    168:1231-1235
40. Hammerschlag MR (1995) Diagnostic methods for intracellular pathogens. Clin
    Microbiol Infect 1[Suppl 1]:S3-S8
41. Hyman CL, Roblin PM, Gaydos CA, Quinn TC, Schachter J, Hammerschlag MR (1995)
    Prevalence of asymptomatic nasopharyngeal carriage of *Chlamydia pneumoniae* in
    subjectively healthy adults: assessment by polymerase chain reaction-enzyme
    immunoassay and culture. Clin Infect Dis 20:1174-1178
42. Maass M, Bartels C, Engel PM, Mamat U, Sievers HH (1998) Endovascular presence of
    viable *Chlamydia pneumoniae* is a common phenomenon in coronary artery disease.
    J Am Coll Cardiol 31:827-832
43. Campbell LA, O'Brien ER, Cappuccio AL, Kuo C-C, Wang S-P, Stewart D, Patton DL,
    Cummings PK, Grayston JT (1995) Detection of *Chlamydia pneumoniae* TWAR in
    human coronary atherectomy tissues. J Infect Dis 172:585-588
44. Juvonen J, Juvonen T, Laurila A, Alakarppa H, Lounatmaa K, Surcel HM, Leinonen M,
    Kairaluoma MI, Saikku P (1997) Demonstration of *Chlamydia pneumoniae* in the
    walls of abdominal aortic aneurysms. J Vasc Surg 25:499-505
45. Lindholt JS, Ostergard L, Henneberg EW, Fasting H, Andersen P (1998) Failure to
    demonstrate *Chlamydia pneumoniae* in symptomatic abdominal aortic aneurysms by
    a nested polymerase chain reaction (PCR). Eur J Vasc Endovasc Surg 15:161-164
46. Weiss SM, Roblin PM, Gaydos CA, Cummings P, Patton DL, Schulhoff N, Shani J,
    Frankel R, Penney K, Quinn TC, Hammerschlag MR, Schachter J (1996) Failure to
    detect *Chlamydia pneumoniae* in coronary atheromas of patients undergoing atherec-
    tomy. J Infect Dis 173:957-962
47. Ong G, Thomas BJ, Mansfield AO, Davidson BR, Taylor-Robinson D (1996) Detection
    and widespread distribution of *Chlamydia pneumoniae* in the vascular system and its
    possible implications. J Clin Pathol 49:102-106

Chlamydia pneumoniae Infections: Applications of Laboratory Methods

R.W. PEELING

Introduction

Since the recognition of *Chlamydia pneumoniae* as a species distinct from *C. psittaci* in 1989, laboratory methods have gradually been developed as tools for the management of *C. pneumoniae* infection, for defining the epidemiology of disease and for research into the pathogenesis of chlamydial infections [1, 2]. These laboratory methods include culture, antigen detection, serology and the polymerase chain reaction (PCR). Early seroepidemiological studies were based on the micro-immunofluorescence (MIF) assay, originally developed for *C. trachomatis*. As the conditions for culture of *C. pneumoniae* become optimised, antigenic and genetic differences of strains from around the world were documented. Antigen detection and PCR assays represent a new generation of tests which can provide rapid diagnosis with ease of specimen transport. The attributes and limitations of each of these laboratory methods will be presented below, followed by a discussion on how these tests can be applied appropriately in different settings.

Laboratory Methods

Laboratory methods for the diagnosis of *C. pneumoniae* infection are summarised in Table 1. The sensitivity shown for many of these methods is low compared to their performance for the diagnosis of *C. trachomatis* infections. This may relate partly to inadequate sampling because of the inaccessibility of the site of colonisation, which is believed to be alveolar macrophages of the lung [1].

Culture

The procedure for culturing *C. pneumoniae* has been adapted from that used for *C. trachomatis*. The inoculum is centrifuged onto the cell monolayer. Cyclohex-imide and 10% fetal calf serum are added to the culture media to inhibit host cell protein synthesis and to stabilise the viability of *C. pneumoniae*, respectively. Yet, few laboratories have been successful in growing *C. pneumoniae*. This is possibly

Table 1. Laboratory diagnosis of *C. pneumoniae* infections

Feature	Culture	DFA	PCR	Serology
Detection	Infectious organism	Antigen	DNA	Antibodies
Specimen/site	Throat swab N/P swab BAL Sputum	Throat swab N/P swab BAL	Throat swab N/P swab BAL Sputum	Blood
Sensitivity	50%–75%	20%–60%	10–100 organisms	60%–80%
Specificity	100%	70%–95%	95%–100%	90%–100%
Processing time	3–12 days	1 h	1–2 days	1–2 days
Specimen transport	4 °C or frozen if > 48 h to lab	Room temperature	Room temperature	Room temperature or 4 °C
Reading of results	Subjective	Subjective	Objective	Subjective

N/P, nasopharyngeal swab; *BAL*, bronchoalveolar lavage; *DFA*, direct fluorescent antibody; *PCR*, polymerase chain reaction

due to specimen quality as well as inherent characteristics of the organism. First, *C. pneumoniae* is easily inactivated during transport. Maass and Dalhoff documented over 80% loss in infectivity of wild strains stored at room temperature over 12 h [3]. Thus cold chain transport is required to preserve specimen viability. Specimens requiring more than 48 h in transport should be frozen, even though some infectivity may be lost on freezing and thawing. Secondly, as discussed previously, specimens are often not collected from the site of colonisation. Thus culture sensitivity may be as low as 50%–60% for throat and nasopharyngeal swabs when serology is used as a gold standard. Higher sensitivity can be obtained with bronchial aspirate or bronchoalveolar lavage (BAL), although invasive procedures are rarely warranted in *C. pneumoniae* infection. Thirdly, *C. pneumoniae* grows poorly in culture, often requiring several blind passages before inclusions can be seen. Different cell lines have been evaluated, and HL and Hep-2 have been found to be better hosts for *C. pneumoniae* than HeLa and McCoy cells [4–6]. The use of trypsin and serum-free media to enhance infectivity has been reported [7, 8]. Culture confirmed by fluorescein-conjugated monoclonal antibodies specific for *C. pneumoniae* should have a specificity of 100%. In spite of the stringent specimen transport requirements and the expense, time and technical expertise required, culture for *C. pneumoniae* is a worthwhile goal for laboratories interested in antigenic variation, antimicrobial susceptibility and research into the pathogenesis of disease.

Antigen Detection

Direct Fluorescent Antibody

The development of monoclonal antibodies specific for *C. pneumoniae* has enabled laboratories to detect elementary bodies (EBs) of *C. pneumoniae* in smears from throat, nasopharyngeal swabs, and bronchial lavage or aspirate specimens. These antibodies are commercially available as either directly or indirectly labelled with fluorescein. Their performance in direct fluorescent antibody (DFA) tests appears to be fairly comparable [9]. Fixation of the smear with acetone is recommended, as methanol may destroy some of the antigens [10]. The sensitivity of DFA is estimated to be 20%–60% compared to culture, and it is higher for specimens from a deep site. The specificity of DFA should approach 95%–99% but it depends very much on the expertise and experience of the technologist, as the reading of results is subjective and there may often be non-specific staining in specimens with mucus. DFA results are available within 30–60 min. This is especially useful in outbreak investigations, where a rapid presumptive diagnosis would allow appropriate treatment of cases and containment of the outbreak. As the smears are fixed with acetone on site, DFA slides can be transported to the laboratory at room temperature.

Enzyme Immunoassay

Enzyme immunoassay (EIA) designed for *C. trachomatis* can be used for the detection of *C. pneumoniae* antigen as well because the capture antibody in *Chlamydia* EIA kits is the genus-specific lipopolysaccharide (LPS). However, the performance of these assays has not been widely evaluated [11].

Polymerase Chain Reaction

Several PCR procedures have been reported for *C. pneumoniae* based on target sequences in the 16S ribosomal DNA, the major outer membrane and others [12–14]. Their lower detection limits are from 5 to 100 EBs, with the performance of most of these protocols being comparable. Nested protocols are generally more sensitive but much more prone to laboratory contamination [15]. PCR is estimated to be at least 25% more sensitive than culture, mainly because stringent specimen transport conditions are not required for PCR [16]. Apart from the sensitivity and the ease of specimen transport, another advantage of PCR is that a multiplex format can be designed to allow the simultaneous detection of several pathogens causing similar clinical syndromes from a single specimen with a single amplification reaction. Hence a PCR multiplex panel for atypical pneumonia can be used to detect *C. pneumoniae*, *Mycoplasma pneumoniae* and *Legionella pneumophila* from a throat swab [17]. Multiplex reaction has also been reported where a target sequence shared by *C. pneumoniae*, *C. trachomatis* and *C. psittaci* is amplified, and then species specificity can be distinguished by restriction fragment length polymorphism patterns [18, 19].

Serology

Given the problems of obtaining an adequate specimen for culture, DFA or PCR, serodiagnosis provides the most convincing evidence of infection if IgM antibodies or a fourfold rise in IgG titres can be shown. However, the need for paired sera to show a fourfold rise in titre is a limitation of serological diagnosis.

Complement Fixation

The target of the antibodies in the complement fixation (CF) test is the genus-specific LPS. Thus it is impossible to determine species-specific antibody response with this test. Although lacking in specificity, the CF test is much less technically demanding than the MIF test and has objective endpoints. Another advantage of the CF test is that LPS antibodies are produced early in primary infection. Hence a serodiagnosis may be reached in sera taken 1 week apart, compared with 3 weeks or more for MIF. For primary infection, the CF test has a sensitivity of 60%. In re-infection, LPS antibodies are rarely detectable, giving CF tests a sensitivity of only approximately 10% [20–23].

Whole Inclusion Fluorescence

Antibody detection kits are available in which the source of antigen is cells infected with a lymphogranuloma strain (LGV) of *C. trachomatis*, fixed on a glass slide. The sensitivity and specificity of these kits for the serodiagnosis of *C. pneumoniae* infection has not been widely evaluated. Thus, antibody titres from these kits should be interpreted with caution.

Micro-immunofluorescence Assay

In the MIF assay, multiple templates of purified EBs from different *Chlamydia* species are fixed onto glass slides as a source of antigen. Fluorescein-conjugated anti-human globulins can be used to detect IgM, IgG and IgA antibodies to all *Chlamydia* species in a single template. Thus cross-reactive antibodies can be easily detected. Properly performed and read, this test provides the most sensitive and specific method for the laboratory diagnosis of *C. pneumoniae* infection. Antibodies against genus-specific antigens such as LPS do not give the apple-green fluorescence typical of antibody response to other outer membrane antigens. As acute *C. pneumoniae* infection generally induces high levels of IgG antibody in MIF, rarely seen in infections with other *Chlamydia* species, these low-level cross-reactive antibodies rarely present a problem in the serodiagnosis of acute *C. pneumoniae* infections for the experienced technologist [21, 24]. Standardisation of this test is an important priority if data from different studies are to be compared. A panel of 22 sera sent to 15 laboratories around the world for MIF resulted in an inter-laboratory agreement of 80% for the serodiagnosis of *C. pneumoniae* [25]. Inter-laboratory variation may be due to the source, quality and concentration of antigens used and reader subjectivity. MIF is now commercially available and awaits performance evaluation.

Enzyme Immunoassay

EIA kits with LPS-extracted EBs or synthetic peptides unique to *C. pneumoniae* as antigen are commercially available for the detection of antibodies to *C. pneumoniae*. Evaluation of these kits is limited, and problems with sensitivity and specificity have been encountered. If the threshold absorbance is raised to increase assay specificity, sensitivity is decreased, and vice versa. Given the objective readout and the availability of technical expertise for EIA in many laboratories, the identification of a highly immunogenic target antigen would be useful for the development of a highly sensitive, specific and technically accessible EIA.

Applications

The appropriate utilisation of the described laboratory methods to diagnose *C. pneumoniae* infection for patient management, outbreak investigations or research depends not only on the test performance but also on conditions of specimen transport and the speed with which test results can be obtained.

Laboratory Diagnosis of Acute *Chlamydia pneumoniae* Infection

C. pneumoniae is rapidly inactivated at room temperature. Hence for specimens where cold chain transport is not available, non-culture tests such as antigen detection or PCR are recommended. Since asymptomatic carriage of *C. pneumoniae* has been documented in 1%–5% of healthy persons, the finding of positive PCR, DFA or culture specimens from the upper respiratory tract should be interpreted in light of the clinical history [26–28]. Table 2 shows a set of criteria

Table 2. Criteria for positivity in the serodiagnosis of *C. pneumoniae* infections

	CF	MIF assay	EIA
Acute infection	Fourfold rise in titre	IgM titre ≥ 16 or IgG titre ≥ 512 or fourfold rise in IgG titre	Cut-off varies according to manufacturer
Past infection		IgG titre 16–256	
Antigen	LPS	EBs	Peptides or EBs
Specificity	Genus specific	Species specific	Genus/species specific
Sensitivity	Primary infection: 60% Re-infection: 10%–40%	60%–80%	Insufficient evaluation

CF, complement fixation; *LPS*, lipopolysaccharide; *MIF*, micro-immunofluorescence; *EBs*, elementary bodies; *EIA*, enzyme immunoassay recommended for the serodiagnosis of *C. pneumoniae* infection based on data from extensive seroepidemiological studies [16]. Serological cross-reactivity to *Bartonella* sp. has been documented [29]. This is possibly due to the presence of shared epitopes on LPS or on various other antigens [30, 31]. Since infection with *Bartonella* sp. is rare, these cross-reactive antibodies rarely present a problem in the interpretation of MIF results. In contrast, with 60% of any adult population being seropositive for *C. pneumoniae*, immunofluorescence assay (IFA) results for *Bartonella* infection should be interpreted in light of the clinical findings. The performance of MIF assays in children appears variable and requires further study [1, 32, 33]. Serodiagnosis based on a single serum sample should be interpreted with caution. This is especially important in sera from the elderly: some older persons may have persistent high IgG titres in the absence of clinically apparent disease or atypical clinical presentation [1, 34] and others may have false-positive IgM results due to the presence of rheumatoid factor in the sera [35].

Antimicrobial Susceptibility Testing and Treatment

No antimicrobial resistance has yet been documented for *C. pneumoniae*, but continuous monitoring is required. Since culture is not widely available and requires stringent transport conditions to preserve specimen viability, many treatment trials for community-acquired pneumonia use the resolution of symptoms as an endpoint, rather than microbiological cure. Reports of persistence of the organism after treatment in both humans and animal models points to possible inadequacy of present treatment regimens for *C. pneumoniae* and the need for more effective treatment trials based on microbiological cure as an endpoint [36, 37]. It may be possible to use non-culture tests to define the aetiology of atypical community-acquired pneumonia in treatment trials, but culture is needed for determining optimal treatment duration and efficacy.

Outbreak Investigations

Many outbreaks of *C. pneumoniae* infection have been reported [1, 38]. The ease of spread of infection within institutions, especially in nursing homes, is a concern. A rapid diagnostic method, such as DFA, would allow rapid presumptive identification of the source of the outbreak within 1 h. Early, appropriate treatment of all infected cases is important to interrupt the chain of transmission. However, DFA often lacks sensitivity. Hence a negative DFA test should not rule out *C. pneumoniae* as a cause of an outbreak. Serology may not provide a timely diagnosis in outbreak investigations, but data on paired sera often provide important information on the extent of an outbreak. The isolation of outbreak strains by culture may provide important information on their phenotype or genotype, which may distinguish them from strains causing milder illness or having a lower frequency of transmission.

Research

In the last decade, studies have shown an association of *C. pneumoniae* infection with coronary heart disease, cerebrovascular disease, asthma and lung cancer [1, 39–45]. It is speculated that persistent or chronic *C. pneumoniae* infection may play a role in initiating or exacerbating an ongoing inflammatory process that leads to adverse outcomes [46]. PCR has been used to document evidence of *C. pneumoniae* in cardiac or other tissues. Culture of infectious organisms from these tissues is not easy as tissue digests are often toxic in cell culture. The question remains of whether viable *C. pneumoniae* is inducing or participating in these inflammatory processes. The lack of access to the presumed site of colonisation hampers the verification of persistent infection in asymptomatic individuals. At present, there is no consensus on serological criteria for defining persistent infection. Gupta et al. used a MIF IgG titre of ≥ 64 as a cut-off for inclusion into a randomised treatment trial of patients with a previous history of myocardial infarction [47]. It has also been proposed that persistent serum IgA titres, are a better marker of chronic chlamydial infection than IgG titres, as IgA has a half-life of 5–7 days in serum and therefore persisting IgA titres, may represent low-level chronic infection as a continuing source of antigenic stimulation. It is important that IgG antibodies be absorbed out before testing sera for IgA [48] in order to avoid false-positive results, since 50%–70% of adult populations worldwide have been shown to be seropositive for *C. pneumoniae*. Immune complexes of antibody with LPS have also been used as a marker of chronic infection, but LPS antibodies are genus-specific, and use of immune complexes may lead to misleading results. Overall, the use of serum antibody response as a marker of susceptibility rather than protection is open to debate. Chiu et al. found that in patients with atherosclerosis who have evidence of *C. pneumoniae* in their plaques, 59% had IgG titres ≥ 128, 22% had IgG titres of 16–64 and 30% had IgA titres ≥ 16, compared with rates of 64%, 23% and 37% for the respective titres in patients with no evidence of *C. pneumoniae* in their plaques [49]. Blasi et al. found that 25 of 26 patients with *C. pneumoniae*-positive plaques were seropositive by IgG and/or IgA, compared with 16 of 25 patients with *C. pneumoniae*-negative plaques [39]. In other studies of the association of *C. pneumoniae* infection with abdominal aortic aneurysm or atherosclerosis, only 60%–75% of those with PCR-confirmed *C. pneumoniae* in their tissue were seropositive by IgG or IgA [42, 50]. Studies of immune responses in animal models of atherosclerosis may be useful in defining markers of persistent infection.

Challenge for the Future

At present MIF serology provides the most sensitive and specific method for the laboratory diagnosis of *C. pneumoniae* infection. However, the MIF test is subjective and technically demanding. A simple rapid test with an objective readout for the laboratory diagnosis of *C. pneumoniae* infection is a priority. A marker for chronic *C. pneumoniae* infection in research studies remains to be defined.

References

1. Kuo C-C, Jackson LA, Campbell LA, Grayston JT (1995) *Chlamydia pneumoniae* (TWAR). Clin Microbiol Rev 8:451-461
2. Peeling RW (1995) Laboratory diagnosis of *Chlamydia pneumoniae* infections. Can J Infect Dis 6:198-203
3. Maass M, Dalhoff K (1995) Transport and storage conditions for cultural recovery of *Chlamydia pneumoniae*. J Clin Microbiol 33:1793-1796
4. Wong KH, Skelton SK, Chan YK (1992) Efficient culture of *Chlamydia pneumoniae* with cell lines derived from the human respiratory tract. J Clin Microbiol 30:1625-1630
5. Roblin PM, Dumornay W, Hammerschlag MR (1992) Use of Hep-2 cells for improved isolation and passage of *Chlamydia pneumoniae*. J Clin Microbiol 30:1968-1971
6. Theunissen JJH, Van Heijst BYM, Wagenvoort JHT, Stolz E, Michel MF (1992) Factors influencing the infectivity of *Chlamydia pneumoniae* elementary bodies on HL cells. J Clin Microbiol 30:1388-1391
7. Maass M, Essig A, Marre R, Henkel W (1993) Growth in serum-free medium improves isolation of *Chlamydia pneumoniae*. J Clin Microbiol 31:3050-3052
8. Kazuyama Y, Lee SM, Amamiya K, Taguchi F (1997) A novel method for isolation of *Chlamydia pneumoniae* by treatment with trypsin or EDTA. J Clin Microbiol 35:1624-1626
9. Montalban GS, Roblin PM, Hammerschlag MR (1994) Performance of three commercially available monoclonal reagents for confirmation of *Chlamydia pneumoniae* in cell culture. J Clin Microbiol 32:1406-1407
10. Wang S-P, Grayston JT (1991) *Chlamydia pneumoniae* elementary body antigenic reactivity with fluorescent antibody is destroyed by methanol. J Clin Microbiol 29:1539-1541
11. Sillis M, White P, Caul EO, Paul ID, Treharne JD (1992) The differentiation of *Chlamydia* species by antigen detection in sputum specimens from patients with community-acquired acute respiratory infections. J Infect 25[Suppl 1]:77-86
12. Campbell LA, Melgosa MP, Hamilton DJ, Kuo C-C, Grayston JT (1992) Detection of *Chlamydia pneumoniae* by polymerase chain reaction. J Clin Microbiol 30:434-439
13. Tong CYW, Sillis M (1993) Detection of *Chlamydia pneumoniae* and *Chlamydia psittaci* in sputum samples by PCR. J Clin Pathol 46:313-317
14. Gaydos CA, Fowler CL, Gill VJ, Eiden JJ, Quinn TC (1993) Detection of *Chlamydia pneumoniae* by polymerase chain reaction–enzyme immunoassay in an immunocompromised population. Clin Infect Dis 17:718-723
15. Black CM, Fields PI, Messmer TO, Berdal BP (1994) Detection of *Chlamydia pneumoniae* in clinical specimens by polymerase chain reaction using nested primers. Eur J Clin Microbiol Infect Dis 13:752-756
16. Grayston JT (1992) Infections caused by *Chlamydia pneumoniae* strain TWAR. Clin Infect Dis 15:757-763
17. Ramirez JA, Ahkee S, Tolentino A, Miller RD, Summersgill JT (1996) Diagnosis of *Legionella pneumophila, Mycoplasma pneumoniae,* or *Chlamydia pneumoniae* lower respiratory infection using the polymerase chain reaction on a single throat swab specimen. Diagn Microbiol Infect Dis 24:7-14
18. Rasmussen SJ, Douglas FP, Timms P (1993) PCR detection and differentiation of *Chlamydia pneumoniae, Chlamydia psittaci, Chlamydia trachomatis*. Mol Cell Probes 6:389-394
19. Messmer TO, Skelton SK, Moroney JF, Daugharty H, Fields B (1997) Application of a multiplex PCR to psittacosis outbreaks. J Clin Microbiol 35:2043-2046

20. Grayston JT, Campbell LA, Kuo C-C et al (1989) A new respiratory tract pathogen: *Chlamydia pneumoniae* strain TWAR. J Infect Dis 161:618-625

21. Grayston JT, Aldous MB, Easton A, Wang S-P et al (1993) Evidence that *Chlamydia pneumoniae* causes pneumoniae and bronchitis. J Infect Dis 163:1231-1235

22. Kauppinen M, Saikku P (1995) Pneumonia due to *Chlamydia pneumoniae*: prevalence, clinical features, diagnosis, and treatment. Clin Infect Dis 21:S244-S252

23. Ekman MR, Leinonen M, Syrjala H, Linnanmaki E, Kujala P, Saikku P (1993) Evaluation of serological methods in the diagnosis of *Chlamydia pneumoniae* during an epidemic in Finland. Eur J Clin Microbiol Infect Dis 12:756-760

24. Li D-K, Daling JR, Wang S-P, Grayston JT (1989) Evidence that *Chlamydia pneumoniae*, strain TWAR, is not sexually transmitted. J Infect Dis 160:328-331

25. Peeling RW, Wang S-P, Grayston JT et al (1998) *Chlamydia* serology: inter-laboratory variation in micro-immunofluorescence results. In: Stephen R, Byrne G, Christiansen G, Clarke IN, Grayston JT, Rank RG, Ridgway GL, Saikku P, Schachter J, Stamm WE (eds) Chlamydial infections. Proceedings of the 9th International Symposium on Human Chlamydial Infection, Napa, CA, 21-28 June, 1998, pp 159-162

26. Gnarpe J, Gnarpe H, Sundelof B (1991) Endemic prevalence of *Chlamydia pneumoniae* in subjectively healthy persons. Scand J Infect Dis 23:387-388

27. Hyman C, Augenbraun MH, Roblin PM, Schachter J, Hammerschlag MR (1991) Asymptomatic respiratory tract infection with *Chlamydia pneumoniae* TWAR. J Clin Microbiol 29:2082-2083

28. Hyman CL, Roblin PM, Gaydos CA, Quinn TC, Schachter J, Hammerschlag MR (1995) Prevalence of asymptomatic nasopharyngeal carriage of *Chlamydia pneumoniae* in subjectively healthy adults: assessment by polymerase chain reaction–enzyme immunoassay and culture. Clin Infect Dis 20:1174-1178

29. Maurin M, Eb F, Etienne J, Raoult D (1997) Serological cross-reactions between *Bartonella* and *Chlamydia* species: implications for diagnosis. J Clin Microbiol 35:2283-2287

30. Knobbloch J, Bialek R, Muller G, Asmus P (1988) Common surface epitopes of *Bartonella bacilliformis* and *Chlamydia psittaci*. Am J Trop Med Hyg 39:427-433

31. Peeling RW, Artsob H, Garvie M, Marrie T (1995) Serologic cross-reactivity between *Bartonella henselae* and *Chlamydia pneumoniae*. In: Proceedings of the 35th Interscience Conference on Antimicrobial Agents and Chemotherapy, San Francisco, p 298 (abstract)

32. Kutlin A, Roblin PM, Hammerschlag MR (1998) Antibody response to *Chlamydia pneumoniae* infection in children with respiratory illness. J Infect Dis 177:720-724

33. Saikku P, Ruutu P, Leinonen M, Panelius J, Tupasi TE, Grayston JT (1988) Acute lower-respiratory tract infection associated with chlamydial TWAR antibody in Filipino children. J Infect Dis 158:1095-1097

34. Orr PH, Peeling RW, Fast M et al (1996) Serological study of responses to selected pathogens causing respiratory tract infection in the institutionalized elderly. Clin Infect Dis 23:1240-1245

35. Verkooyen RP, Hazenberg MA, Van Haaren GH et al (1992) Age-related interference with *Chlamydia pneumoniae* microimmunofluorescence serology due to circulating rheumatoid factor. J Clin Microbiol 30:1287-1290

36. Hammerschlag MR, Chirgwin K, Roblin PM et al (1992) Persistent infection with *Chlamydia pneumoniae* following acute respiratory illness. Clin Infect Dis 14:178-182

37. Malinverni R, Kuo C-C, Campbell LA, Lee A, Grayston JT (1995) Effects of two antibiotic regimens on course and persistence of experimental *Chlamydia pneumoniae* TWAR pneumonitis. Antimicrob Agents Chemother 39:45-49

38. Troy C, Peeling R, Ellis A et al (1997) *Chlamydia pneumoniae* as a new source of infectious outbreaks in nursing homes. JAMA 277:1214-1218
39. Blasi F, Denti F, Erba M et al (1996) Detection of *Chlamydia pneumoniae* but not *Helicobacter pylori* in atherosclerotic plaques of aortic aneurysms. J Clin Microbiol 34:2766-2769
40. Wimmer MLJ, Sandmann-Strupp R, Saikku P, Haberl RL (1996) Association of chlamydial infection with cerebrovascular disease. Stroke 27:2207-2210
41. Laurila A, Anttila T, Laara E et al (1997) Serological evidence of an association between *Chlamydia pneumoniae* infection and lung cancer. Int J Cancer 74:31-34
42. Juvonen J, Juvonen T, Laurila A et al (1997) Demonstration of *Chlamydia pneumoniae* in the walls of abdominal aortic aneurysms. J Vasc Surg 25:499-505
43. Juvonen J, Juvonen T, Laurila A et al (1998) Can degenerative aortic valve stenosis be related to persistent *Chlamydia pneumoniae* infection? Ann Intern Med 128:741-744
44. Von Hertzen L, Alakarppa H, Koskinen R et al (1997) *Chlamydia pneumoniae* infection in patients with chronic obstructive pulmonary disease. Epidemiol Infect 118:155-164
45. Hahn D, Anttila T, Saikku P (1996) Association of *Chlamydia pneumoniae* IgA antibodies with recent symptomatic asthma. Epidemiol Infect 117:513-517
46. Danesh J, Collins R, Peto R (1997) Chronic infections and coronary heart disease: is there a link? Lancet 350:430-436
47. Gupta S, Leatham EW, Carrington D, Mendall M, Kaski JC, Camm AJ (1997) Elevated *Chlamydia pneumoniae* antibodies, cardiovascular events, and azithromycin in male survivors of myocardial infarction. Circulation 96:404-407
48. Jauhianen T, Tuomi T, Leinonen M, Kark D, Saikku P (1994) Interference of immunoglobulin G (IgG) antibodies in IgA antibody determinations for *Chlamydia pneumoniae* by microimmunofluorescence test. J Clin Microbiol 32:839-840
49. Chiu B, Viira E, Tucker W, Fong IW (1997) *Chlamydia pneumoniae*, cytomegalovirus and herpes simplex virus in atherosclerosis of the carotid artery. Circulation 96:2144-2148
50. Puolakkainen M, Kuo C-C, Shor A, Wang S-P, Grayston JT, Campbell LA (1993) Serological response to *Chlamydia pneumoniae* in adults with coronary arterial fatty streaks and fibrolipid plaques. J Clin Microbiol 31:2212-2214

Chlamydia pneumoniae:
How to Document Respiratory Infection

M.R. HAMMERSCHLAG

Introduction

As *Chlamydia pneumoniae* is an obligate intracellular parasite capable of causing prolonged, often subclinical infection, diagnosis of *C. pneumoniae* infection is somewhat complicated. Although isolation of the organism implies infection, it may not imply that the organism is causing pneumonia or other respiratory infection in the patient. It is also unclear whether colonization or asymptomatic infection without disease elicits an antibody response. Multiple diagnostic methods have been evaluated, but there is no "gold standard" for determining whether disease occurring in an individual is due to *C. pneumoniae*. Although it has been suggested that there are differences in the antibody response to primary infection, reinfection and reactivated infection, there are limited data correlating serology with culture. This is further complicated by the lack of standardized methods for serology and nonculture methods such as polymerase chain reaction (PCR).

Diagnosis of Respiratory Infection Due to *Chlamydia pneumoniae*

C. pneumoniae can be isolated from nasopharyngeal (NP) and throat swabs, sputum and pleural fluid of patients with pneumonia, bronchitis and asthma [1–3]. *C. pneumoniae* has also been isolated from middle ear fluids of children with acute otitis media [4]. The nasopharynx appears to be the optimum site for isolation of the organism, especially in children [2]. The relative yield from sputum is not known. Sputum can be toxic to cells; also, many patients with *C. pneumoniae* infection may not have productive cough. This is especially true in children.

Initial studies suggested that *C. pneumoniae* was much more difficult to isolate in tissue culture than *C. trachomatis*. Originally the same methods were used, namely HeLa or McCoy cells pretreated with dextran diethyl-aminoethyl (DEAE). Multiple passages were needed, the inclusions were very small and difficult to see, and in general the yield was very poor. *C. pneumoniae* grows more readily in other cell lines derived from respiratory tissue, specifically HEp-2 and HL cells [5–7].

Omission of pretreatment with dextran DEAE results in much larger inclusions and specimens need only be passed once. Culture with an initial inoculation and one passage should take 4–7 days.

NP specimens for culture can be obtained with Dacron-tipped wire-shafted swabs. Each lot of swabs should be tested in a mock infection system as the adhesive used can differ from lot to lot, and some adhesives can be inhibitory to growth of chlamydiae or toxic to the cells. Specimens for culture should be placed in appropriate transport media, usually a sucrose-phosphate buffer with antibiotics and fetal calf serum, and stored immediately at –70 °C. Viability decreases if specimens are held at room temperature. After 72 h incubation, culture confirmation can be performed by staining with either a *C. pneumoniae* species-specific or a *Chlamydia* genus-specific [anti-lipopolysaccharide (LPS)] fluorescein-conjugated monoclonal antibody [8]. Unfortunately, there are no commercially produced *C. pneumoniae*-specific reagents available in the United States, and availability is limited in Europe. Performance of these reagents has not been extensively evaluated. Preliminary studies suggest that staining characteristics can vary depending on strain of organism and method of fixation [8, 9]. If a genus-specific antibody is used, *C. pneumoniae* should be confirmed by differential staining with a specific *C. trachomatis* antibody; if the latter is negative, then the isolate is either *C. pneumoniae* or *C. psittaci*. If there has been no avian exposure, psittacosis is highly unlikely.

Limited studies have suggested that various PCR methods are at least as sensitive as culture for detection of *C. pneumoniae* in respiratory specimens. The performance and utility are covered in detail in another chapter in this volume.

As isolation of *C. pneumoniae* was difficult and initially limited, initial emphasis was placed on serologic diagnosis. Grayston et al. [1] proposed a set of criteria for serologic diagnosis of *C. pneumoniae* infection with the microimmunofluorescence (MIF) test that is used by many laboratories and clinicians. For acute infection the patient should have a fourfold increase in IgG titer, a single IgM titer of 1:16 or greater, or a single IgG titer of 1:512 or higher. Past or pre-existing infection is defined as an IgG titer of 1:16 or higher but less than 1:512. It was further proposed that the pattern of antibody response in primary infection differed from that seen in reinfection. In initial infection, the IgM response appears about 3 weeks after the onset of illness and the IgM response appears at 6–8 weeks. In reinfection, the IgM response may be absent and the IgG occurs earlier, within 1–2 weeks [2]. A fourfold titer rise or a titer ≥ 1:64 with the complement fixation (CF) test is also felt to be diagnostic. Initially, Grayston et al. [10] found that fewer than one third of hospitalized patients with suspected *C. pneumoniae* infection had detectable CF antibody. However, in a recent report of a small outbreak of *C. pneumoniae* infections among University of Washington students, all seven patients with pneumonia had CF titers of 1:64 or greater [11].

Because of the relatively long period until the development of a serologic response in primary infection, the antibody response may be missed if convalescent sera are obtained too soon, i.e. earlier than 3 weeks after the onset of illness. Use of paired sera also only affords a retrospective diagnosis, which is of little

Table 1. Correlation of *C. pneumoniae* serology and culture in pneumonia treatment studies

Study	Age range	n	Positive test for *C. pneumoniae*		
			Culture	Serology[a]	Culture and serology
Block et al. [2]	3–12 years	260	34 (13%)	48 (18%)	8 (3%)
Harris et al. [13]	6 months to 16 years	456	31 (6.7%)	32 (7%)	5 (1.1%)
Hammerschlag et al. [14]	12–93 years	48	10 (20.8%)	11 (23%)	6 (12.5%)

[a] Fourfold rise in specific IgM or IgM, single IgM $\geq 1{:}16$, or single IgG $\geq 1{:}512$

help in deciding how to treat the patient. The criteria for use of a single serum sample have not been correlated with the results of culture and are based mainly on data from adults. The antibody response in acute infection may take longer than 3 months to develop. Acute, culture-documented infection can also occur without seroconversion, especially in children [2, 12]. The correlation of culture and serology in three pneumonia treatment studies is summarized in Table 1. As part of a multicenter pneumonia treatment study in children 3–12 years of age, Block et al. isolated *C. pneumoniae* from 34 (13.1%) of the 260 children enrolled. Serologic evidence of acute infection was found in 48 (18.5%), but only 8 (23%) of the culture-positive children met the serologic criteria for acute infection, most had no detectable antibody by the MIF test even after 3 months of follow-up [2]. The majority of the "positive" serologic results in the culture-negative children were stable high IgG titers ($\geq$ 1:512). Seroconversions were infrequent. None of the children had CF antibody. Similar results were reported in another pediatric pneumonia treatment study by Harris et al. [13]: only 5 (16%) of 31 culture-positive children met the serologic criteria for acute infection. The children in this multicenter study were 6 months to 16 years of age, and the isolation rate of *C. pneumoniae* was 7.8%. In another study in children [12], *C. pneumoniae* was isolated from 13 (11%) of 118 children 5–15 years of age who were initially evaluated for either new or acute exacerbations of asthma. Only 5 of the children with culture-confirmed infection had detectable IgG antibody to *C. pneumoniae*. One child who was noncompliant with his antibiotic therapy was culture-positive on five occasions over a 3-month period, but no anti-*C. pneumoniae* antibody was present at any time.

When sera from culture-positive, but MIF-negative children with respiratory infection were examined by immunoblotting, over 89% of these children had antibody to a number of *C. pneumoniae* proteins but only 24% reacted with the major outer membrane protein (MOMP)[15]. These results were similar to those reported by others using sera from adults [16–19]. The MOMP does not appear to be immunodominant in the immune response to *C. pneumoniae* infection although it has been demonstrated to be immunodominant in *C. trachomatis* infection [16, 17, 20]. Monoclonal antibodies to specific epitopes of the MOMP are neutralizing for *C. trachomatis* but not *C. pneumoniae* [21]. The MOMP is the major surface-exposed antigen of *C. trachomatis* and may be the major antigen in the MIF assay. The lack of reactivity in the MIF assay observed in children may be secondary to the lack of reactivity to the MOMP. Unfortunately, there was no reactivity to any *C. pneumoniae* protein or combination of proteins that could readily differentiate infected from uninfected children [15]. When paired sera were examined, the band patterns remained the same for over 70% of the children [15]. In the remaining children, changes in the immunoblots of acute phase sera compared with convalescent sera were unique for each patient. When the same sera were immunoblotted against recent clinical isolates of *C. pneumoniae*, there were differences in the intensity of reaction and the band patterns, indicating possible antigenic diversity between the isolates. This was also observed by Black et al. [18] with sera from adults.

The correlation between culture and serology is higher in adults, but culture-documented infection in adults with pneumonia can also occur in the absence of seroconversion or detectable antibody by MIF [14] (Table 1). Background rates of seropositivity can also be very high in some adult populations. Hyman et al. [22], in a study of asymptomatic *C. pneumoniae* infection among subjectively healthy adults in Brooklyn, New York, found 81% to have IgG or IgM titers of 1:16 or greater. Seventeen percent had evidence of "acute infection": IgG equal to or greater than 1:512 and/or IgM equal to or greater than 1:16. However, none of these individuals were culture or PCR positive. Similar results were reported by Kern et al. [23] among healthy firefighters and policemen in Rhode Island. The specificity of the MIF IgM assay can be affected by the presence of rheumatoid factor. A study from the Netherlands found that there was an increased probability of false positives due to rheumatoid factor with increasing age [24]. Sera should be routinely absorbed before MIF IgM testing. Hyman et al. [22] absorbed all the IgM-positive sera; the titers did not change. Some IgG antibody may result from a heterotypic response to other chlamydial species as there are cross-reactions with the MOMP between the three species as well as cross-reactions due to the genus LPS antigen [25]. Moss et al. reported that antibodies to *C. pneumoniae* and *C. psittaci* accounted for up to half of all chlamydial IgG-positive persons attending a sexually transmitted disease clinic [26].

The MIF test is not standardized: there can be a significant subjective component in performing the assay. A recent study by Peeling et al. [27] attempted to address the problem of interlaboratory variation in the performance of the MIF test by sending a panel of 22 acute and convalescent sera to 14 different laboratories. Some used an in-house MIF, while several laboratories used one of two commercially available kits. The overall agreement of all laboratories was 80%, using one laboratory as the "gold standard". The range was 50%–100% depending on the isotype. Agreement for serodiagnostic criteria were 69% for negative, 68% for "chronic" and 87% for a fourfold increase of IgG.

An important confounding variable in the diagnosis of *C. pneumoniae* infection is the presence of asymptomatic infection. Several small studies have revealed a rate of asymptomatic infection ranging from 2% to 5% in adults and children [4, 12, 22, 28]. These individuals were usually seronegative or had MIF IgG ≥ 1:256 [12, 22]. There are no large, population-based studies that have examined the relationship of asymptomatic infection to age or serologic status. Persistent *C. pneumoniae* infection following acute respiratory infection has been reported and may last for several months to years [29]. In two patients with persistent infection for up to 9 years, IgM and IgG titers fluctuated widely [30]. Combined with the observation that coinfections with other organisms, such as *Mycoplasma pneumoniae* and *Streptococcus pneumoniae*, are frequent in individuals with respiratory infection and positive *C. pneumoniae* cultures [2, 11, 13, 31], it is possible that *C. pneumoniae* may be a cofactor or innocent bystander. Block et al. [2] reported that 20% of the children with culture-documented *C. pneumoniae* infection were coinfected with *M. pneumoniae*; these children could not be differentiated clinically from those who were infected with either agent alone. It has been suggested that the identification of the *C. pneumoniae* in a respiratory specimen by culture or PCR combined with the demonstration of seroconversion be used for the definitive diagnosis of *C. pneumoniae* infection in adults [31].

Diagnosis of Respiratory Infection: Implications for Therapy

Data on the treatment of *C. pneumoniae* infection are very limited. There are few reported controlled studies. Considering the ambiguity concerning the diagnosis, confounding variables such as mixed infections and colonization, the results are often difficult to interpret. Most published studies have small numbers of patients and rely on serologic diagnosis, which in essence only gives a clinical endpoint. Plouffe et al. [32] compared ofloxacin to standard therapy, which was usually a β-lactam antibiotic plus a macrolide for the treatment of community-acquired pneumonia in adults. Using the Grayston criteria [1], 40 patients were considered to have *C. pneumoniae* infection: 20 (83%) of 24 who were treated with ofloxacin and 12 (75%) of 16 who received standard therapy were considered to have had a satisfactory clinical response. In a subsequent larger multicenter study, File et al. [33] compared levofloxacin to ceftriaxone and/or cefuroxime. Erythromycin or doxycycline could be added to the latter regimen at the discretion of the physician. Clinical success was observed in 46 (98%) of 47 patients with serologic evidence of acute *C. pneumoniae* infection, compared to 50 (93%) of 54 patients who were treated with ceftriaxone and/or cefuroxime. There was no difference in clinical response when the patients with serologic evidence of *C. pneumoniae* were stratified by having a fourfold rise in IgG or IgM (definite infection), a single IgG ≥ 1:512 or IgM ≥ 1:256 (probable infection), or addition of erythromycin or doxycycline. These results were surprising in that previous reports had suggested that β-lactams were ineffective in treating *C. pneumoniae* infection [1]. An alternate explanation questions the specificity of the serologic criteria.

Anecdotally, we have observed several patients who have remained persistently culture-positive and clinically symptomatic despite 7- to 30-day courses of doxycycline, tetracycline and erythromycin [29]. Only four published treatment studies have utilized culture to evaluate the microbiologic eradication of *C. pneumoniae* in relation to the clinical response. Block et al. [2], in a multicenter treatment study in children with pneumonia, found that *C. pneumoniae* was eradicated from the nasopharynx of 15 (79%) of the 19 children who received clarithromycin compared to 12 (79%) of 14 who received erythromycin. However, all the children improved clinically with complete resolution of their chest radiographs despite persistence of the organism. Emre et al. [12] treated 12 children, 5–16 years of age, with acute exacerbations of asthma who were culture positive for *C. pneumoniae,* with erythromycin or clarithromycin for 10–14 days. The organism was eradicated in all six children who were treated for 14 days with erythromycin and in five of six treated for 10 days with clarithromycin. Overall, nine (75%) of these children demonstrated dramatic improvement in their reactive airway disease associated with eradication of the organism. In a subsequent pediatric pneumonia treatment study [13], children were randomized (2:1) to receive pediatric suspensions of either azithromycin or the comparative agent (amoxicillin-clavulanate if < 5 years; erythromycin if ≥ 5 years of age). Cultures were obtained at baseline and again 15–19 days after the initiation of treatment. A total of 456 children with pneumonia from 27 sites in 20 US states were enrolled; *C. pneumoniae* was isolated from 36 (7.9%) of the children. *C. pneumoniae* was eradicated after treatment from the nasopharynx of 19 (83%) of 23 evaluable patients who received azithromycin, four of four, who received amoxicillin-clavulanate and seven of seven who received erythromycin ($p = 0.9$, chi square). In an open, noncomparative multicenter pneumonia treatment study [34], adolescents and adults ≥ 12 years of age were given 1.5 g of azithromycin orally over 5 days. Cultures were started at baseline, at 10–14 days and six weeks after the initiation of treatment. *C. pneumoniae* was isolated from 10 (20.8%) of 48 patients with pneumonia who were enrolled in this study. *C. pneumoniae* was eradicated from the nasopharynx of 7 (70%) of the 10 culture-positive patients after treatment. The minumum inhibitory concetrations (MICs) and minimum chlamydicidal concentrations (MCCs) of three of nine isolates obtained after treatment from two of seven persistently infected patients in both studies who were treated with azithromycin increased fourfold after treatment, although they were still within the range considered susceptible to the antibiotic [34]. It is not clear if this is an isolated event or suggestive of possible development of resistance. All patients improved clinically despite persistence of the organism. In the previous pneumonia treatment study comparing clarithromycin and erythromycin [35], there was no change in MICs or MCCs of isolates of *C. pneumoniae* despite persistence of the organism in eight children with pneumonia, two of whom were treated with erythromycin and six with clarithromycin. Although relative resistance of *C. trachomatis* to erythromycin and doxycycline has been reported, the relationship to treatment failure is unclear [36, 37]. If diagnosis of respiratory infection due to *C. pneumoniae* is limited to serology, emergence of resistance as well as microbiologic efficacy cannot be assessed.

References

1. Grayston JT, Campbell LA, Kuo C-C, Modhorst CH, Saikku P, Thom DH, Wang S-P (1990) A new respiratory tract pathogen: *Chlamydia pneumoniae* strain TWAR. J Infect Dis 161:618-625
2. Block S, Hedrick J, Hammerschlag MR, Cassell GH (1995) *Mycoplasma pneumoniae* and *Chlamydia pneumoniae* in community-acquired pneumonia in children: comparative safety and efficacy of clarithromycin and erythromycin suspensions. Pediatr Infect Dis J 14:471-477
3. Augenbraun MH, Roblin PM, Mandel LJ, Hammerschlag MR, Schachter J (1991) *Chlamydia pneumoniae* pneumonia with pleural effusion: diagnosis by culture. Am J Med 91:437-438
4. Block S, Hammerschlag MR, Hedrick J, Tyler R, Smith A, Roblin PM, Gaydos C, Pham D, Quinn TC, Palmer R, McCarty J (1997) *Chlamydia pneumoniae* in acute otitis media. Pediatr Infect Dis J 16:858-862
5. Cles L, Stamm WE (1990) Use of HL cells for improved isolation and passage of *Chlamydia pneumoniae*. J Clin Microbiol 28:938-940
6. Wong KH, Skelton SK, Chan YK (1992) Efficient culture of *Chlamydia pneumoniae* with cell lines derived from the human respiratory tract. J Clin Microbiol 30:1625-1630
7. Roblin PM, Dumornay W, Hammerschlag MR (1992) Use of HEp-2 cells for improved isolation and passage of *Chlamydia pneumoniae*. J Clin Microbiol 30:1968-1971
8. Montalban GS, Roblin PM, Hammerschlag MR (1994) Performance of three commercially available monoclonal reagents for confirmation of *Chlamydia pneumoniae* in cell culture. J Clin Microbiol 32:1406-1407
9. Wang S-P, Grayston JT (1991) *Chlamydia pneumoniae* elementary body antigenic reactivity with fluorescent antibody is destroyed by methanol. J Clin Microbiol 29:1539-1541
10. Grayston JT, Kuo C-C, Wang S-P, Altman J (1986) A new *Chlamydia psittaci* strain, TWAR, isolated in acute respiratory tract infections. N Engl J Med 315:161-168
11. Grayston JT, Aldous MB, Easton A, Wang SP, Kuo C-C, Campbell LA, Altman J (1993) Evidence that *Chlamydia pneumoniae* causes pneumonia and bronchitis. J Infect Dis 168:1231-1235
12. Emre U, Roblin PM, Gelling M, Dumornay W, Rao M, Hammerschlag MR, Schachter J (1994) The association of *Chlamydia pneumoniae* infection and reactive airway disease in children. Arch Pediatr Adolesc Med 148:727-731
13. Harris JA, Kolokathis A, Campbell M, Cassell HG, Hammerschlag MR (1998) Safety and efficacy of azithromycin in the treatment of community-acquired pneumonia in children. Pediatr Infect Dis J 17:865-871
14. Hammerschlag MR, Gregory W, Schwartz DB, Pistorious BJ, Inverso JA, Kolokathis A (1997) Azithromycin in the treatment of community-acquired pneumonia (CAP) due to *Chlamydia pneumoniae*. In: Abstracts of the 37th Interscience Conference on Antimicrobial Agents and Chemotherapy, September 28-October 1, 1997. American Society for Microbiology, Washington, DC, abstr K-138, p 352
15. Kutlin A, Roblin P, Hammerschlag MR (1998) Antibody response to *Chlamydia pneumoniae* infection in children with respiratory illness. J Infect Dis 177:720-724
16. Campbell LA, Kuo C-C, Wang S-P, Grayston JT (1990) Serologic response to *Chlamydia pneumoniae* infection. J Clin Microbiol 28:1261-1264
17. Iijima Y, Miyashita N, Kishimoto T, Kanamoto Y, Soejima R (1994) Characterization of *Chlamydia pneumoniae* species-specific protein immunodominant in humans. J Clin Microbiol 32:583-588

18. Black CM, Jonson JE, Farshy CE, Brown TM, Berdal BP (1991) Antigenic variation among strains of *Chlamydia pneumoniae*. J Clin Microbiol 29:1312-1316
19. Jantos CA, Heck S, Roggendorf R, Sen-Gupta M, Hegemann J (1997) Antigenic and molecular analysis of different *Chlamydia pneumoniae* strains. J Clin Microbiol 35:620-623
20. Glassick T, Gifard P, Timms P (1996) Outer membrane protein 2 gene sequences indicate that *Chlamydia pecorum* and *Chlamydia pneumoniae* cause infections in koalas. Syst Appl Microbiol 19:457-464
21. Peterson EM, Cheng X, Qu Z, de la Maza LM (1996) Characterization of the murine antibody response to peptides representing the variable domains of the major outer membrane protein of *Chlamydia pneumoniae*. Infect Immun 64:3354-3359
22. Hyman CL, Roblin PM, Gaydos CA, Quinn TC, Schachter J, Hammerschlag MR (1995) The prevalence of asymptomatic nasopharyngeal carriage of *Chlamydia pneumoniae* in subjectively healthy adults: assessment by polymerase chain reaction–enzyme immunoassay and culture. Clin Infect Dis 20:1174-1178
23. Kern DG, Neill MA, Schachter J (1993) A seroepidemiologic study of *Chlamydia pneumoniae* in Rhode Island. Chest 104:208-213
24. Verkooyen RP, Hazenberg MA, Van Haaren GH, Van Den Bosch JM, Snijder RJ, Van Helden HP, Verbrugh HA (1992) Age-related interference with *Chlamydia pneumoniae* microimmunofluorescence serology due to circulating rheumatoid factor. J Clin Microbiol 30:1287-1290
25. Carter MW, Al-Mahdwawi SAH, Giles IG, Treharne JD, Ward ME, Clarke IN (1991) Nucleotide sequence and taxonomic value of the major outer membrane protein gene of *Chlamydia pneumoniae* IOL-207. J Gen Microbiol 137:465-475
26. Moss TR, Darougar S, Woodland RM et al (1993) Antibodies to *Chlamydia* species in patients attending a genitourinary clinic and the impact of antibodies to *C. pneumoniae* and *C. psittaci* on the sensitivity and the specificity of *C. trachomatis* serology tests. Sex Transm Dis 20:61-65
27. Peeling RW, Wang SP, Grayston JT, Blasi F, Boman J, Clad A, Freidank H, Gaydos CA, Gnarpe J, Hagiwara T, Jones RB, Orfila J, Persson K, Poulakkainen M, Saikku P, Schachter J (1998) *Chlamydia* serology: inter-laboratory variation in microimmunofluorescence results. In: Stephens RS, Byrne GI, Christiansen G, Clarke IN, Grayston JT, Rank RG, Ridgway GL, Saikku P, Schachter J, Stamm WE (eds) *Chlamydia* infections. Proceedings of the 9th International Symposium on Human *Chlamydia* Infections, 21-28 June, 1998. University of California, San Francisco, pp 159-162
28. Gnarpe J, Gnarpe H, Sundelof B (1991) Endemic prevalence of *Chlamydia pneumoniae* in subjectively healthy persons. Scand J Infect Dis 23:387-388
29. Hammerschlag MR, Chirgwin K, Roblin PM, Gelling M, Dumornay W, Mandel L, Smith P, Schachter J (1992) Persistent infection with *Chlamydia pneumoniae* following acute respiratory illness. Clin Infect Dis 14:178-182
30. Dean D, Roblin P, Mandel L, Schachter J, Hammerschlag MR (1998) Molecular evaluation of serial isolates from patients with persistent *Chlamydia pneumoniae* infections. In: Stephens RS, Byrne GI, Christiansen G, Clarke IN, Grayston JT, Rank RG, Ridgway GL, Saikku P, Schachter J, Stamm WE (eds) *Chlamydia* infections. In: Proceedings of the 9th International Symposium on Human Chlamydial Infections, 21-28 June, 1998. University of California, San Francisco, pp 219-222
31. Bartlett JG, Breiman RF, Mandell LA, File TM (1998) Community-acquired pneumonia in adults: guidelines for management. Clin Infect Dis 26:811-838
32. Plouffe JF, Herbert MT, File TM, Baird I, Parsons JN, Kahn JB, Reilly-Gauvin KT, The Pneumonia Study Group (1996) Ofloxacin versus standard therapy in treatment of

community-acquired pneumonia requiring hospitalization. Antimicrob Agents Chemother 40:1175-1179

33. File TM, Segreti J, Dunbar L, Player R, Kohler R, Williams RR, Kojak C, Rubin A (1997) A multicenter, randomized study comparing the efficacy and safety of intravenous and/or oral levofloxacin versus ceftriaxone and/or cefuroxime axetil in the treatment of adults with community-acquired pneumonia. Antimicrob Agents Chemother 41:1965-1972

34. Roblin PM, Hammerschlag MR (1998) Microbiologic efficacy of azithromycin and susceptibility to azithromycin of isolates of *Chlamydia pneumoniae* from adults and children with community-acquired pneumonia. Antimicrob Agents Chemother 42:194-196

35. Roblin PM, Montalban G, Hammerschlag MR (1994) Susceptibility to clarithromycin and erythromycin of isolates of *Chlamydia pneumoniae* from children with pneumonia. Antimicrob Agents Chemother 38:1588-1589

36. Mourad AM, Sweet RC, Sugg N, Schachter J (1980) Relative resistance to erythromycin in *Chlamydia trachomatis*. Antimicrob Agents Chemother 18:696-698

37. Jones, RB, Van der Pol B, Martin DH, Shepard MK (1990) Partial characterization of *Chlamydia trachomatis* isolates resistant to multiple antibiotics. J Infect Dis 162:1309-1315

Chlamydia pneumoniae: Epidemiology

F. Blasi, C. Arosio, R. Cosentini

Introduction

In 1989, the *Chlamydia* strain previously labelled TWAR was recognized as a third species of the *Chlamydia* genus on the basis of ultrastructural and DNA homology analysis and named *Chlamydia pneumoniae* [1].

Like the other *Chlamydia* species, this agent is an obligate intracellular, Gram-negative bacterium present in two developmental forms: infective elementary bodies (EBs) and reproductive reticulate bodies (RBs). Chlamydiae possess a specific replication cycle which differs from conventional bacteria. They multiply within membrane-bound vacuoles in eukaryotic host cells but are unable to generate adenosine triphosphate (ATP) and are therefore dependent on the host cell ATP deposits for all energy requirements. Moreover, they are incapable of de novo nucleotide biosynthesis and are dependent on host nucleotide pools [2].

C. pneumoniae has been recognized as a cause of respiratory tract infections and is considered the most common nonviral intracellular human respiratory pathogen [3, 4]. *C. pneumoniae* is involved in a wide spectrum of respiratory infections of the upper respiratory tract (pharyngitis, sinusitis and otitis) and lower respiratory tract (acute bronchitis, exacerbations of chronic bronchitis and asthma, and community-acquired pneumonia) in both immunocompetent and immunocompromised hosts [5–22].

This agent has also been associated with other diseases, both pulmonary (sarcoidosis) [23, 24] and extrapulmonary (coronary artery diseases, erythema nodosum, Guillain-Barré syndrome, culture-negative endocarditis, thyroiditis, arthritis, encephalitis) [25–35].

Population Antibody Prevalence

Since the isolation of *C. pneumoniae* and the development of a specific microimmunofluorescence test, several seroepidemiological studies have been conducted both prospectively and retrospectively [9, 10].

These data have shown a worldwide diffusion of *C. pneumoniae* infection. In developed countries the infection seems to be rather uncommon before the age of

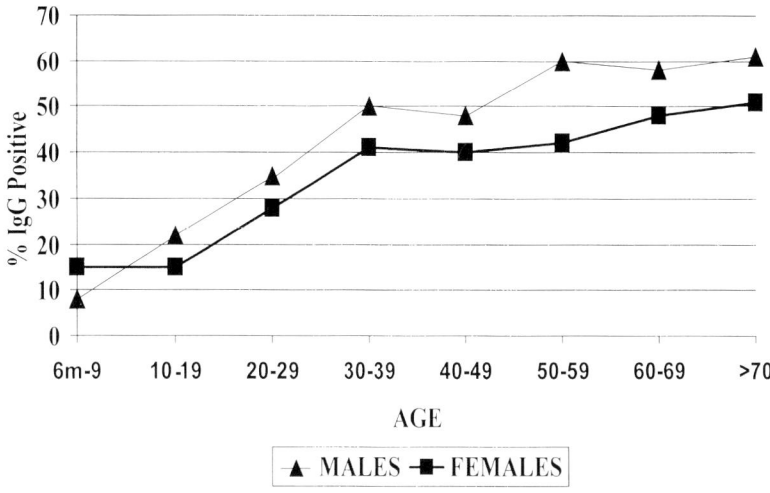

Fig. 1. *C. pneumoniae* seroprevalence in a sample of an immunocompetent population in Milan, Italy

5 years. Seroprevalence increases during school age and reaches over 50% in adults. Males usually show a higher seropositivity rate [18] (Fig. 1).

Seroepidemiological data from developing countries show an overall higher prevalence of *C. pneumoniae* infection [36]. In these populations pre-school-age infection seems to be rather frequent and seroprevalence reaches more than 70% in adults.

Antibody seroprevalence to *C. pneumoniae* is higher both in immunocompromised adults and children than in immunocompetent hosts [18].

Periodicity

According to seroepidemiologic surveys performed in western countries, *C. pneumoniae* infection seems to be both endemic and epidemic [37]. Peaks of incidence during epidemics generally last 2–3 years, although shorter outbreaks have been reported. Periods of low incidence last 3–4 years, suggesting a new cycle of *C. pneumoniae* infection approximately every 6 years [3]. No evidence of seasonal periodicity in *C. pneumoniae* infection has been observed [3], and this has been recently confirmed in a population-based active surveillance study on community-acquired pneumonia [38].

Immunity

The serological response to *C. pneumoniae* infection is characterized by two different patterns. Primary infection shows an IgM titer rise followed by IgG increase, whereas reinfection shows IgG and IgA titer rise without IgM increase.

Table 1 shows the timing of antibody response to *C. pneumoniae* infection. IgM antibodies are usually undetectable after 2–6 months from acute infection, whereas IgA may persist longer and could represent indirect evidence of persistent infection [39]. In immunocompetent subjects IgG antibodies may be detectable for more than 2 years [3]. Conversely, in immunocompromised subjects with HIV infection we have observed shorter persistence (less than 1 year), probably due to impaired antibody synthesis [22].

Asymptomatic carriage of *C. pneumoniae* in subjectively healthy adults appears to be relatively uncommon, ranging from 2% to 4% of the general population [40, 41]. In certain subjects, namely COPD patients, a higher rate of chronic carriage/infection has been found [42, 43].

A recent study by Normann et al. [44], conducted on children attending day-care centers in Sweden, found that 22.7% of the children had a positive PCR test for *C. pneumoniae* on throat swab specimens. It is interesting to note that a similar rate was recorded among the attending personnel (23.2%). PCR positivity for *C. pneumoniae* was also high among family members of the index children. These data are in contrast with previous reports and seem to indicate a higher rate of carriage than previously suspected, even if this study was carried out during an incidence peak.

Table 1. Timing (weeks) of antibody response to *C. pneumoniae* infection

	IgM	IgG	IgA
First infection	2–4	6–8	–
Reinfection	–	1–3	1–2

Transmission

Current available data suggest that *C. pneumoniae* is primarily transmitted by human-to-human contact without any animal reservoir [9, 45]. Wang and Grayston found no serological evidence of cat or dog infection during the Finnish military epidemics [46].

C. pneumoniae infection spreads slowly, with a case-to-case interval of about 30 days. Serological data show that the duration of epidemics varies from 5 to 8 months, suggesting a relatively long incubation period.

Family transmission, from child to child, was observed in Japan in 1990 [14]; Mordhorst et al. [15] described an outbreak of *C. pneumoniae* infections in four farm families living close together in Denmark with an unusually high incidence of symptomatic infection, particularly lower respiratory tract infection, among family members. These data support the human-to-human contact spread of *C. pneumoniae* infection and underline the role of this agent in family cluster respiratory infections, although Aldous et al. [16], in a serological study of family serum samples carried out between 1966 and 1979, reported that acute infections more often affected a single family member than multiple members. We reported two family outbreaks where we recorded a high rate (75%) of symptomatic infections [17]. These data are in contrast with the low incidence of infection recorded during epidemics in military trainees in Finland [9] and in the serological study of Aldous et al. [16], while they are consistent with those reported by Mordhorst et al. [15].

The time span of infection spread in both families was unusually short, ranging from 5 to 18 days; this may be explained by the living habits. Both families lived in small flats with high person-to-person contact.

This finding has been recently confirmed by Normann et al. [44], who report that *C. pneumoniae* seems to be easily communicable among individuals living in close proximity.

C. pneumoniae has recently been identified as a source of infection in nursing home infectious outbreaks, causing serious morbidity and mortality among residents and morbidity among nursing staff [47].

Acute *Chlamydia pneumoniae* Respiratory Infections

C. pneumoniae is an important cause of human respiratory tract diseases (Table 2). This agent is involved in upper respiratory tract infections (pharyngitis, sinusitis etc.), acute bronchitis and exacerbations of chronic bronchitis [5–7, 55].

C. pneumoniae is now known to be a relevant cause of community-acquired pneumonia, being involved in 6% to more than 20% of cases [48]. Most recent reports rank this agent among the three most common etiologic agents, generally presenting a mild, and in some cases self-limiting, clinical course. It has been

Table 2. Incidence of *C. pneumoniae* infections

Disease	Range of incidence	References
Asymptomatic infection	Common	[1, 3]
Flu-like syndrome	Common	[1, 3]
Community-acquired pneumonia	6%–25%	[3–5, 10, 45, 48–52]
Outbreaks in close communities	–	[9, 13, 47]
Family outbreaks	–	[14–17]
Upper respiratory tract infections	5%–10%	[1, 3, 5, 8]
COPD exacerbations	4%–5%	[6, 7, 42, 43]
Asthma attacks	1%–18%	[11, 12, 44, 53, 54]

shown to cause severe forms of pneumonia, particularly in elderly patients and in the presence of chronic cardiopulmonary diseases [49, 50]. A recent prospective study on community-acquired pneumonia in elderly patients by Riquelme et al. [51] also identified *C. pneumoniae* as the second most common pathogen, occurring in 9% of patients. As previously suggested by Torres and El-Ebiary [52], identification of *C. pneumoniae* in mixed infections may indicate that this pathogen could facilitate infections by other microrganisms.

The potential role of *C. pneumoniae* as a respiratory pathogen in immunocompromised patients has recently been suggested on the basis of seroprevalence studies and both culture and PCR identification of the micro-organism in patients with lower respiratory tract infections [18, 19, 21, 22, 56, 57]. However, the pathogenetic role of *C. pneumoniae* in this population is still debated.

A possible role for *C. pneumoniae* in asthma has been recently hypothesized. In several patients the infection is associated with wheezing and asthma onset [11, 53]. Hahn et al. reported a dose-response relationship between specific antibody titers and wheezing prevalence [11]. In that study four patients with acute infection subsequently developed asthma and four others experienced an exacerbation of previously diagnosed asthma. Other groups demonstrated that *C. pneumoniae* causes asthma exacerbations. Allegra et al. [12] found that about 10% of asthma exacerbations in adults were due to this pathogen. Emre et al. [53] reported similar results in a pediatric population. Moreover, they demonstrated that treatment with macrolide may improve the course of reactive airway disease.

A recent study [54] involving 108 children with asthma symptoms, aged 9–11 years, showed that chronic *C. pneumoniae* infection is common in school-age children and immune responses to *Chlamydia* are positively associated with frequency of asthma exacerbations. The authors suggest that the immune response to chronic *C. pneumoniae* infection may interact with allergic inflammation to increase asthma symptoms.

Furthermore, the number of episodes reported by each child during the 13 months of the study was used to assess the possible relationship between asthma exacerbations and sIgA to *C. pneumoniae*.

The results of these and other studies lead to the hypothesis that *C. pneumoniae* chronic infection may play a part in the natural history of asthma conditioning at least in part the chronic inflammation and hyper-responsiveness which characterize bronchial asthma. Only large epidemiological studies and therapeutic intervention, double-blind studies versus placebo, will clarify the role of this interesting pathogen in the aetiopathogenesis of bronchial asthma.

Cardiovascular Diseases

Known risk factors, i.e. smoking, hypercholesterolemia, Lp(a) levels, hypertension etc., explain 50%–70% of the cases of myocardial infarction. Recent evidence indicates the possible role of viral and bacterial infections in the development of atherosclerosis and their association with myocardial infarction [25, 58, 59].

Seroepidemiological evidence indicates that the majority of patients with CHD present an anti-*C. pneumoniae* antibody pattern consistent with chronic infection [26–29]. Furthermore, *C. pneumoniae* has been detected in atherosclerotic coronary plaques by several methods, including immunocytochemistry, transmission electron microscopy and molecular biology techniques [30–33].

Recently, we detected *C. pneumoniae* DNA in a high proportion of aortic aneurysm plaques [60]. Furthermore, our serological data support the hypothesis that chronic *C. pneumoniae* antibody pattern may be a possible risk factor marker for atherosclerosis.

Recently, *C. pneumoniae* has been isolated by culture from the coronary artery of a patient with coronary atherosclerosis and from a carotid endarterectomy specimen, providing direct evidence of the presence of viable organism in atheromatous lesions [61, 62].

We recently found a high incidence of acute *C. pneumoniae* infection in patients with acute myocardial infarction (AMI) [63]. A significantly higher prevalence of IgG titers was observed in patients with acute myocardial infarction (35/61) than in blood donors (18/61) ($p = 0.003$). These findings add further evidence to the hypothesis that *C. pneumoniae* infection may act as a trigger for acute myocardial infarction. *C. pneumoniae* reinfection could lead to instability within atherosclerotic plaques via reactivation of a chronic or latent infection and/or immune-mediated endothelial damage. The demonstration of an association between *C. pneumoniae* reinfection and acute myocardial infarction is a new aspect that may be linked to the previously suggested role of chronic infection in the pathogenesis of atherosclerosis.

C. pneumoniae was frequently found in advanced carotid atherosclerotic lesions, and although these findings do not establish a causal relationship between infection and atherosclerosis, they represent another piece of the puzzle that links *C. pneumoniae* to atherosclerosis development [64]. This study confirmed a previous report based on seroepidemiological evidence that showed a significant cross-sectional association between past *C. pneumoniae* infection and asymptomatic carotid atherosclerosis [65].

Moreover, a recent study found an association between *C. pneumoniae* chronic infection, diagnosis based on serological pattern, and increased risk of cerebrovascular disease, namely stroke and transient ischemic event [66].

Conclusions

The role of *C. pneumoniae* infection in acute respiratory infections, such as pneumonia and chronic bronchitis exacerbations, is well established. Data regarding the importance of this pathogen in immunocompromised subjects are still insufficient to draw definitive conclusions, but suggest that *C. pneumoniae* may also have a role as a pathogen in this patient population.

A further field of great interest is the possible role of *C. pneumoniae* in the pathogenesis of asthma. In patients with asthma this micro-organism is undoubtedly a cause of exacerbations, whereas further studies are needed to define whether infection with this agent alters the natural history of the disease.

Lastly, a recent line of research of great future interest is the association between chronic *C. pneumoniae* infection and atherosclerosis. Should this association be confirmed, the correct treatment of *C. pneumoniae* infection may have a strong impact on public health.

References

1. Grayston JT, Kuo C-C, Campbell LA et al (1989) *Chlamydia pneumoniae* sp. nov. for *Chlamydia* sp. strain TWAR. Int J Syst Bacteriol 39:88-90
2. Leinonen M (1993) Pathogenetic mechanisms and epidemiology of *Chlamydia pneumoniae*. Eur Heart J 14:57-61
3. Thom DH, Grayston JT (1991) Infections with *Chlamydia pneumoniae* strain TWAR. Clin Chest Med 12:245-256
4. Marrie TJ (1993) *Chlamydia pneumoniae*. Thorax 48:1-4
5. Grayston JT Campbell LA, Kuo C-C et al (1990) A new respiratory tract pathogen *Chlamydia pneumoniae* strain TWAR. J Infect Dis 161:618-625
6. Beaty CD, Grayston JT, Wang S-P et al (1991) *Chlamydia pneumoniae*, strain TWAR, infection in patients with chronic obstructive pulmonary disease. Am Rev Respir Dis 144:1408-1410
7. Blasi F, Legnani D, Lombardo VM et al (1993) *Chlamydia pneumoniae* infection in acute exacerbations of COPD. Eur Respir J 6:19-22
8. Saikku P (1992) The epidemiology and significance of *Chlamydia pneumoniae*. J Infect 25:27-34
9. Kleemola M, Saikku P, Visakorpi R et al (1988) Epidemics of pneumonia caused by TWAR, a new chlamydial organism, in military trainees in Finland. J Infect Dis 157:230-236
10. Marrie TJ, Grayston JT, Wang S-P et al (1987) Pneumonia associated with TWAR strain of *Chlamydia*. Ann Intern Med 106:507-511
11. Hahn DL, Dodge RW, Golubjatnikov R (1991) Association of *Chlamydia pneumoniae* (strain TWAR) infection with wheezing, asthmatic bronchitis, and adult-onset asthma. JAMA 266:225-230
12. Allegra L, Blasi F, Centanni S et al (1994) Acute exacerbations of asthma in adults: role of *Chlamydia pneumoniae* infection. Eur Respir J 7:2165-2168
13. Pether JVS, Wang S-P, Grayston JT (1989) *Chlamydia pneumoniae* strain TWAR as the cause of an outbreak in a boys' school previously called *Psittacosis*. Epidemiol Infect 103:395-400
14. Yamazaki T, Nakada H, Sakurai N et al (1990) Transmission of *Chlamydia pneumoniae* in young children in a Japanese family. J Infect Dis 162:1390-1392
15. Mordhorst CH, Wang S-P, Grayston JT (1992) Outbreak of *Chlamydia pneumoniae* infection in four farm families. Eur J Clin Microbiol Infect Dis 11:617-620
16. Aldous MB, Grayston JT, Wang S-P (1992) Seroepidemiology of *Chlamydia pneumoniae* TWAR infection in Seattle families, 1966-1979. J Infect Dis 166:646-649
17. Blasi F, Cosentini R, Denti F et al (1994) Two family outbreaks of *Chlamydia pneumoniae* infection. Eur Respir J 7:102-104
18. Blasi F, Cosentini R, Clerici Schoeller M et al (1993) *Chlamydia pneumoniae* seroprevalence in immunocompetent and immunocompromised populations in Milan. Thorax 48:1261-1263

19. Augenbraun MH, Roblin MR, Chirwing K et al (1991) Isolation of *Chlamydia pneumoniae* from lungs of patients infected with the human immunodeficiency virus. J Clin Microbiol 29:401-402

20. Clark R, Mushatt D, Fazal B (1991) Case report: *Chlamydia pneumoniae* pneumonia in HIV-infected man. Eur J Med Sci 302:155-156

21. Gaydos CA, Flower CL, Gill BJ et al (1993) Detection of *Chlamydia pneumoniae* by polymerase chain reaction-enzyme immunoassay in an immunocompromised population. Clin Infect Dis 17:718-723

22. Blasi F, Boschini A, Cosentini R et al (1994) Outbreak of *Chlamydia pneumoniae* infection in an ex injection-drug users community. Chest 105:812-815

23. Grönhagen-Riska C, Saikku P, Riska H et al (1992) Antibodies to a TWAR – a novel type of *Chlamydia* – in sarcoidosis. In: Grassi C, Rizzato G, Pozzi E (eds) Sarcoidosis and other granulomatous disorders. Elsevier, Amsterdam, pp 297-301

24. Poulakkainen M, Campbell LA, Kuo C-C et al (1996) Serological response to *Chlamydia pneumoniae* in patients with sarcoidosis. J Infect 33:199-205

25. Dahlen GH, Boman J, Birgander LS, Lindblom B (1995) Lp(a) lipoprotein, IgG, IgA, and IgM antibodies to *Chlamydia pneumoniae* and HLA class II genotype in early coronary artery disease. Atherosclerosis 114:165-174

26. Saikku P, Leinonen M, Mattila K et al (1988) Serological evidence of an association of a novel chlamydia, TWAR, with chronic coronary heart disease and acute myocardial infarction. Lancet 29:983-986

27. Thom DH, Wang S-P, Grayston JT et al (1991) *Chlamydia pneumoniae* strain TWAR antibody and angiographically demonstrated coronary artery disease. Arterioscler Thromb 11:547-551

28. Saikku P, Leinonen M, Tenkanen L et al (1992) Chronic *Chlamydia pneumoniae* infection as a risk factor for coronary heart disease in the Helsinki Heart Study. Ann Intern Med 116:273-278

29. Linnanmaki E, Leinonen M, Mattila K (1993) *Chlamydia pneumoniae*-specific circulating immune complexes in patients with chronic coronary heart disease. Circulation 87:1130-1134

30. Shor A, Kuo C-C, Patton DL (1992) Detection of *Chlamydia pneumoniae* in coronary arterial fatty streaks and atheromatous plaques. S Afr Med J 82:158-161

31. Kuo C-C, Shor A, Campbell LA et al (1993) Demonstration of *Chlamydia pneumoniae* in atherosclerotic lesions of coronary arteries. J Infect Dis 167:841-849

32. Campbell LA, O'Brien ER, Cappuccio AL et al (1995) Detection of *Chlamydia pneumoniae* TWAR in human coronary atherectomy tissues. J Infect Dis 172:585-588

33. Kuo C-C, Grayston JT, Campbell LA et al (1995) *Chlamydia pneumoniae* (TWAR) in coronary arteries of young adults (15-34 years old). Proc Natl Acad Sci USA 92:6911-6914

34. Haidl S, Ivarsson S, Bjerre I et al (1992) Guillain-Barré syndrome after *Chlamydia pneumoniae* infection. N Engl J Med 326:576-577

35. Socan M, Veovic B, Kese D (1994) *Chlamydia pneumoniae* and meningoencephalitis. N Engl J Med 331:406 (letter)

36. Saikku P, Ruutu P, Leinonen M et al (1988) Acute lower respiratory tract infection associated with Chlamydia TWAR antibodies in Filipino children. J Infect Dis 158:1095-1097

37. Grayston JT (1992) Infections caused by *Chlamydia pneumoniae* strain TWAR. Clin Infect Dis 15:757-763

38. Marston BJ, Plouffe JF, File TM et al (1997) Incidence of community-acquired pneumonia requiring hospitalization. Arch Intern Med 157:1709-1718

39. Saikku P (1991) Problems in diagnosis of *Chlamydia pneumoniae* infections. In: Vaheri A, Tilton RC, Balows A (eds) Rapid methods and automation in microbiology and immunology. Springer, Berlin Heidelberg New York, pp 309-313

40. Gnarpe J, Gnarpe H, Sundelof BO (1991) Endemic prevalence of *Chlamydia pneumoniae* in subjectively healthy persons. Scand J Infect Dis 23:387-388

41. Hyman CL, Roblin PM, Gaydos CA et al (1995) Prevalence of asymptomatic nasopharyngeal carriage of *Chlamydia pneumoniae* in subjectively healthy adults: assessment by polymerase chain reaction–enzyme immunoassay and culture. Clin Infect Dis 20:1174-1178

42. von Hertzen L, Isohao R, Leinonen M et al (1996) *Chlamydia pneumoniae* antibodies in chronic obstructive pulmonary disease. Int J Epidemiol 25:658-664

43. Blasi F, Cosentini R, Damato S et al (1997) *Chlamydia pneumoniae* chronic infection increases the risk of bacterial colonization in chronic bronchitis. Am J Crit Care Respir Med 155:A592

44. Normann E, Gnarpe J, Gnarpe H et al (1998) *Chlamydia pneumoniae* in children attending day-care centers in Gävle, Sweden. Pediatr Infect Dis J 17:474-478

45. Saikku P, Wang S-P, Kleemola M et al (1985) An epidemic of mild pneumonia due to an unusual *Chlamydia psittaci* strain. J Infect Dis 151:832-839

46. Wang S-P, Grayston JT (1986) Microimmunofluorescence serological studies with TWAR organism. In: Oriel JD, Ridgway G, Schachter J, Taylor-Robinson D, Ward M (eds) Chlamydial infections. Cambridge University Press, Cambridge, UK, pp 329-332

47. Troy CJ, Peeling RW, Ellis AG et al (1997) *Chlamydia pneumoniae* as a new source of infectious outbreaks in nursing homes. JAMA 277:1214-1218

48. Almirall J, Morató I, Riera F et al (1993) Incidence of community-acquired pneumonia and *Chlamydia pneumoniae* infection: a prospective multicentre study. Eur Respir J 6:14-18

49. Cosentini R, Blasi F, Raccanelli R et al (1996) Severe community-acquired pneumonia: a possible role for *Chlamydia pneumoniae*. Respiration 63:61-65

50. Pacheco A, Gonzales SJ, Aroncena C et al (1991) Community-acquired pneumonia caused by *Chlamydia pneumoniae* strain TWAR in chronic cardiopulmonary disease in the elderly. Respiration 58:316-320

51. Riquelme R, Torres A, El-Ebiary M et al (1996) Community-acquired pneumonia in the elderly. Am J Respir Crit Care Med 154:1450-1455

52. Torres A, El-Ebiary M (1993) Relevance of *Chlamydia* TWAR in community-acquired respiratory infections. Eur Respir J 6:7-8

53. Emre U, Roblin PM, Gelling M et al (1994) The association of *Chlamydia pneumoniae* infection and reactive airway disease in children. Arch Pediatr Adolesc Med 148:727-732

54. Cunningham AF, Johnston SL, Julious SA et al (1998) Chronic *Chlamydia pneumoniae* infection and asthma exacerbations in children. Eur Respir J 11:345-349

55. von Hertzen L, Alakarppa H, Koskinen R et al (1997) *Chlamydia pneumoniae* infection in patients with chronic obstructive pulmonary disease. Epidemiol Infect 118:155-164

56. Boschini A, Smacchia C, Di Fine M et al (1996) Community acquired pneumonia in a cohort of former injection-drug users with and without human immunodeficiency virus infection: incidence etiologies and clinical aspects. Clin Infect Dis 23:107-113

57. Dalhoff K, Maass M (1996) *Chlamydia pneumoniae* pneumonia in hospitalised patients. Clinical characteristics and diagnostic value of polymerase chain reaction detection in BAL. Chest 110:351-356

58. Pesonen E, Siitonen O (1981) Acute myocardial infarction precipitated by infectious disease. Am Heart J 101:512-513

59. Spodick DH, Flessas AP, Johnson MM (1984) Association of acute respiratory symptoms with the onset of acute myocardial infarction: prospective investigation of 150 consecutive patients and matched control patients. Am J Cardiol 53:481-482

60. Blasi F, Denti F, Erba M et al (1996) Detection of *Chlamydia pneumoniae* and not of *Helicobacter pylori* in atherosclerotic plaques of aortic aneurysms. J Clin Microbiol 34:2766-2769

61. Ramirez JA, Ahkee S, Summersgill JT et al (1996) Isolation of *Chlamydia pneumoniae* from the coronary artery of a patient with coronary atherosclerosis. Ann Intern Med 125:979-982

62. Jackson LA, Campbell LA, Kuo C-C et al (1997) Isolation of *Chlamydia pneumoniae* from a carotid endoarterectomy specimen. J Infect Dis 176:292-295

63. Blasi F, Cosentini R, Raccanelli R et al (1997)A possible association of *Chlamydia pneumoniae* infection and acute myocardial infarction in patients younger than 65 years of age. Chest 112:309-312

64. Grayston JT, Kuo C-C, Coulson AS et al (1995) *Chlamydia pneumoniae* (TWAR) in atherosclerosis of the carotid artery. Circulation 92:3397-3400

65. Melnick SL, Shahar E, Folsom AR et al (1993) Past infection by *Chlamydia pneumoniae* strain TWAR and asymptomatic carotid atherosclerosis Am J Med 945:499-504

66. Wimmer MLJ, Sandmannstrupp R, Saikku P et al (1996) Association of chlamydial infection with cerebrovascular disease. Stroke 27:2207-2210

Pharmacological and Pharmacokinetic Basis of *Chlamydia pneumoniae* Treatment

G. GIALDRONI GRASSI

Introduction

Chlamydia pneumoniae, like other *Chlamydia* species, is an obligate intracellular parasite. For its growth to be inhibited the antimicrobial agent must penetrate cells and be able to interfere with protein synthesis of the micro-organism. Therefore, antibiotics that are likely to be active against *C. pneumoniae* are macrolides, tetracyclines, chloramphenicol, quinolones and rifampicin, which have demonstrated the capacity to enter cells and develop antimicrobial activity intracellularly for *C. psittaci* and *C. trachomatis*, as well as for other pathogens.

Drugs

In order to exert their antibacterial activity, antibiotics must reach the infectious focus. Infection can be localized in the interstitial spaces of tissues or inside the cells. The physicochemical properties of drugs are the main factors conditioning their distribution in tissues and penetration in cells. For the therapy of infection in the respiratory tree, according to localization, it is necessary that antibiotics reach adequate concentration in lung parenchyma, bronchial tissue, and bronchial secretions, and inside the cells if the infection is intracellular. The behavior of all classes of antibiotics at level of respiratory tract has been thoroughly investigated [1]. The recently developed microlavage technique performed by fiberoptic bronchoscopy allows one to obtain specimens of alveolar epithelial lining fluid and alveolar macrophages in which it is possible to measure antibiotic concentrations after systemic administration in man [2]. The availability of this information about the pharmacokinetic behavior of antibiotics at the level of the respiratory tract has been of great importance in anticipating and assessing their clinical efficacy in respiratory infection.

Clindamycin, rifampicin, tetracyclines, macrolides and fluoroquinolones accumulate in phagocytes [3, 4]. Macrolides show the greatest capacity for accumulation in cells, where they are localized in cytosol and lysosomes. In polymorphonuclear neutrophils (PMN), the cellular/extracellular (C/E) ratio varies from

2 to 14 for erythromycin and josamycin and reach the highest values for dirithromycin, clarithromycin and azithromycin [5–10]. In alveolar macrophages the C/E ratio of dirithromycin is about 80, that of clarithromycin can range according to the time of sample collection from about 40 to > 100 [10, 11]. Peculiar behavior is shown by azithromycin: it has a very long half-life of about 50 h accompanied by very low serum levels and extremely high tissue and intracellular levels, particularly in PMN, alveolar macrophages and fibroblasts, from which it is slowly released. The C/E ratio in alveolar macrophages is about 300 after 48 h, but it can reach values > 1000 3–4 days following administration, because of the extremely low serum levels (≤ 0.01 µg/ml) [12–16].

Correlation between intracellular accumulation and antimicrobial activity has been submitted to careful analysis. A large amount of antibiotics in cells does not always ensure higher antibacterial activity. Cell penetration of macrolides correlates with extracellular concentration and antimicrobial activity correlates with intracellular accumulation in experimental models. Fluoroquinolones, which accumulate in cells to a lesser extent than macrolides, nevertheless show an excellent antimicrobial activity, while clindamycin, which shows a C/E ratio somewhat superior to fluoroquinolones, displays low activity against intracellular *Staphylococcus aureus* [5]. Evidently the nature of the parasite, its growth rate, the different experimental conditions and the mechanism of action of the antibiotic can greatly influence the outcome of experiments performed in vitro and in animal models. The clinical efficacy against intracellular infections shown by antibiotics with the capacity to enter the cell has confirmed, at least in the majority of cases, the good predictive properties of some experimental models.

In Vitro Activity

Due to the obligate intracellular localization of *C. pneumoniae* the in vitro antibiotic susceptibility testing must be performed in tissue cultures. The determinations have been most commonly carried out on cultures of Hep-2 and HeLa 229 cells, but McCoy and HL cells have also been employed. The test is usually performed in 96-well microtiter plates, the inoculum being 0.1 ml of the test strain diluted to obtain 10^3–10^4 inclusion-forming units/ml. After incubation at 35 °C for 72 h, cultures are fixed and stained for inclusions with fluorescein-conjugated antibody to the lipopolysaccharide genus antigen. The minimal inhibitory concentration (MIC) is the lowest antibiotic concentration at which no inclusion is seen. The minimal chlamydicidal concentration (MCC) can be determined by aspirating the antibiotic-containing medium from cell culture, carefully washing wells and adding-antibiotic-free medium. Cultures are then frozen at –70 °C, thawed and passed onto new cells, incubated at 35 °C for 72 h and then fixed and stained to detect inclusions. The MCC is the lowest antibiotic concentration at which no inclusion is detectable after passage [17, 18].

Data on in vitro activity of antibiotics against *C. pneumoniae* are relatively limited, due to the difficulty in isolating the agent and performing the susceptibility

Table 1. In vitro susceptibility of *C. pneumoniae* to tetracyclines, macrolides and ketolides

Drug	MIC (µg/ml)	MCC (µg/ml)	References
Tetracycline	0.05–1	0.05–4	[18, 19, 22, 25, 26]
Doxycycline	0.01–0.5	0.12–2	[25, 27–30]
Minocycline	0.016–0.06	0.06–0.125	[31]
Erythromycin	0.01–0.5	0.01–0.25	[18, 19, 22, 25, 26, 28, 32]
Clarithromycin	0.004–0.25	0.004–0.25	[25, 26, 27, 28, 30, 32, 33]
14-OH clarithromycin	0.03	0.25	[19]
Azithromycin	0.01–2	0.06–0.25	[18, 19, 25, 26, 28, 34]
Roxithromycin	0.05–2	0.06–2	[25, 26, 27, 32]
Ketolide HMR 3647	0.01–2	0.03–2	[35]
Ketolide RU 64004	0.01–0.5	0.01–1	[35, 36]

MIC, minimal inhibitory concentration; *MCC*, minimal chlamydicidal concentration: ranges of values reported in literature (values are given as range against clinical isolates or against type strains of *C. pneumoniae*)

test. Moreover, the data in the literature are often discrepant: probably the results are influenced by the experimental conditions. The timing of addition of the antibiotic to the culture seems to be crucial in some cases: if it is added before inoculating *C. pneumoniae* in culture cells, MIC and MCC can be up to eight times lower than if it is added after *C. pneumoniae* inoculation. It has been pointed out that the tests in which cells are infected before being exposed to antibiotics are likely to be closer to conditions existing in vivo, where infection always precedes the administration of antibiotics. However, not all antibiotics are affected to the same extent by the way the experiment is conducted [19, 20]. Even studies apparently carried out in very similar conditions often show evident discrepancies, the reason for which has not been clarified. The use of in vitro kinetic models mimicking the variation of concentration occurring in vivo could give more information on this problem [20, 21].

Tetracyclines and erythromycin show good in vitro activity and have been so far the drugs most commonly employed in the treatment of *C. pneumoniae* infection. Doxycycline and minocycline seem to be a little more active than tetracycline [19, 22–26] (Table 1). The most active macrolide seems to be clarithromycin [19, 25–28, 32, 37]. This finding has recently been confirmed by the determination of susceptibility to clarithromycin in the largest series of recent clinical isolates of *C. pneumoniae* so far tested, during the course of a multicenter study carried out in the USA, comparing clarithromycin and erythromycin in the treatment of community-acquired pneumonia in children (3–12 years of age). *C. pneumoniae* was isolated in 42 (16%) of the 260 children enrolled. MIC_{90} and MCC_{90} of the 49 isolates tested were both 0.031 µg/ml for clarithromycin and 0.125 µg/ml for erythromycin, respectively [33]. The 14-hydroxymetabolite of clarithromycin also maintains good activity, comparable to roxithromycin, azithromycin and ery-

Table 2. In vitro susceptibility of *C. pneumoniae* to quinolones

Drug	MIC (µg/ml)	MCC (µg/ml)	References
Ciprofloxacin	0.25–4[a]	2–8	[25, 26, 35, 37, 38]
Ofloxacin	0.25–2	0.5–2	[25, 29–31, 34, 37, 39]
Levofloxacin	0.125–0.5	0.125–0.5	[28]
Lomefloxacin	0.25	–	[25, 38, 39]
Sparfloxacin	<0.01–0.25	0.125–0.5	[39, 40]
Fleroxacin	2–8	2–8	[40]
Tosufloxacin	0.125	–	[28, 41]
Grepafloxacin	0.06–0.12	–	[29]
Trovafloxacin	0.5–1	–	[30, 31]
Moxifloxacin (BAY 12-8039)	0.06	0.125	[42]
BAY 3118	0.015	0.015	[43]
OPC-71116	0.25–0.5	0.5–2	[40]

MIC, minimal inhibitory concentration; *MCC*, minimal chlamydicidal concentration: ranges of values reported in literature (values are given as range against clinical isolates or against type strains of *C. pneumoniae*)
[a] MIC and MCC $\geq$ 16 µg/ml have been reported by only one group [23]

thromycin. Fifteen isolates of *C. pneumoniae* from ten patients with community-acquired pneumonia were tested for susceptibility to azithromycin. MICs and MCCs were 0.25 µg/ml both for 50% and 90% of the strains (range 0.0125-0.25 µg/ml). The MIC and MCC of one isolate were four times higher after treatment, although it remained susceptible to azithromycin [34].

The ketolides are a new class of macrolide antibiotics with a 3-keto function instead of the cladinose sugar, endowed with good activity against a broad range of respiratory pathogens. Either MIC and MCC of the derivative HMR 3647, at which 90% of recent isolates were inhibited, showed to be 0.25 µg/ml (range 0.0125-2 µg/ml). However, the activity of HMR 3647 against older isolates passaged intensively in laboratory was ten times lower. This variability was not observed with the other macrolides or quinolones tested [35]. The activity of another ketolide derivative, RU 64004, was tested only against a few strains of *C. pneumoniae*. In one study MICs and MCCs were $\leq$ 0.01 and 0.05 µg/ml, respectively, while in another study the values of these parameters were 0.5 µg/ml and 1 µg/ml, respectively [35, 36]. The observed discrepancies could be related to differences in tissue culture methods.

Fluoroquinolones show good activity (Table 2). The most active compounds are sparfloxacin and BAY 3118 (a compound now discarded because of toxicity problems) followed by tosufloxacin and l-ofloxacin (levofloxacin). Levofloxacin is more active than ofloxacin [19, 26, 28, 37–40, 43]. Susceptibility of *C. pneumoniae* to ciprofloxacin and fleroxacin is lower than to other tested derivatives, but the MIC of $\geq$ 16 µg/ml reported for ciprofloxacin by some authors [19] seems excessively high. The most recent quinolone derivatives show good activity against *C. pneumoniae*. Grepafloxacin was some 8–16 times more active than ofloxacin, showing MIC_{90} of 0.12 μg/ml (range 0.06-0-12), and 2–4 times less active than clarithromycin. MCC was 0.25 μg/ml [29]. MICs for trovafloxacin ranged from 0.12 μg/ml to 1 μg/ml, MIC_{90} and MCCs being 1 μg/ml [30, 31]. The MICs of moxifloxacin (BAY 12-8039) against three strains of *C. pneumoniae* were 0.6 μg/ml and MCCs ranged from 0.06 to 0.125 [42].

Beta-lactams and aminoglycosides which do not enter cells or enter very poorly and have as target the bacterial cell wall, a structure lacking in chlamydiae, are inactive. However, Kuo and Grayston [22] observed that penicillin and ampicillin, while showing no effect on *Chlamydia* viability, could inhibit infectivity. Rifampicin, clindamycin, chloramphenicol and co-trimoxazole, which show some in vitro activity against *C. trachomatis* and *C. psittaci,* might also be active against *C. pneumoniae,* but no data are yet available.

Animal Models

The availability of a reliable animal model for *C. pneumoniae* infection would be of great importance in better understanding the immunopathology of the disease and the value in vivo of antimicrobials that are active in vitro. So far only three animal models have been developed, in monkeys, rabbits and mice [44]. In rabbits and mice, a respiratory disease consisting in pneumonia with different characteristics according to methods of inoculation and inoculum size was obtained. The systemic spreading of the organism in infected animals could be ascertained by the demonstration of its DNA by polymerase chain reaction in spleen tissue and blood monocytes [45, 46].

So far very few studies have been performed to evaluate the possible role of in vitro-active antibiotics in experimental *C. pneumoniae* infection. Sparfloxacin, one of the most active fluoroquinolones, showed excellent activity, superior to those of minocycline, tosufloxacin, clarithromycin and ofloxacin, in experimental pneumonia caused by *C. pneumoniae* in leukopenic mice [41].

Clinical Relevance of Experimental Findings

The clinical efficacy of the different antibiotics in the treatment of *C. pneumoniae* infection is extensively treated in another chapter in this volume. It is worthwhile to observe that a good correlation between experimental data and clinical results seems to exist. Tetracyclines have so far been the most frequently prescribed drugs, leading to satisfactory clinical results [23, 24].

Some of the most recent fluoroquinolones and macrolide derivatives have shown an excellent activity in vitro but, at present, it is not possible to give any clinical comparative evaluation. There is limited clinical experience with clarithromycin, azithromycin, ofloxacin and sparfloxacin: results were satisfactory [33, 34, 37, 47–49].

References

1. Bergogne-Bérézin E, Valleé E (1994) Pharmacokinetics of antibiotics in respiratory tissues and fluids. In: Pennington JE (ed) Respiratory infections: diagnosis and management (3rd edn). Raven Press, New York, pp 715-740
2. Baldwin DR, Honeybourne D, Wise R (1992) Pulmonary disposition of antimicrobial agents: methodological consideration. Antimicrob Agents Chemother 36:1171-1175
3. Johnson JD, Hand WL, Francis JB, King-Thompson NK, Corwin RW (1980) Antibiotic uptake by alveolar macrophages. J Lab Clin Med 95:429-439
4. Prokesch RC, Hand WL (1982) Antibiotic entry into polymorphonuclear leukocytes. Antimicrob Agents Chemother 21:373-380
5. Tulkens PM (1991) Intracellular pharmacokinetics and localization of antibiotics as predictors of their efficacy against intraphagocytic infections. Scand J Infect Dis Suppl 74:209-217
6. Tulkens PM (1991) Intracellular distribution and activity of antibiotics. Eur J Clin Infect Dis 102:100-106
7. Peters DH, Clissod SP (1992) Clarithromycin. A review of its antimicrobial activity, pharmacokinetic property and therapeutic potential. Drugs 44:117-164
8. Carlier MB, Zenebergh A, Tulkens PM (1987) Cellular uptake and subcellular distribution of roxithromycin and erythromycin in phagocytic cells. J Antimicrob Chemother 20[Suppl B]:47-56
9. Fraschini F, Scaglione F, Pintucci G, Maccarinelli G et al (1991) The diffusion of clarithromycin and roxithromycin into nasal mucosa, tonsil and in lung in humans. J Antimicrob Chemother 27[Suppl A]:61-65
10. Bergogne-Bérézin E (1993) Tissue distribution of dirithromycin: comparison with erythromycin. J Antimicrob Chemother 31[Suppl C]:77-87
11. Anderson R, Joone G, van Rensburg CEJ (1988) An in vitro evaluation of the cellular uptake and intraphagocytic bioactivity of clarithromycin (A-56268, TE-031), a new macrolide antimicrobial agent. J Antimicrob Chemother 22:923-933
12. MacDonald PJ, Pruul H (1991) Phagocyte uptake and transport of azithromycin. Eur J Clin Microbiol Infect Dis 10:828-833
13. Foulds G, Shepard RM, Johnson RB (1990) The pharmacokinetics of azithromycin in human serum and tissues. J Antimicrob Chemother 25[Suppl A]:73-82
14. Baldwin DR, Honeybourne D, Wise R (1992) Pulmonary disposition of antimicrobial agents: in vivo observations and clinical relevance. Antimicrob Agents Chemother 36:1176-1180
15. Baldwin DR, Wise R , Andrews JM, Ashby JP et al (1990) Azithromycin concentrations at the sites of pulmonary infection. Eur Respir J 3:886-890
16. Patel KB, Xuan D, Nightingale CH, Tessier PR, Russomanno JH, Quintiliani R (1997) A comparison of the bronchopulmonary pharmacokinetics of clarithromycin and azithromycin. In: Zinner SH, Young LS, Acar JF, Neu HC (eds) Expanding indications for the new macrolides, azalides and streptogramins. Dekker, New York, pp 439-446
17. Gump DW (1991) Antimicrobial susceptibility testing for some atypical microorganisms: chlamydiae, mycoplasms, rickettsia, and spirochetes. In: Lorian V (ed) Antibiotic in laboratory medicine (3rd edn). Williams & Wilkins, Baltimore, pp 279-294
18. Welsh LE, Gaydos CA, Quinn TC (1992) In vitro evaluation of activities of azithromycin, erythromycin and tetracyclines against *Chlamydia trachomatis* and *Chlamydia pneumoniae*. Antimicrob Agents Chemother 36:291-294

19. Cooper MA, Baldwin D, Matthews RS, Andrews JM, Wise R (1991) In vitro susceptibility of *Chlamydia pneumoniae* (TWAR) to seven antibiotics. J Antimicrob Chemother 35:407-413

20. Hjelm E, Hulten K, Nystrom-Rosander C, Gustafsson J, Engstrand L, Cars O (1997) Assay of antibiotic susceptibility of *Chlamydia pneumoniae*. Scand J Infect Dis Suppl 104:13-14

21. Lowdin E, Odenholt I, Cars O (1994) A new in vitro model for pharmacodynamic studies of antibiotics. 34th Interscience Conference on Antimicrobial Agents and Chemotherapy, Orlando, FL, 4-7 October, 1994, Abstr 100

22. Kuo C-C, Grayston JT (1988) In vitro drug susceptibility of *Chlamydia* sp. strain TWAR. Antimicrob Agents Chemother 32:257-258

23. Atmar RL, Greenberg SB (1989) Pneumonia caused by *Mycoplasma pneumoniae* and the TWAR agent. Semin Respir Infect 4:19-31

24. Bourke SJ (1993) Chlamydial respiratory infections. BMJ 306:1219-1220

25. Fenelon LE, Mumtaz G, Ridgway GL (1990) The in vitro susceptibility of *Chlamydia pneumoniae*. J Antimicrob Chemother 26:763-767

26. Chirwing K, Roblin PM, Hammerschlag MR (1989) In vitro susceptibilities of *Chlamydia pneumoniae* (*Chlamydia* sp. strain TWAR). Antimicrob Agents Chemother 33:1634-1635

27. Orfila J, Haider F (1992) In vitro susceptibilities of *Chlamydia pneumoniae* strain IOL 207 against clarithromycin, compared to different molecules. In: Adam D, Lode H, Rubinstein E (eds) Recent advances in chemotherapy. Proceedings of the 17th International Congress of Chemotherapy, Berlin, 23-28 June, 1991. Futuramed, Munich, pp 2454-2455

28. Hammerschlag MR, Qumei KK, Roblin PM (1992) In vitro activities of azithromycin, clarithromycin, l-ofloxacin and other antibiotics against *Chlamydia pneumoniae*. Antimicrob Agents Chemother 36:1573-1574

29. Ridgway GL, Salman H, Robbins MJ, Dencer C, Felmingham D (1997) The in vitro activity of grepafloxacin against *Chlamydia* spp, *Mycoplasma* spp, *Ureaplasma urealyticum* and *Legionella* spp. J Antimicrob Chemother 40[Suppl A]:31-36

30. Roblin PM, Hammerschlag MR (1997) In vitro activity of trovafloxacin against *Chlamydia pneumoniae*. Antimicrob Agents Chemother 41:2033-2034

31. Felmingham D, Robbins MJ, Ingley K, Mathias I, Bhogal H, Leakey A, Ridgway GL, Gruneberg RN (1997) In vitro activity of trovafloxacin, a new fluoroquinolone, against recent clinical isolates. J Antimicrob Chemother 39[Suppl B]:43-49

32. Ridgway GL, Mumtaz C, Fenelon L (1991) In vitro activity of clarithromycin and other macrolides against the type strain of *Chlamydia pneumoniae*. J Antimicrob Chemother 27[Suppl A]:43-45

33. Roblin PM, Montalban G, Hammerschlag MR (1994) Susceptibilities to clarithromycin and erythromycin of isolates of *Chlamydia pneumoniae* from children with pneumonia. Antimicrob Agents Chemother 36:1573-1574

34. Roblin PM, Sokolovskaya N, Hammerschlag MR (1997) Susceptibility to azithromycin to isolates of *Chlamydia pneumoniae* from patients with community-acquired pneumonia. In: Zinner SH, Young LR, Acar JF, Neu HC (eds) Expanding indications for the new macrolides, azalides, and streptogramins. Dekker, New York, pp 322-325

35. Roblin PM, Hammerschlag MR (1998) In vitro activity of a new ketolide antibiotic, HMR 3647, against *Chlamydia pneumoniae*. Antimicrob Agents Chemother 42:1515-1516

36. Haider F, Eb F, Orfila J (1995) Ketolides and *Chlamydia*: in vitro evaluation of RU 004. 35th International Conference on Antimicrobial Agents and Chemotherapy. American Society for Microbiology, WashingtonDC, 17-20 September, 1995, abstr F 165, p 142

37. Soejima R, Niki Y, Kishimoto T, Kimura M, Kubota Y (1994) Anti-chlamydial activities of newly developed fluoroquinolones and their clinical usefulness for *Chlamydia* respiratory infections. 5th International Symposium on New Quinolones, Singapore, 25-27 August, 1994, abstr 135, p 178

38. Hammerschlag MR, Hyman CL, Roblin PM (1992) In vitro activities of five quinolones against *Chlamydia pneumoniae*. Antimicrob Agents Chemother 36:682-683

39. Orfila J, Haider F (1992) In vitro susceptibility of *Chlamydia pneumoniae* strain IOL 207 against temafloxacin compared to different other molecules. In: Adam D, Lode H, Rubinstein E (eds) Recent advances in chemotherapy. Proceedings of the 17th International Congress of Chemotherapy, Berlin, 23-26 June, 1991. Futuramed, Munich, pp 2344-2345

40. Roblin PM, Montalban G, Hammerschlag MR (1994) In vitro activities of OPC-17116, a new quinolone, ofloxacin and sparfloxacin against *Chlamydia pneumoniae*. Antimicrob Agents Chemother 38:1402-1403

41. Nakata K, Okazaki Y, Hattori H, Nakamura S (1994) Protective effect of sparfloxacin in experimental pneumonia caused by *Chlamydia pneumoniae* in leukopenic mice. Antimicrob Agents Chemother 38:1757-1762

42. Donati M, Rumpianesi F, Pavan G, Sambri V, Cevenini R (1997) In vitro activity of Bay12-8039 against *Chlamydia trachomatis* and *Chlamydia pneumoniae*. 37th International Conference on Antimicrobial Agents and Chemotherapy, Toronto, September 28-October 1, 1997, abstr F 142, p 170

43. Andrews JM, Wise R, Brenwald N (1993) In vitro activity of BAY3118. 6th European Congress of Clinical Microbiology and Infectious Diseases, Seville, 28-31 March, 1993, Abstr 4, p 71

44. Laitinen K, Alakarppa H, Laurila A, Leinonen M (1997) Animal models for *Chlamydia pneumoniae* infection. Scand J Infect Dis Suppl 104:15-17

45. Kuo C-C, Jackson LA, Campbell LA, Grayston JT (1995) *Chlamydia pneumoniae* (TWAR). Clin Microbiol Res 8:451-461

46. Yang ZP, Kuo C-C, Grayston JT (1995) Systematic dissemination of *Chlamydia pneumoniae* following intranasal inoculation of mice. J Infect Dis 171:736-738

47. Kobayashi H (1986) Clinical evaluation of ofloxacin in lower respiratory tract infections. Infection 14[Suppl 4]:S279-S282

48. Lipsky BA, Tack KJ, Kuo C-C, Wang S-P (1990) Ofloxacin treatment of *Chlamydia pneumoniae* (strain TWAR) lower respiratory tract infections. Am J Med 89:722-724

49. Lode H, Garau J, Grassi C, Hosie G, Huchon G, Legakis N, Segev S, Wijnands G (1998) Treatment of community-acquired pneumonia: a randomized comparison of sparfloxacin, amoxycillin-clavulanic acid and erythromycin. Eur Respir J 8:1999-2007

Chlamydia pneumoniae: Clinical Characteristics of Acute Respiratory Infections

R. Cosentini, P. Tarsia, F. Blasi

Introduction

Chlamydia pneumoniae appears to be an important cause of human respiratory tract disease. Several reports show a high incidence of infection in community-acquired pneumonia, ranging from 6% to 25%, and a remarkable role in pneumonia outbreaks in closed communities such as military garrisons, schools, and families [1–7]. Furthermore, *C. pneumoniae* is involved in upper respiratory tract infections (pharyngitis, sinusitis and otitis), acute bronchitis and exacerbations of chronic bronchitis [8, 9]. Several authors report a possible aetiologic role of this pathogen in adult onset asthma and in asthma exacerbations [10–13]. Several other diseases associated with *C. pneumoniae* infection, such as erythema nodosum, Guillain-Barré syndrome, culture-negative endocarditis, arthritis and encephalitis, have been sporadically reported [14–16]. Seroepidemiological evidence of a possible association between *C. pneumoniae* infection and sarcoidosis has also been suggested [17–19].

Upper Respiratory Tract Infections

Involvement of *C. pneumoniae* infection in pharyngitis, otitis and sinusitis has been described with an incidence ranging from 5% to 10% [20–22]. Shortly after the first identification of this micro-organism Huovinen et al. described *C. pneumoniae* as the third most common pathogen following β-haemolytic streptococci and *Mycoplasma pneumoniae* in a population of 106 adult patients with pharyngitis [21].

Generally, no specific clinical manifestations have been shown for upper respiratory tract infections caused by *C. pneumoniae*. Sore throat, plugged ears, swollen throat, mucus in the throat, hoarseness, cough, headache and fatigue may be present alone or in combination. Sore throat in particular is a symptom commonly associated with *C. pneumoniae* infections of both upper and lower respiratory tract [21, 23, 24].

In humans chlamydial infections are often chronic, and persistent infection is a fairly common finding following acute respiratory infection with *C. pneumoniae*

[24, 25]. Falck et al. recently identified this agent both serologically and by PCR in patients with chronic pharyngitis [26]. Interestingly, pharyngeal examination of these patients commonly revealed granulations (islands of lymphoid tissue) on the retropharyngeal mucosal membrane or abundant brick-red rice-like lymph follicles at the back of the throat. The authors suggest this might be a manifestation of *C. pneumoniae* infection in the same way that genital and eyelid lymph follicles are a typical finding of *C. trachomatis* infection. Retropharyngeal granulations disappeared following antibiotic treatment but were present during relapses. Most patients treated with macrolides or tetracyclines for 2–9 weeks showed clinical remission but one or more relapses occurred after weeks or a few months in all but one patient.

A biphasic pattern in the clinical manifestations of *C. pneumoniae* infections has been observed. Upper respiratory tract infections such as pharyngitis often herald or are associated with infections of the lower respiratory tract that may appear 1–3 weeks later [20].

Lower Respiratory Tract Infections

C. pneumoniae infection of the lower respiratory tract is often associated with persistent cough. A recent prospective study on 65 patients with cough lasting more than 2 weeks showed that 20% had serological evidence of acute *C. pneumoniae* infection, an incidence comparable to that of *Bordetella pertussis* in the same population [27]. In this study, a higher body temperature was more common in patients with *C. pneumoniae* infection than in other patients, although this was not clinically significant.

Acute Bronchitis

Different reports indicate that approximately 5% of cases of acute bronchitis are caused by *C. pneumoniae* infection [20, 28]. The clinical manifestations, although generally mild, are often prolonged. In a prospective study [24], 19 of 96 patients seeking medical attention for acute respiratory infections were found to have acute bronchitis caused by *C. pneumoniae*. Four of these patients experienced a relapse despite prolonged treatment with doxycycline.

Serial sputum examinations in a patient with acute bronchitis caused by *C. pneumoniae* identified an intense inflammatory response, initially lymphocytic and then neutrophilic [29]. In the same study, sputum flow cytometry showed an absolute T-lymphocyte predominance with a decrease in the CD4/CD8 ratio and activation of cytotoxic lymphocytes, suggesting activation of the Th1 pathway. The results of this study, although carried out in a single patient, are consistent with previous reports on the inflammatory modifications during *C. pneumoniae* respiratory tract infection in animal models [30].

Asthma

Up to not long ago it was commonly thought that bacterial infections play a minor role in asthma attacks [31]. Since the early 1990s the role of *C. pneumoniae* in exacerbations of asthma has been investigated. Hahn et al. [10] first reported a possible association between *C. pneumoniae* infection and adult-onset asthma. Later studies confirmed the aetiological role of *C. pneumoniae* infection in asthma exacerbations in both adults and children [11–13]. In adults *C. pneumoniae* is reported to cause approximately 10% of asthma exacerbations [11, 32]. Most studies described patients with mild to moderate exacerbations, whereas a recent study by our group, while confirming the role of this pathogen in mild to moderate asthma exacerbations, suggests that *C. pneumoniae* must also be considered as a cause of severe asthma attacks [33] (Table 1).

The role of *C. pneumoniae* infection in acute asthma exacerbations is further suggested by the fact that in asthma patients antibiotic treatment with clarithromycin reduces airway hyper-responsiveness [12, 34].

Table 1. Demographic, functional, serological and PCR data on patients with acute asthma exacerbations

	Severe asthma exacerbations (PEF ≤ 50% of predicted) ($n = 15$)	Mild to moderate asthma exacerbations (PEF > 50% of predicted) ($n = 20$)
Mean age	32.7 ± 9.9	32.2 ± 10.5
Males/females	9/6	11/9
Mean FEV_1 on admission	0.58 ± 0.10 l/s	1.71 ± 0.33 l/s
Mean PEF on admission	147 ± 42.3 l/min	463 ± 85.2 l/min
Acute infection (serology)	9/15	2/20
C. pneumoniae PCR positivity on pharyngeal swab specimens in acute infection cases	6/9	1/2

FEV_1, forced expiratory volume in 1 s; *PEF*, peak espiratory flow

Chronic Bronchitis

The onset of chronic obstructive pulmonary disease (COPD) is primarily associated with cigarette smoking, although it is not clear whether the inflammatory changes found in the airways of smokers are sufficient to explain the severe limitations on airflow typical of the late stages of this disease [35]. Therefore, it has been suggested that other factors, including infections, may interact with cigarette smoking in the natural history of the disease [36]. Given that *C. trachomatis* infection is known to cause tissue derangement in chronic pelvic inflammatory dis-

Table 2. Culture positivity in *C. pneumoniae* PCR-positive and -negative stable COPD patients

PCR for *C. pneumoniae*	No. of samples	No. of bacteria	Total
Positive* (12 patients)	61	70	131
Negative (27 patients)	115	47	162
Total	176	117	293

* Chi-square test $p < 0.001$

ease, it may be supposed that chronic *C. pneumoniae* infection may promote similar tissue scarring mechanisms in the airways.

The association between *C. pneumoniae* infection and chronic bronchitis has been investigated, and it appears that approximately 5% of COPD acute exacerbations are sustained by this pathogen [9]. In the same study Blasi et al. found a significantly higher frequency of IgG anti-*C. pneumoniae* antibodies in patients with COPD exacerbations than in controls [9]. It was suggested that this could be due either to chronic *C. pneumoniae* infection or to a higher rate of acute infections in these patients. Von Hertzen et al. [37] found no differences in serum IgG antibodies between patients and controls, whereas the difference in serum IgA prevalence was significant. Moreover, local sputum IgA antibodies against *C. pneumoniae*, absent in the majority of pneumonia patients, were a common finding in the sputa of chronic bronchitis patients, along with local antibodies towards bacteria more commonly associated with COPD such as *Haemophilus influenzae* and *Branhamella catarrhalis*.

A later study by von Hertzen et al. [38] on consecutive patients with COPD gave further proof of chronic *C. pneumoniae* infection in these patients, given the stable IgA levels, the almost complete absence of seroconversions and the frequent presence of circulating immunocomplexes. In a later review [39], von Hertzen suggested that the elevated serum antibody levels and the presence of specific antibodies in sputum that are characteristic of *C. pneumoniae* involvement in COPD may indicate a biased Th2-type immune response with increased IL-4 and IL-10 production. IL-10 has been shown to induce IgA antibody production, and the high IgA levels found in COPD patients may reflect a defence mechanism to mitigate airway inflammation.

Although most of the above studies contained patients with mild to moderate COPD exacerbations, a recent study by Soler et al. investigated the aetiological pattern of severe COPD exacerbations requiring mechanical ventilation [40]. Evidence of *C. pneumoniae* infection was found in 18% of patients, although in almost a third of cases a mixed infection was present.

Whereas in healthy subjects the lower respiratory tract is usually sterile, in COPD patients bacterial colonisation of the airways is common. In a recent study Blasi et al. (unpublished data) evaluated clinically stable COPD patients by obtaining at least three sputum samples from each patient at 4-week intervals. Quantitative culture was performed on sputum samples and a nested PCR was applied for the detection of C. pneumoniae DNA (Table 2). Sputum cultures in patients with C. pneumoniae infection yielded a significantly higher number of pathogens than in C. pneumoniae-negative patients. These data indicate that C. pneumoniae chronic infection may increase susceptibility to airway colonisation by other pathogens.

Pneumonia

In numerous epidemiological studies on pneumonia carried out during this decade C. pneumoniae has appeared to be a relevant cause of community-acquired pneumonia, being associated in 6% to more than 20% of cases, and often ranking among the three most common aetiologic agents [41–44].

The clinical course of the disease may vary. During early reports C. pneumoniae pneumonia was described as generally presenting a mild, and in some cases self-limiting, clinical course [41, 42]. However, more recently this agent has been shown to cause severe forms of pneumonia, particularly in elderly patients, and in presence of underlying chronic cardiopulmonary diseases [45–47].

Presenting symptoms most frequently reported by patients with C. pneumoniae pneumonia are sore throat and hoarseness [20] (Table 3). After a period of up to a week, dry persistent cough often sets in [23]. In some cases sinusitis is present together with C. pneumoniae pneumonia. Body temperature is generally slightly increased, seldom going higher than 38–39 °C. Fever therefore often missed if the patient is not seen early in the course of infection.

Physical examination does not often show abnormalities and, if present, physical findings are generally not specific. Pulmonary rales, rhonchi or signs of pulmonary consolidation are sometimes found.

Chest X-ray generally reveals small pulmonary infiltrates, sublobar or segmental in presentation (Table 4). Multiple infiltrates may sometimes be seen and are

Table 3. Common symptoms in C. pneumoniae pneumonia and frequency of presentation

Symptom	Frequency of presentation
Headache	60%–70%
Hoarseness	65%–75%
Sore throat	70%–80%
Dry cough	75%–90%
Fever (>37.8 °C)	25%–45%
Abnormal breath sounds	65%–78%
Leucocytes >10 000/mm	15%–25%
Sedimentation rate >15 mm/h	50%–70%

Table 4. Most commonly occurring radiographic presentations of *C. pneumoniae* pneumonia

Radiographic involvement	Frequency of presentation
Normal	0–6%
Single sublobar lesion	70%–85%
Lobar	4%–7%
Bilateral involvement	7%–14%

often bilateral. Extensive lobar involvement is uncommon, whereas pleural effusion may be present in up to 20% of cases.

Blood testing is unspecific: a high erythrocyte sedimentation rate is commonly present (35–60 mm), whereas leucocytosis is often absent. Increased alkaline phosphate levels were described in a Swedish population of patients with *C. pneumoniae* pneumonia [48], although a later Finnish study was unable to confirm this finding [49].

The symptoms of *C. pneumoniae* pneumonia recede within 3 weeks, but recovery may be reached earlier following adequate antibiotic treatment. In some cases recurrences of pneumonia have been described weeks after symptoms have disappeared.

Community-acquired pneumonia often occurs in patients with comorbid conditions. Among these, COPD is the most common underlying disease in patients with pneumonia requiring hospitalisation [50]. In a recent Spanish multicentre study on community-acquired pneumonia in COPD patients [51], *C. pneumoniae* was found to be the second most important aetiologic agent of pneumonia after *Streptococcus pneumoniae*.

Although initially considered to run with a mild clinical course, sporadic cases of severe *C. pneumoniae* community-acquired pneumonia were reported in the early 1990s [2, 52]. A recent study by Cosentini et al. [45] reported that *C. pneumoniae* was identified as aetiologic agent in 10% of patients with severe community-acquired pneumonia. Marik et al. [46] described a case of severe community-acquired pneumonia associated with shock and multiorgan dysfunction caused by *C. pneumoniae* infection in a previously healthy 24-year-old woman.

Numerous reports have shown that *C. pneumoniae* infection is increasingly recognised as a cause of pneumonia in elderly patients [43, 46, 53–55]. In a study by Riquelme et al. [54] on community-acquired pneumonia in the elderly, *C. pneumoniae* was found to be the second most common aetiologic agent (36% of cases) following *Streptococcus pneumoniae* (42% of cases). In a recent study carried out to determine the cause of outbreaks of acute respiratory illness among elderly residents of three nursing homes in Canada, evidence of *C. pneumoniae* infection was sought for by micro-immunofluorescence testing on paired serum samples, culture, and direct fluorescent antibody assays [55]. This organism was found to cause serious morbidity and mortality among residents (16 cases of pneumonia, 6 deaths) and also morbidity among staff (hoarseness, sore throat and cough). It appeared that among residents hoarseness and pharyngitis were common presenting symptoms, although often overlooked. A new non-productive cough was present in 100% of residents with documented *C. pneumoniae* infection.

Numerous studies have identified *C. pneumoniae* as a cause of pneumonia in HIV-infected adults and children [56–61]. Evidence of *C. pneumoniae* infection in these patients was gathered by culture [56, 61], antibody seroconversion [57, 59, 60], and PCR [58, 61]. Clinically, pneumonia caused by this agent may take a more severe course in HIV-positive patients than in HIV-negative subjects [59], although in some cases the clinical picture may be indistinguishable [60].

References

1. Kleemola M, Saikku P, Visakorpi R et al (1988) Epidemics of pneumonia caused by TWAR, a new chlamydial organism, in military trainees in Finland. J Infect Dis 157:230-236
2. Marrie TJ, Grayston JT, Wang S-P et al (1987) Pneumonia associated with TWAR strain of Chlamydia. Ann Intern Med 106:507-511
3. Pether JVS, Wang S-P, Grayston JT (1989) *Chlamydia pneumoniae* strain TWAR as the cause of an outbreak in a boys' school previously called *Psittacosis*. Epidemiol Infect 103:395-400
4. Yamazaki T, Nakada H, Sakurai N et al (1990) Transmission of *Chlamydia pneumoniae* in young children in a Japanese family. J Infect Dis 162:1390-1392
5. Mordhorst CH, Wang S-P, Grayston JT (1992) Outbreak of *Chlamydia pneumoniae* infection in four farm families. Eur J Clin Microbiol Infect Dis 11:617-620
6. Aldous MB, Grayston JT, Wang S-P (1992) Seroepidemiology of *Chlamydia pneumoniae* TWAR infection in Seattle families, 1966-1979. J Infect Dis 166:646-649
7. Blasi F, Cosentini R, Denti F et al (1994) Two family outbreaks of *Chlamydia pneumoniae* infection. Eur Respir J 7:102-104
8. Beaty CD, Grayston JT, Wang S-P et al (1991) *Chlamydia pneumoniae*, strain TWAR, infection in patients with chronic obstructive pulmonary disease. Am Rev Respir Dis 144:1408-1410
9. Blasi F, Legnani D, Lombardo VM et al (1993) *Chlamydia pneumoniae* infection in acute exacerbations of COPD. Eur Respir J 6:19-22
10. Hahn DL, Dodge RW, Golubjatnikov R (1991) Association of *Chlamydia pneumoniae* (strain TWAR) infection with wheezing, asthmatic bronchitis, and adult-onset asthma. JAMA 266:225-230
11. Allegra L, Blasi F, Centanni S et al (1994) Acute exacerbations of asthma in adults: role of *Chlamydia pneumoniae* infection. Eur Respir J 7:2165-2168
12. Emre U, Roblin PM, Gelling M et al (1994) The association of *Chlamydia pneumoniae* infection and reactive airway disease in children. Arch Pediatr Adolesc Med 148:727-732
13. Cunningham AF, Johnston SL, Julious SA et al (1998) Chronic *Chlamydia pneumoniae* infection and asthma exacerbations in children. Eur Respir J 11:345-349
14. Haidl S, Ivarsson S, Bjerre I et al (1992) Guillain-Barré syndrome after *Chlamydia pneumoniae* infection. N Engl J Med 326:576-577
15. Socan M, Veovic B, Kese D (1994) *Chlamydia pneumoniae* and meningoencephalitis. N Engl J Med 331:406

16. Marrie TJ, Harczy M, Mann OE (1990) Culture negative endocarditis probably due to *Chlamydia pneumoniae.* J Infect Dis 161:127-129
17. Black CM, Bullard JC, Staton GW Jr et al (1992) Seroprevalence of *Chlamydia pneumoniae* antibodies in patients with pulmonary sarcoidosis in North Central Georgia. In: Mårdh PA, La Placa M, Ward M (eds) Proceedings of the European Society for *Chlamydia* Research, Stockholm, 2-7 September, 1992. The University of Uppsala, Uppsala, p 175 (abstract)
18. Grönhagen-Riska C, Saikku P, Riska H et al (1992) Antibodies to a TWAR – a novel type of *Chlamydia* – in sarcoidosis. In: Grassi C, Rizzato G, Pozzi E (eds) Sarcoidosis and other granulomatous disorders. Elsevier, Amsterdam pp 297-301
19. Poulakkainen M, Campbell LA, Kuo C-C et al (1996) Serological response to *Chlamydia pneumoniae* in patients with sarcoidosis. J Infect 33:199-205
20. Grayston JT (1989) *Chlamydia pneumoniae,* strain TWAR. Chest 95:664-669
21. Huovinen P, Lahtonen R, Ziegler T et al (1989) Pharyngitis in adults: the presence and the coexistence of viruses and bacterial organisms. Ann Intern Med 110:612-616
22. Ogawa H, Fujisawa T, Kazuyama Y (1990) Isolation of *Chlamydia pneumoniae* from middle ear aspirates of otitis media with effusion: a case report. J Infect Dis 162:1000-1001
23. Grayston JT, Campbell LA, Kuo C-C et al (1990) A new respiratory tract pathogen: *Chlamydia pneumoniae* strain TWAR. J Infect Dis 161:618-625
24. Hammerschlag MR, Chirgwin K, Roblin PM et al (1992) Persistent infection with *Chlamydia pneumoniae* following acute respiratory illness. Clin Infect Dis 14:178-182
25. Schachter J (1992) The pathogenesis of chlamydial infection. In: Mårdh PA, La Placa M, Ward M (eds) Proceedings of the European Society for *Chlamydia* Research, Stockholm, 2-7 September, 1992. The University of Uppsala, Uppsala, p 67-72
26. Falck G, Engstrand I, Gad A, Gnarpe J, Gnarpe H, Laurila A (1997) Demonstration of *Chlamydia pneumoniae* in patients with chronic pharyngitis. Scand J Infect Dis 29:585-589
27. Wright SW, Edwards KM, Decker MD et al (1997) Prevalence of positive serology for acute *Chlamydia pneumoniae* infection in emergency department patients with persistent cough. Acad Emerg Med 4:179-183
28. Grayston JT, Kuo C-C, Wang S-P et al (1986) Clinical findings in TWAR respiratory tract infections. In: Oriel JD (ed) Chlamydial infections. Cambridge University Press, Cambridge, UK, pp 329-332
29. Pizzichini MMM, Pizzichini E, Efrhimiavis A et al (1997) Markers of inflammation in induced sputum in acute bronchitis caused by *Chlamydia pneumoniae.* Thorax 52:929-931
30. Yang XP, Kuo C-C, Grayston T (1993) A mouse model of *Chlamydia pneumoniae* strain TWAR pneumonia. Infect Immun 61:2037-2040
31. Frick WE, Busse WW (1988) Respiratory infections: their role in airway responsiveness and pathogenesis of asthma. Clin Chest Med 9:539-549
32. Miyashita N, Kubota Y, Nakajiama M et al (1998) *Chlamydia pneumoniae* and exacerbations of asthma in adults. Ann Allergy Asthma Immunol 80:405-409
33. Cosentini R, Gandino A, Tarsia P et al (1998) Severe asthma exacerbations: role of acute *Chlamydia pneumoniae* infection. Thorax (submitted)
34. Allegra L, Blasi F, Cosentini R et al (1998) Treatment with clarithromycin in exacerbations of asthma caused by *Chlamydia pneumoniae.* 4th International Conference on the macrolides, azalides, streptogramins and ketolides, Barcelona, 21-23 January, 1998, p 45

35. Lamb D (1995) Pathology. In: Calverly P, Pride N (eds) Chronic obstructive pulmonary disease. Chapman and Hall, London pp 9-34

36. Murphy TF, Sethi S (1992) Bacterial infection in chronic obstructive pulmonary disease. Am Rev Respir Dis 146:1067-1083

37. von Hertzen L, Leinonen M, Koskinen R et al (1994) Evidence of persistence of *Chlamydia pneumoniae* infection in patients with COPD. In: Orfila J, Byrne Gl, Cherneskey MA et al (eds) Chlamydial infections. Esculapio, Bologna, pp 473-476

38. von Hertzen L, Alakarppa H, Koskinen R et al (1997) *Chlamydia pneumoniae* infection in patients with chronic obstructive pulmonary disease. Epidemiol Infect 118:155-164

39. von Hertzen L (1998) *Chlamydia pneumoniae* and its role in chronic obstructive pulmonary disease. Ann Med 30:27-37

40. Soler N, Torres A, Ewig S et al (1998) Bronchial microbial patterns in severe exacerbation of chronic obstructive pulmonary disease (COPD) requiring mechanical ventilation. Am J Respir Crit Care Med 157:1498-1505

41. Thom DH, Grayston JT (1991) Infections with *Chlamydia pneumoniae* strain TWAR. Clin Chest Med 12:245-256

42. Almirall J, Moratò I, Riera F et al (1993) Incidence of community-acquired pneumonia and *Chlamydia pneumoniae* infection: a prospective multicentre study. Eur Respir J 6:14-18

43. Steinhoff D, Lode H, Ruckdeschel G et al (1996) *Chlamydia pneumoniae* as a cause of community-acquired pneumonia in hospitalized patients in Berlin. Clin Infect Dis 22:958-964

44. Blasi F, Cosentini R, Legnani D et al (1993) Incidence of community-acquired pneumonia caused by *Chlamydia pneumoniae* in Italian patients. Eur J Clin Microbiol Infect Dis 12:696-699

45. Cosentini R, Blasi F, Raccanelli R et al (1996) Severe community-acquired pneumonia: a possible role for *Chlamydia pneumoniae*. Respiration 63:61-65

46. Marik PE, Iglesias J (1997) Severe community-acquired pneumonia, shock and multiorgan dysfunction syndrome caused by *Chlamydia pneumoniae*. J Intern Med 241:441-444

47. Pacheco A, Gonzales SJ, Aroncena C et al (1991) Community-acquired pneumonia caused by *Chlamydia pneumoniae* strain TWAR in chronic cardiopulmonary disease in the elderly. Respiration 58:316-320

48. Sundelof B, Gnarpe J, Gnarpe H et al (1993) *Chlamydia pneumoniae* in Swedish patients. Scand J Infect Dis 25:429-433

49. Kauppinen MT, Saikku P, Kujala P et al (1996) Clinical picture of community-acquired *Chlamydia pneumoniae* pneumonia requiring hospital treatment: a comparison between chlamydial and pneumococcal pneumonia. Thorax 51:185-189

50. Marrie JT, Durant H, Yates L (1989) Community-acquired pneumonia requiring hospitalisation: 5-year prospective study. Rev Infect Dis 11:586-599

51. Torres A, Dorca J, Zalacaìn R et al (1996) Community-acquired pneumonia in chronic obstructive pulmonary disease – a Spanish multicenter study. Am J Crit Care Med 154:1456-1461

52. Rumbak MJ, Baselski V, Belenchia JM et al (1993) Case report: acute postoperative respiratory failure caused by *Chlamydia pneumoniae* and diagnosed by bronchoalveolar lavage. Am J Med Sci 305:390-393

53. Thom DH, Grayston JT, Campbell LA et al (1994) Respiratory infection with *Chlamydia pneumoniae* in middle-aged and older adult outpatients. Eur J Clin Microbiol Infect Dis 13:785-792

54. Riquelme R, Torres A, El-Ebiary M et al (1997) Community-acquired pneumonia in the elderly – clinical and nutritional aspects. Am J Crit Care Med 156:1908-1914
55. Troy CJ, Peeling RW, Ellis AG et al (1997) *Chlamydia pneumoniae* as a new source of infectious outbreaks in nursing homes. JAMA 277:1214-1218
56. Augenbraun MH, Roblin MR, Chirwing K et al (1991) Isolation of *Chlamydia pneumoniae* from lungs of patients infected with the human immunodeficiency virus. J Clin Microbiol 29:401-402
57. Clark R, Mushatt D, Fazal B (1991) Case report: *Chlamydia pneumoniae* pneumonia in HIV-infected man. Eur J Med Sci 302:155-156
58. Gaydos CA, Flower CL, Gill BJ et al (1993) Detection of *Chlamydia pneumoniae* by polymerase chain reaction–enzyme immunoassay in an immunocompromised population. Clin Infect Dis 17:718-723
59. Blasi F, Boschini A, Cosentini R et al (1994) Outbreak of *Chlamydia pneumoniae* infection in an ex injection-drug users community. Chest 105:812-815
60. Boschini A, Smacchia C, Di Fine M et al (1996) Community acquired pneumonia in a cohort of former injection-drug users with and without human immunodeficiency virus infection: incidence etiologies and clinical aspects. Clin Infect Dis 23:107-113
61. Dalhoff K, Maass M (1996) *Chlamydia pneumoniae* pneumonia in hospitalised patients. Chest 110:351-356

Are Atypical Pathogens Important for Patients with Community-Acquired Pneumonia?

M.S. NIEDERMAN

Introduction

The term "atypical pathogens" refers to a variety of organisms, including *Mycoplasma pneumoniae, Chlamydia pneumoniae,* and *Legionella* spp., that can cause community-acquired pneumonia (CAP). This designation was developed when investigators realized that some patients with pneumonia had a clinical picture and natural history that differed from that seen in patients with pneumococcal infection. The syndrome, initially associated with *M. pneumoniae* [1], is characterized by gradual onset of illness, with low-grade fever, mucoid sputum and a non-toxic presentation, with a chest radiograph that shows more severe involvement than indicated by the patient's findings. Over the years, the frequency of pneumonia due to atypical pathogens has been widely variable in clinical series, the need for therapy of these pathogens has been questioned, the role of these organisms in severe ICU-treated CAP has been controversial, and the definition of the patient most at risk has been uncertain. In addition, there has been debate about whether identifying the presence of the "atypical pneumonia syndrome" has any diagnostic value and whether clinicians should use the presence or absence of this syndrome to guide initial empiric antibiotic therapy of CAP [2-4].

In 1993 the American Thoracic Society (ATS) published guidelines for the therapy of CAP [4], and discussed the role of atypical pathogens in this illness, coming to several conclusions: (1) The frequency of these organisms is generally low, and most patients with CAP do not need therapy directed at them. (2) When these organisms are present, it is mostly in the outpatient setting, in young patients without serious comorbidity; they are rarely of concern in older outpatients with comorbid illness. (3) In hospitalized patients, *Legionella* is the major organism of concern, and one that should be empirically treated in all ICU-admitted CAP patients; however, most other hospitalized patients do not need coverage for atypical pathogens. (4) Clinical features are not useful for predicting the presence of these organisms, since the "atypical" presentation of pneumonia can occur even with bacterial pathogens, for example in a host who has an impaired inflammatory response. In addition, *Legionella* can present with features that overlap both typical and atypical pneumonia syndromes. Several recent studies have emphasized that clinical features are not generally useful for predicting the microbial etiology of CAP, and radiographic studies may be equally unhelpful [2–5].

Are Atypical Pathogens Common in CAP?

Shortly after the ATS guidelines were published, a group of investigators from Johns Hopkins Hospital reported data from 205 non-HIV-infected patients with CAP admitted from the emergency department. A very low frequency of atypical pathogen infection was documented. Of the group, only 9.8% had any atypical pathogen infection documented, although nearly 40% had no identified organism [6]. Diagnostic testing was reportedly aggressive, including *Legionella* testing with urinary antigen, direct fluorescent antibody (DFA) or culture of respiratory secretions, examination for acute titer increases, and observation for convalescent titer rises; *Mycoplasma* testing with convalescent titers; and *C. pneumoniae* testing with polymerase chain reation, enzyme immunoassay, or culture. Based on the relatively low frequency of atypical pathogen infection, the authors concluded that the ATS view of these organisms was correct and that empiric therapy should involve a β-lactam with selective use of a macrolide.

Recently, the same authors reported a re-evaluation of these data [7]. In this report, it was clear that very few patients had acute and convalescent titers collected for *Chlamydia*, and only half had these studies for *Mycoplasma* and *Legionella*. Of this group, only 29 patients had atypical pathogens identified, and in 16 patients (55%) this was part of a mixed infection (including mixed infection in 71% with *C. pneumoniae*), while mixed infection occurred in less than 10% of those patients with bacterial pathogen infection. When clinical and radiographic features were examined, there was no distinctive pattern for patients with atypical pathogens compared with those with conventional bacterial pathogens. Of patients with atypical pathogens, only four received appropriate therapy, and no patient without specific therapy against these pathogens died. These findings led the authors to conclude, again, that macrolide therapy is not routinely needed for patients with CAP. In addition, the authors concluded that atypical pathogen infection is often part of a mixed infection and that patients with this type of infection cannot be identified on the basis of clinical features.

In spite of these observations, other recent studies have reported a much higher incidence of infection with atypical pathogens and have found these organisms to be part of a mixed infection, often with bacterial pathogens. The first of these studies, reported by Lieberman et al. [8], involved 346 patients admitted to a hospital in Israel. The remarkable finding in this study was that 39% of the patients had mixed infection, usually with an atypical pathogen and a bacterial organism, and this accounted for the observation that over 60% of the population had a reported atypical pathogen involved in their illness (Fig. 1). Overall, 29% had *Mycoplasma* infection , 16% *Legionella*, and 18% *C. pneumoniae*. These organisms were not confined to young and healthy individuals, with *Legionella* and *C. pneumoniae* being common in all age groups. In fact, 50% of the *C. pneumoniae*

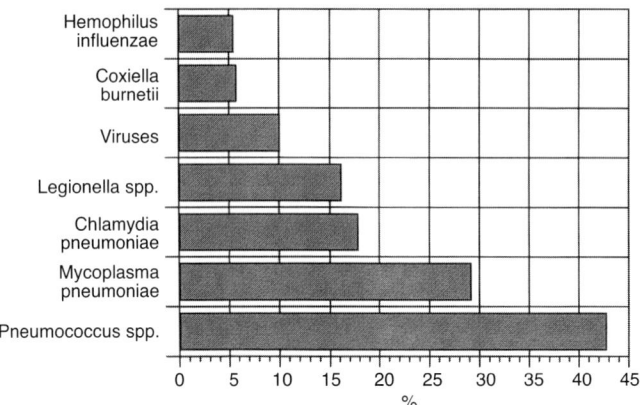

Fig. 1. Pathogens in 346 patients with community-acquired pneumonia admitted to a hospital in Israel. Although *Pneumococcus* was the most commonly identified pathogen, atypical organisms were present in over 60% of the patients, because over 40% had mixed infection involving these organisms. (Data from [8])

patients were above the age of 65 [8]. There was a general trend for *M. pneumoniae* to be found more commonly in patients without comorbid illness than in those with such diseases (36% vs 15%). In this study, criteria for diagnosing the presence of atypical pathogens depended mostly on serologic findings, using not only IgG antibodies, but also IgM and sometimes IgA responses, comparing acute and convalescent titers. The implication of these findings for therapy was uncertain, since only 48.7% of the patients with atypical pathogen infection received appropriate therapy, yet outcomes were generally good.

In a study conducted in the United States, a high frequency of atypical pathogens was also documented in a cohort of 2776 patients, representing all admitted CAP patients in two Ohio counties observed over a 1-year period [9]. Patients had extensive diagnostic testing, with 69% having serologic samples collected and 44% having both acute and convalescent titers evaluated. In this group, a possible etiologic diagnosis was made in 44% of the population, with *M. pneumoniae* being most common, accounting for 32.5% of all such diagnoses, followed by *S. pneumoniae* in 12.6% and *C. pneumoniae* in 8.9% of cases. Infections with *Mycoplasma* and *Legionella* were more common with increasing age, while *Chlamydia* was seen more commonly in patients aged 18–34 years.

In another study of CAP in Germany [10], 236 hospitalized patients were evaluated and many had antibodies to *C. pneumoniae* (48%); nearly 20% met serologic criteria for the diagnosis of acute infection, but only 11.4% had both a clinical and serologic picture of infection with this pathogen. The study findings are interesting in documenting that some patients with serologic findings of *C. pneumoniae* may not really have the clinical illness of pneumonia due to this organism. Still, the high frequency of antibodies and rising titers to this organism means that coinfection with this pathogen may be common, or that acute infection with another organism promotes a non-specific rise in antibody titers to *C. pneumoniae*. In the patients with both serologic and clinical findings of infection with the organism, the mean age was 58 years, and the clinical picture varied from mild to severe, with 11% being admitted to the ICU, but with no patients dying. The chest radiograph showed interstitial infiltrates in 18% of patients, and 26% had pleural effusion.

In a recent epidemic of infection in three Canadian nursing homes investigators did not observe *C. pneumoniae* infection to be free of mortality [11]. In that study, 16 patients with CAP due to *C. pneumoniae* were documented and 6 died. The important conclusions from this study were that infection with this pathogen could occur in all patient populations, including the institutionalized elderly, and that the infection could be associated with serious morbidity, with an observed mortality rate of > 30%. Interestingly, some epidemiologic data in the study suggested the possibility of person-to-person spread of the organism to account for the epidemic.

Atypical pathogens have been well documented, as described above, in hospitalized patients with CAP, but they may also be important among outpatients. Marrie et al. documented CAP by chest radiograph in 149 outpatients and found that atypical pathogens or viruses accounted for half of all the infections observed [12]. Overall, *M. pneumoniae* was present in 23% of patients, while *C. pneumoniae* was present in 11%, *Legionella* in 1%, and viruses in 10% (Fig. 2).

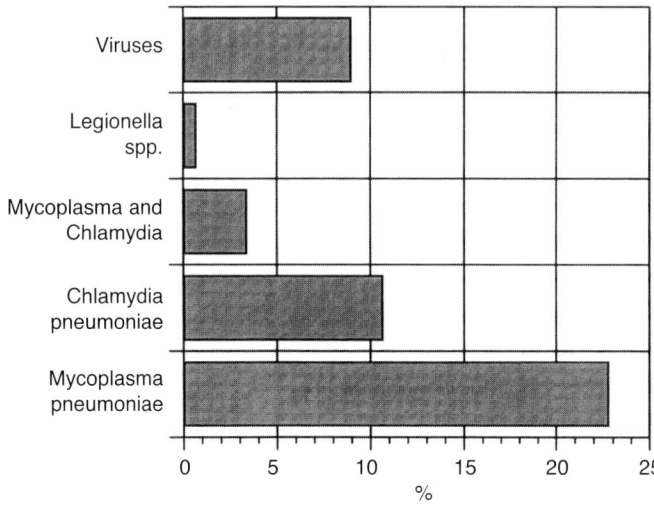

Fig. 2. In a study of 149 outpatients in Canada, atypical pathogens and viruses were present in nearly half of all patients with radiographic pneumonia. (Data from [12])

Table 1. The role of atypical pathogens in community-acquired pneumonia

- Atypical pathogens may be present in 40%-60% of all CAP patients
- Serologic diagnoses of atypical pathogen infection are common in CAP, but not always confirmed by clinical symptoms and response to therapy
- Atypical pathogens are commonly present along with bacterial pathogens in CAP (coinfection)
- Atypical pathogens are present in patients of all ages and comorbid illness states, and in all degrees of severity of CAP
- Routine therapy of CAP with a macrolide is associated with improved outcome: do all patients need therapy of atypical pathogens?
- CAP with atypical pathogens can lead to death

Putting all of the recent studies together, I reach the following conclusions about atypical pathogens in CAP (Table 1): (1) Using careful serologic testing, the incidence of atypical pathogens in CAP may not be as low as previously thought, with anywhere from 40% to 60% of both inpatients and outpatients having evidence for CAP involving these organisms. (2) Many of the studies documenting a high incidence of these organisms have relied on serologic testing, and not all patients who meet the serologic criteria for infection have clinical evidence of pneumonia due to these organisms. Further studies are needed to define whether these serologic diagnoses are accurate, and whether the presence of these organisms can be confirmed by other methods. (3) Often atypical pathogens are present as part of a coinfection involving bacterial agents. (4) The impact of these organisms on therapy is uncertain, as many patients with CAP improve without specific therapy for atypical pathogens. (5) Patients of all ages and comorbidities can be infected with these organisms, and their presence is not confined to young and otherwise healthy individuals. (6) Infection with these organisms is not always benign, and some patients, even those with *C. pneumoniae* infection, may die when they develop CAP due to atypical pathogens.

Should Patients with CAP Be Routinely Treated for Atypical Pathogens?

Although the findings of the group from Johns Hopkins suggest that routine therapy of atypical pathogens in CAP is not needed, this view is not necessarily substantiated by other studies. In an evaluation of the role of coinfection, Kauppinen et al. [13] evaluated three groups of patients: those with pure *C. pneumoniae* pneumonia ($n = 24$), those with pure pneumococcal pneumonia ($n = 9$), and those with infection involving both organisms ($n = 13$). The authors found that when *C. pneumoniae* was present alone, only 36% of patients received adequate therapy, yet the course was relatively benign, with a length of stay of 8.4 days. With pneumococcal infection, all patients received adequate therapy, and length of stay was 10.5 days. However, if mixed infection was present, all patients were treated for *Pneumococcus*, none for *Chlamydia*, and the length of stay was prolonged to

21.9 days. The findings in this study suggest that *C. pneumoniae* may potentiate the severity of pneumococcal infection and that routine therapy of this pathogen could possibly have some benefit for patients with mixed infection.

Unfortunately, there are sparse outcome data to directly support the need for routine therapy of atypical pathogens and to tie such therapy to bacteriologic or serologic data. However, there are outcome studies of CAP that show that the use of a macrolide is associated with a better outcome, for both inpatients and outpatients, than if no macrolide is used [14, 15]. Although these observations could be explained by a beneficial anti-inflammatory effect of macrolides, their antibacterial effect is equally likely to account for the improved outcome. If this latter possibility is correct, then this is indirect evidence of an important role for atypical pathogens in CAP, often as copathogens.

Gordon et al. [14] retrospectively examined the records of 4448 patients admitted to the hospital, but not the ICU, with CAP. Patients were divided into five groups: those who received monotherapy with a β-lactam recommended by the ATS guidelines ($n = 1938$), those who received one of these β-lactams with a macrolide ($n = 784$), those who received a mixture of recommended and non-recommended therapy according to the guidelines ($n = 383$), those who received therapy not in accordance with the guidelines ($n = 1027$), and 207 patients who had inappropriately long delays (generally > 36 h) before receiving therapy. The study found that patients who received guideline-recommended therapy had a significantly lower chance of dying than those who received non-recommended therapy, but that the lowest mortality rate of all was in those patients who received both a β-lactam and a macrolide. In another data set, the same general findings emerged (Peter Houck, Health Care Financing Agency Western states, personal communication). In that study, 8918 Medicare patients hospitalized for CAP were evaluated and only 17.5% received macrolide therapy, either alone or in combination with a β-lactam. Mortality significantly lower than with regimens not recommended by the ATS guidelines was seen only in the 184 patients who received macrolide monotherapy and in the 1127 patients who received a recommended β-lactam combined with a macrolide.

In the outpatient setting, one validation study also showed great value for macrolides in both young patients without comorbid illness as well as in older patients with or without comorbid illness [15]. In that study, both outpatient groups achieved better outcomes at lower costs with the use of a macrolide than with to other regimens. Although there were no bacteriologic data to explain these findings, it was surprising that even in the older population with comorbid illness, there was a trend toward lower hospitalization rates and mortality in patients who received macrolide monotherapy than in those who received β-lactam monotherapy. These findings again suggest that routine therapy directed at atypical pathogens may be beneficial for all types of outpatients with CAP.

If atypical pathogen coinfection is indeed common in patients with CAP, then it may have implications not only for therapy, but also for diagnostic testing. For example, if pneumococcal pneumonia is documented by a suggestive sputum Gram stain and/or a positive blood culture, what therapy should be used? Should antibiotics be directed only at *Pneumococcus*, or should atypical pathogens (as part of a coinfection) also be treated? If the answer to the latter question is yes, then the value of diagnostic information (in terms of focusing antibiotic therapy), is very limited.

What Studies Are Needed for the Future?

As described above, a lot of circumstantial evidence now suggests that atypical pathogens are important in patients with CAP: they are commonly present when looked for, they often coexist with bacterial pathogens, they may lead to a more complicated course when not treated in the presence of bacterial copathogens, and outcomes (including mortality) are improved if macrolides are incorporated in CAP therapy regimens.

In the future, it will be necessary to document the role of these organisms more clearly. This will require routine serologic testing, along with cultures to substantiate the high frequency of infection with these organisms. In addition, it will be necessary to conduct outcome studies that correlate the use of therapy for atypical pathogens with improved outcomes in patients who are actually documented to have CAP due to these organisms. If these findings can be supplemented with pathogenesis studies that document a plausible mechanism for atypical pathogens to potentiate the severity of infection with common bacteria, then the data will be even stronger. In the meantime, it is my belief that all patients with CAP should be routinely treated for atypical pathogens, using a macrolide either alone or in combination with a β-lactam, depending on the presence of risk factors for other specific bacterial agents. Alternatively, monotherapy with a new fluoroquinolone (grepafloxacin, levofloxacin, sparfloxacin, or trovafloxacin) would also provide adequate coverage for atypical pathogen infection coexisting with bacterial pathogens.

References

1. Chanock RM, Hayflick L, Barile MF (1961) Growth on artificial medium of an agent associated with atypical pneumonia and its identification as a PPLO. Proc Natl Acad Sci USA 478:41
2. Woodhead MA, MacFarlane JT (1987) Comparative clinical laboratory features on legionella with pneumococcal and mycoplasma pneumonias. Br J Dis Chest 81:133-139
3. Farr BM, Kaiser DL, Harrison BDW, Connolly CK (1989) Prediction of microbial aetiology at admission to hospital for pneumonia from the presenting clinical features. Thorax 44:1031-1035
4. Niederman MS, Bass JB, Campbell GD, Fein AM, Grossman RF, Mandell LA, Marrie TJ, Sarosi GA, Torres A, Yu VL (1993) Guidelines for the initial management of adults with community-acquired pneumonia: diagnosis, assessment of severity, and initial antimicrobial therapy. Am Rev Respir Dis 148:1418-1426

5. Sopena N, Sabria-Leal M, Pedro-Botet ML, Padilla E, Dominguez J, Morera J, Tudela P (1998) Comparative study of the clinical presentation of *Legionella pneumonia* and other community-acquired pneumonias. Chest 113:1195-1200

6. Mundy LM, Auwaerter PG, Oldach D, Warner ML, Burton A, Vance E et al (1995) Community-acquired pneumonia: impact of immune status. Am J Respir Crit Care Med 152:1309-1315

7. Mundy LM, Oldach D, Autwaerter PG, Gaydos CA, Moore RD, Bartlett JG et al (1998) Implication for macrolide treatment in community-acquired pneumonia. Chest 113:1201-1206

8. Lieberman D, Schlaeffer F, Boldur I, Lieberman D, Horowith S, Friedman MG et al (1996) Multiple pathogens in adult patients admitted with community-acquired pneumonia: a one year prospective study of 346 consecutive patients. Thorax 51:179-184

9. Marston BJ, Plouffe JF, File TM, Hackman BA, Salstrom SJ, Lipman HB et al (1997) Incidence of community-acquired pneumonia requiring hospitalization. Arch Intern Med 157:1709-1718

10. Steinhoff D, Lode H, Ruckdeschel G, Heidrich B, Rolfs A, Fehrenbach FJ, Mauch H, Hoffken G, Wagner J (1996) *Chlamydia pneumoniae* as a cause of community-acquired pneumonia in hospitalized patients in Berlin. Clin Infect Dis 22:958-964

11. Troy CJ, Peeling RW, Ellis AG et al (1997) *Chlamydia pneumoniae* as a new source of infectious outbreaks in nursing homes. JAMA 277:1214-1218

12. Marrie TJ, Peeling RW, Fine MJ et al (1996) Ambulatory patients with community-acquired pneumonia: the frequency of atypical agents and clinical course. Am J Med 101:509-515

13. Kauppinen MT, Saikku P, Kujala P, Herva E, Syrjala H (1996) Clinical picture of *Chlamydia pneumoniae* requiring hospital treatment: a comparison between chlamydial and pneumococcal pneumonia. Thorax 51:185-189

14. Gordon GS, Throop D, Berberian L, Niederman M, Bass J, Alemayehu D, Mellis S (1996) Validation of the therapeutic recommendations of the American Thoracic Society (ATS) guidelines for community-acquired pneumonia in hospitalized patients. Chest 110:55S

15. Gleason PP, Kapoor WN, Stone RA, Lave JR, Obrosky DS, Schulz R et al (1997) Medical outcomes and antimicrobial costs with the use of the American Thoracic Society Guidelines for outpatients with community-acquired pneumonia. JAMA 278:32-39

Immunology of *Chlamydia pneumoniae*

M. Leinonen

Introduction

Chlamydiae are obligate intracellular parasites and at their simplest they can be regarded as highly specialised Gram-negative bacteria. Both the structural components of the chlamydial cell (virulence factors) and the host cell factors – i.e. how the host resists chlamydial infection – play a role in the immunological mechanisms associated with chlamydial infections. At the moment, not much is known about the immunology of *Chlamydia pneumoniae* infection, but evidently most immunological mechanisms associated with other chlamydial infections are also involved in *C. pneumoniae* infections.

All chlamydial species have a tendency to cause chronic infections. Persistent *C. psittaci* infections in birds and mammals have been known for years, and infections caused by lymphogranuloma venereum (LGV) and *C. psittaci* may persist in humans for 10–20 years. Generally, the mostly mild acute infections caused by *C. trachomatis* resolve without sequels, but they may also progress to severe chronic inflammation leading to blindness (trachoma) even 50 years after the primary infection, as well as to infertility, ectopic pregnancies and reactive arthritis. *C. pneumoniae* is also able to cause chronic infections and it has been associated with several chronic disease conditions, most importantly with chronic lung processes and atherosclerosis. The immunopathological mechanisms by which chlamydiae cause inflammation and subsequent chronic sequels remains unclear.

Different chlamydial species and even biovars display different tissue tropism and infect different cell types. Most *C. trachomatis* biovars infect mucosal epithelium and tend to remain localised or to spread along mucosal epithelium (e.g., in trachoma and pelvic inflammatory disease). However, *C. psittaci* and the LGV biovar of *C. trachomatis* are able to cause infections in a variety of cell types, including mononuclear phagocytes. *C. pneumoniae* is also able to multiply in monocytes and macrophages and in vascular endothelial cells as well as in smooth muscle cells and can induce the production of cytokines, adhesion molecules and procoagulant activity in these cells [1–7]. It has been shown recently that in mice *C. pneumoniae* can disseminate inside the monocytes from respiratory tract into circulation [8]. This may evidently happen in humans, too, because persons with chronic infection frequently have *C. pneumoniae* DNA in their peripheral blood monocytes [9]. Monocytes and macrophages are important for immunological defence, and the survival and multiplication of *C. pneumoniae* inside these cells may contribute to the immunological features of *C. pneumoniae* infections. It has been shown recently that *C. pneumoniae* induces foam cell formation of human macrophages and is thus able to initiate or promote atheroma development [10]. When *C. pneumoniae* is present in macrophages and vascular endothelial cells, bacteria and their structural components – either shed from infected cells or liberated when host cells are destroyed – have an easy access to circulation. These components are able to bind to antibodies present in circulation, forming immune complexes which may maintain inflammatory reactions in the vascular system [11–13].

Antibody Response to *Chlamydia pneumoniae* Infections

Being a Gram-negative bacterium, *Chlamydia* has a typical cell wall component, lipopolysaccharide (LPS). Chlamydial LPS is of the deep-rough type, having only an acidic ketodeoxyoctonate (KDO) trisaccharide unit linked to lipid A part of the molecule [14]. The endotoxin activity of chlamydial LPS seems to be much lower than that of Gram-negative bacteria [15]. The decreased toxicity might be an advantage to *Chlamydia*. When it is shed from infected cells, high endotoxin activity could immediately lead to a deleterious response in the host. Symptoms reminiscent of endotoxin shock have never been described in connection with chlamydial infections. The antibody response to LPS seems to be rapid in acute *C. pneumoniae* infections [16], and the measurement of LPS antibodies might thus be helpful in diagnosis, if the interval between the acute and convalescent sera is less than 2 weeks. In chronic *C. pneumoniae* infections, infected macrophages or endothelial cells are in close contact with the circulation, which means that LPS shed from these cells should be present in the circulation. The demonstration of an antibody response to chlamydial LPS in patients after acute myocardial infarction actually led to the discovery of the association of *C. pneumoniae* infection with cardiovascular diseases [17]. Furthermore, circulating chlamydial LPS-containing immune complexes [11, 13] have been demonstrated in patients with cardiovascular diseases.

The outer membrane proteins (OMPs) of *C. pneumoniae* seem to be somewhat different from those of the other chlamydial species. The major outer membrane protein (MOMP) of *C. trachomatis* is highly immunogenic and also responsible for serotype specificity. The MOMP of *C. pneumoniae* seems to be only poorly immunogenic, and no differences in the amino acid sequences of MOMPs of different *C. pneumoniae* isolates have thus far been found [18, 19]. When the antibody responses to different isolates of *C. pneumoniae* are compared, the kinetics of responses seem to be different, suggesting that there are different immunotypes among *C. pneumoniae* strains [18] (our unpublished data). At the moment, however, we do not know exactly which structural components may confer to the serotype specificity of *C. pneumoniae,* although it has been suggested that serovar-specific antigenic determinants may reside within the 65-kDa protein [20].

The serum antibody response to the surface proteins of *C. pneumoniae* can be demonstrated by the micro-immunofluorescence (MIF) method during acute infections. Primary infections are characterised by a rapid IgM response and delayed IgG responses, which can be demonstrable as late as 6 weeks after the onset of the disease [21, 22]. However, it is possible that the delayed IgG response may simply be due to the fact that most laboratories use as a MIF antigen two original *C. pneumoniae* strains, TW 183 and IOL 207, rather than their own strains circulating in their population. No IgM antibodies are found in reinfections, and the IgG and IgA responses are more rapid than in primary infections [16, 21, 22]. Complement-fixing chlamydial group-specific antibodies are formed in primary infections, especially in young adults, but they are not generally seen in reinfections [16, 21, 22]. However, patients with both primary infection and reinfection show an antibody response to LPS [16].

Immunoblotting analyses of sera from infected humans have shown the antibody responses to be directed against several structural proteins, most of them species-specific [23–25]. In contrast to the other chlamydial species, antibody responses to *C. pneumoniae* MOMP are seen only seldom. Sera from patients with *C. pneumoniae* infection from USA have been reported to contain antibodies most frequently to a high-molecular-weight 98-kDa protein which has been considered *C. pneumoniae*-specific [23], while in chronic infections the antibodies frequently recognise 43-kDa and 52-kDa proteins [26]. Two of these proteins, the 98-kDa and 43-kDa proteins, are also recognised by immune complex-bound antibodies in the sera of Finnish patients with chronic coronary heart disease [12]. Recent studies in Germany have also suggested that patients with cardiovascular diseases have antibodies against 98-kDa and 40-kDa proteins more frequently than controls (odds ratio 2.3 and 29.4, respectively) [27]. In contrast, only 14% of the acute German sera reacted with the 98-kDa protein, whereas another species-specific 54-kDa protein was recognised by 93% of the sera with *C. pneumoniae* antibodies [24]. The great variation in the prevalences of antibodies against different proteins cannot possibly be explained only by individual responsiveness to different antigens; epidemic and regional variation of *C. pneumoniae* strains must also play a part. Protein analyses of several *C. pneumoniae* isolates have proved that quantitative differences can be detected in the relative amounts of structural proteins [25].

Cell-mediated Immunity to *Chlamydia pneumoniae*

Since chlamydiae are obligate intracellular parasites, T-cell-mediated immunological mechanisms have been suggested to play a role both in the protection and in the destructive immunopathology associated with chlamydial infections. Both humoral and cell-mediated types of immunity have been shown to be involved in the resolution of chlamydial infection, although antibodies do not appear to be essential. Congenitally athymic mice are unable to resolve infection [28], whereas B-cell-deficient mice are able to do so [29], implying that cell-mediated immunity is important in resolution. The role of T-cells is further emphasised by the clearance of infection by adoptive transfer of a *Chlamydia*-specific T-cell line to athymic mice [30]. Both CD4+ and CD8+ cells are activated in the primary response to chlamydial infection [31]. CD4+ cells secrete cytokines, which activate other lymphocytes, whereas CD8+ cells lyse infected target cells, which mechanism has also been shown to be important in immunity against other intracellular bacteria [32].

In *C. trachomatis* infections, cell-mediated immunity is thought to be responsible for the chronic scarring processes leading to trachoma and tubal obstruction. The most direct evidence of a delayed hypersensitivity reaction has been obtained from experiments in which crude extracts of *Chlamydia* elicit severe ocular inflammation in immune animals with similar histopathology as in trachoma or *Chlamydia*-induced infertility [33, 34]. The hypersensitivity has been shown to be closely associated with the 57-kDa protein, the chlamydial heat shock protein, hsp60 [35]. Wick et al. [36] proposed that hsp60 might promote atherosclerosis by stimulating autoimmunity. Recently, Kol et al. have shown that *C. pneumoniae* hsp60 colocalises with human hsp60 in plaque macrophages in human atherosclerotic lesions. Furthermore, the rabbits which develop aortic arteriosclerotic changes after intranasal challenge [37] also develop antibodies to *C. pneumoniae* hsp60 which cross-react with mycobacterial hsp60 (Huittinen et al., unpublished). These findings suggest that chlamydial hsp60, by antigenic mimicry, might provoke an autoimmune reaction against human hsp60.

T-cell-mediated immunity against *C. pneumoniae* has been studied in persons with acquired laboratory infections caused by *C. pneumoniae* [38]. They showed a definite antigen-specific lymphocyte proliferation response, which started to increase at 3 weeks and had a peak value at 8–9 weeks after the onset of symptoms. In healthy individuals, lymphocyte proliferative responses are similar in males and females, and there is no clear correlation with humoral responses. However, individuals with persistently elevated IgA antibodies to *C. pneumoniae* as a possible marker of chronic infection tend to have a decreased lymphocyte response suggesting deficient or suppressed cell-mediated immunity [39]. In contrast to healthy individuals, in whom T-cell reactivity is specific to the *C. pneumoniae* antigen, patients with severe coronary heart disease elicit a T-cell response cross-reactive with different chlamydial species, which might be directed against conservative protein epitopes in MOMP or chlamydial heat shock proteins shared by different chlamydial species [40]. These results suggest that T-cell immunity might be important in protection against *C. pneumoniae,* and in chronic infections or reinfections T-cells may also be responsible for the immunopathology associated with the disease.

The role of cytokines in the growth of chlamydiae has been elucidated in several in vitro studies. Interferon-γ (IFN-γ)-mediated activation of host cells to restrict chlamydial replication has been proposed as a mechanism for establishing persistent *C. trachomatis* infection in vivo. IFN-γ-mediated persistence involves the induction of indolamine-2,3-dioxygenase which leads to degradation of tryptophan, an amino acid essential for chlamydial growth [41]. In vitro, this leads to the formation of large aberrant replicative forms and a persistent infection. *C. pneumoniae* growth is also inhibited by IFN-γ [42, 43], which implies that this mechanism may be involved in the development of chronic *C. pneumoniae* infections.

C. pneumoniae is able to induce the secretion of interleukin-1 (IL-1), IL-6 and tumour necrosis factor-α (TNF-α) in human peripheral monocytes [5], and these cytokines may confer the resistance to infection [44, 45]. However, cytokines also participate in the inflammatory reaction, and it has been indicated that several reactivities associated with endotoxin shock can be induced by replacing LPS with TNF-α. Furthermore, TNF-α inhibits lipoprotein lipase, leading to mobilisation of lipids and to elevated serum triglyceride and lowered HDL levels [46]. We have shown that in acute *C. pneumoniae* pneumonia, triglyceride levels are significantly higher and HDL levels, especially those of HDL_2, significantly lower than in either viral or pneumococcal pneumonia [47]. It can be speculated that, in chronic *C. pneumoniae* infections, continuous cytokine production might lead to the serum lipid pattern considered a risk factor for coronary heart disease [48].

References

1. Kaukoranta-Tolvanen SS, Laitinen K, Saikku P, Leinonen M (1994) *Chlamydia pneumoniae* multiplies in human endothelial cells in vitro. Microb Pathog 16:313-319
2. Godzik KL, O'Brien ER, Wang SK, Kuo C-C (1995) In vitro susceptibility of human vascular wall cells to infection with *Chlamydia pneumoniae*. J Clin Microbiol 33:2411-2414
3. Gaydos CA, Summersgill JT, Sahney NN, Ramirez JA, Quinn TC (1996) Replication of *Chlamydia pneumoniae* in vitro in human macrophages, endothelial cells, and aortic artery smooth muscle cells. Infect Immun 64:1614-1620
4. Kaukoranta-Tolvanen SS, Ronni T, Leinonen M, Saikku P, Laitinen K (1996) Expression of adhesion molecules on endothelial cells stimulated by *Chlamydia pneumoniae*. Microb Pathog 21:407-411
5. Kaukoranta-Tolvanen SS, Teppo AM, Laitinen K, Saikku P, Linnavuori K, Leinonen M (1996) Growth of *Chlamydia pneumoniae* in cultured human peripheral blood mononuclear cells and induction of a cytokine response. Microb Pathog 21:215-221
6. Fryer RH, Schwobe EP, Woods ML, Rodgers GM (1997) *Chlamydia* species infect human vascular endothelial cells and induce procoagulant activity. J Invest Med 45:168-174
7. Knoebel E, Vijayagopal P, Figueroa JE II, Martin DH (1997) In vitro infection of smooth muscle cells by *Chlamydia pneumoniae*. Infect Immun 65:503-506
8. Moazed TC, Kuo C-C, Grayston JT, Campbell LA (1998) Evidence of systemic dissemination of *Chlamydia pneumoniae* via macrophages in the mouse. J Infect Dis 177:1322-1325
9. Boman J, Söderberg S, Forsberg J, Birgander LS, Allard A, Persson K, Jidell E, Kumlin U, Juto P, Waldenström A, Wadell G (1998) High prevalence of *Chlamydia pneumoniae* DNA in peripheral blood mononuclear cells in patients with cardiovascular disease and in middle-aged blood donors. J Infect Dis 178:274-277

10. Kalayoglu MV, Byrne GI (1998) Induction of macrophage foam cell formation by *Chlamydia pneumoniae*. J Infect Dis 177:725-729

11. Leinonen M, Linnanmäki E, Mattila K, Nieminen MS, Valtonen V, Leirisalo-Repo M, Saikku P (1990) Circulating immune complexes containing chlamydial lipopolysaccharide in acute myocardial infarction. Microb Pathog 9:67-73

12. Linnanmäki E, Leinonen M, Mattila K, Ekman MR, Nieminen MS, Valtonen V, Saikku P (1993) Presence of *Chlamydia pneumoniae* specific antibodies in circulating immune complexes in coronary heart disease. Circulation 87:1130-1134

13. Saikku P, Leinonen M, Tenkanen L, Ekman MR, Linnanmäki E, Manninen V, Mänttäri M, Frick MH, Huttunen JK (1992) Chronic *Chlamydia pneumoniae* infection as a risk factor for coronary heart disease in the Helsinki Heart Study. Ann Int Med 116:273-278

14. Nurminen M, Rietschel ET, Brade H (1985) Chemical characterisation of *Chlamydia trachomatis* lipopolysaccharide. Infect Immun 48:573-575

15. Brade L, Schramek S, Schade U, Brade H (1986) Chemical, biological and immunochemical properties of *Chlamydia psittaci* lipopolysaccharide. Infect Immun 54:568-574

16. Ekman MR, Leinonen M, Syrjälä H, Linnanmäki E, Kujala P, Saikku P (1993) Evaluation of serological methods in the diagnosis of *Chlamydia pneumoniae* during an epidemic in Finland. Eur J Clin Microbiol 12:756-760

17. Saikku P, Leinonen M, Mattila K, Ekman MR, Nieminen MS, Mäkelä PH, Huttunen J, Valtonen V (1988) Serologic evidence of an association of a novel *Chlamydia*, TWAR, with chronic coronary heart disease and acute myocardial infarction. Lancet ii:983-985

18. Black CM, Johnson JE, Farshy CE, Brown TM, Berdal BP (1991) Antigenic variation among strains of *Chlamydia pneumoniae*. J Clin Microbiol 29:1312-1316

19. Gaydos CA, Quinn TC, Bobo LD, Eiden JJ (1992) Similarity of *Chlamydia pneumoniae* strains in the variable domain IV region of the major outer membrane protein gene. Infect Immun 60:5319-5323

20. Jantos CA, Heck S, Roggendorf R, Sen-Gupta M, Hegemann JH (1997) Antigenic and molecular analyses of different *Chlamydia pneumoniae* strains. J Clin Microbiol 35:620-623

21. Grayston JT, Campbell LA, Kuo C-C, Mordhorst CH, Saikku P, Thom D, Wang S-P (1990). A new respiratory tract pathogen: *Chlamydia pneumoniae*, strain TWAR. J Infect Dis 161:618-625

22. Ekman MR, Grayston JT, Visakorpi R, Kleemola M, Kuo C-C, Saikku P (1993) An epidemic of infections due to *Chlamydia pneumoniae* in military conscripts. Clin Infect Dis 17:420-425

23. Campbell LA, Kuo C-C, Wang S-P, Grayston JT (1990) Serological response to *Chlamydia pneumoniae* infection. J Clin Microbiol 28:1261-1264

24. Freidank, HM, Herr AS, Jacobs E (1993) Identifications of *Chlamydia pneumoniae* specific protein antigens in immunoblots. Eur J Clin Microbiol Infect Dis 12:947-951

25. Iijima Y, Miyashita N, Kishimoto T, Kanamoto Y, Soejima R, Matsumoto A (1994) Characterisation of *Chlamydia pneumoniae* species-specific proteins immunodominant in humans. J Clin Microbiol 32:583-588

26. Puolakkainen M, Kuo C-C, Shor A, Wang S-P Grayston JT, Campbell LA (1993) Serological response to *Chlamydia pneumoniae* in adults with coronary arterial fatty streaks and fibrolipid plaques. J Clin Microbiol 31:2212-2214

27. Maass M, Gieffers J (1997) Cardiovascular disease risk from prior *Chlamydia pneumoniae* infection can be related to certain antigens recognised in the immunoblot profile. J Infect 35:171-176

28. Rank RG, Söderberg LS, Barron AL (1985) Chronic chlamydial genital infections in congenitally athymic nude mice. Infect Immun 48:847-849
29. Ramsey KH, Söderberg LS, Rank RG (1988) Resolution of chlamydial infection in B-cell deficient mice and immunity to reinfection. Infect Immun 56:1320-1325
30. Ramsey KH, Rank RG (1991) Resolution of chlamydial genital infection with antigen specific T-cell lines. Infect Immun 59: 925-931
31. Stagg AJ, Elsley WA, Pickett MA, Ward ME, Knight SC (1993) Primary human T-cell responses to the major outer membrane protein of Chlamydia trachomatis. Immunology 79:1-9
32. Kaufman SH (1988) CD8+ T lymphocytes in intracellular microbial infections. Immunol Today 9:168-174
33. Watkins NG, Hadlow WJ, Moos AB, Caldwell HD (1986) Ocular delayed hypersensitivity: a pathogenetic mechanism of chlamydial conjunctivitis in guinea pigs. Proc Natl Acad Sci USA 83:7480-7487
34. Moller BR, Weström L, Ahrons S, Ripa T, Swensson L, Mecklenburg C, Henrikson H, Mårdh PA (1979) Chlamydia trachomatis infection of the Fallopian tubes. Br J Vener Dis 55:422-429
35. Morrison RP, Belland RJ, Lyng K, Caldwell HD (1989) Chlamydial disease pathogenesis. The 57-kDa chlamydial hypersensitivity antigen is a stress response protein. J Exp Med 170:1271-1283
36. Wick G, Kleindienst R, Schett G, Amberger A, Xu Q (1995) Role of heat shock protein 60/65 in the pathogenesis of atherosclerosis. Int Arch Allergy Immunol 107:130-131
37. Kol A, Sukhova GK, Lichtman AH, Libby P (1998) Chlamydial heat shock protein 60 localises in human atheroma and regulates macrophage tumor necrosis factor α and matrix metalloproteinase expression. Circulation 98:300-307
38. Laitinen K, Laurila A, Pyhälä L, Leinonen M, Saikku P (1997) Chlamydia pneumoniae infection induces inflammatory changes in the aortas of rabbits. Infect Immun 65:4832-4835
39. Surcel HM, Syrjälä H, Leinonen M, Saikku P, Herva E (1993) Cell-mediated immunity to Chlamydia pneumoniae measured as lymphocyte blast transformation in vitro. Infect Immun 61:2196-2199
40. Halme S, von Herzen L, Kaprio J, Koskenvuo M, Leinonen M, Saikku P, Surcel H-M (1998) Chlamydia pneumoniae-specific cell-mediated and humoral immunity in healthy people. Scand J Immunol 47:517-520
41. Halme S, Syrjälä H, Saikku P, Leinonen M, Airaksinen J, Surcel H-M (1997) Lymphocyte responses to chlamydial antigens in patients with coronary heart disease. Eur Heart J 18:1095-1101
42. Beatty WL, Belanger TL, Desai AA, Morrison RP, Byrne GI (1994) Tryptophan depletion as a mechanism of γ-interferon mediated chlamydial persistence. Infect Immun 62:3705-3711
43. Mehta SJ, Miller RD, Ramirez JA, Summersgill JT (1998) Inhibition of Chlamydia pneumoniae replication in Hep-2 cells by interferon-γ: role of tryptophan catabolism. J Infect Dis 177:1326-1331
44. Holtman H, Shemer-Avni Y, Wessel K, Sarov I, Wallach D (1990) Inhibition of growth of Chlamydia trachomatis by tumour necrosis factor is accompanied by increased prostaglandin synthesis. Infect Immun 58:3168-3172
45. Williams DM, Magee DM, Bonewald LF, Smith JG, Bleicker CA, Byrne GI, Schachter J (1990) A role in vivo for tumour necrosis factor alpha in host defence against Chlamydia trachomatis. Infect Immun 58:1572-1576

46. Kawakami M, Pekala PH, Lance MD, Cerami A (1983) Lipoprotein lipase suppression in 3T3 L1 cells by an endotoxin-induced mediator from exudate cells. Proc Natl Acad Sci USA 9:912-916

47. Leinonen M (1993) Pathogenetic mechanisms and epidemiology of *Chlamydia pneumoniae*. Eur Heart J 14:57-61

48. Laurila A, Bloigu A, Näyhä S, Hassi J, Leinonen M, Saikku P (1997) Chronic *Chlamydia pneumoniae* infection is associated with a serum lipid profile known to be a risk factor for atherosclerosis. Arterioscler Thromb Vasc Biol 17:2910-2913

Chronic *Chlamydia pneumoniae* Infections

P. Saikku

Introduction

Chronic infections are the most important chlamydial infections. Moreover, with the rising average lifetime, the incidence and importance of chronic infections with late sequelae tend to rise. *Chlamydia trachomatis* infections may take tens of years for blindness to develop in trachoma; grave symptoms of lymphogranuloma venereum (LGV) are seen after years of progression, and it takes years to develop complications of chronic silent pelvic inflammatory disease (PID), such as ectopic pregnancy and infertility.

The discovery of *C. pneumoniae,* an extremely common *Chlamydia*, which readily invades the lungs, prompted studies of chronic pulmonary involvement. The lungs also provide a pathogen with an opportunity for easy dissemination into the body, and *C. pneumoniae* has been associated with non-respiratory chronic diseases, too (Table 1).

Table 1. Chronic diseases associated or suggested as associated with *C. pneumoniae*

Respiratory tract diseases	Cardiovascular diseases
Chronic pharyngitis	Coronary arteriosclerosis
Chronic otitis media	AMI
Chronic bronchitis	Carotid arteriosclerosis
Asthma	TIAs
COPD	Stroke
Sarcoidosis	Periferal arteriosclerosis
Lung cancer	Vasculitides
	Hypertonia
Other	Cardiomyopathy
Arthritis	
Dyslipidaemia	

COPD, chronic obstructive pulmonary disease; *AMI*, acute myocardial infarction; *TIAs*, transient ischaemic attacks

Diagnosis

Although the diagnosis of acute *C. pneumoniae* infection is difficult, the diagnosis of the chronic diseases it might cause is a real problem. The amount of infective agent in acute *C. pneumoniae* infection seems to be in most cases quite low, and it could be even smaller in chronic infections. The most difficult possibility is a "hit-and-run" situation, where the agent has triggered an abnormal reaction, a self-supporting process causing progression of the disease, although the inducer itself has disappeared.

Culture

It is a well-known phenomenon, from *C. trachomatis* studies, that chlamydial culture is insensitive in chronic infections, although the agent is relatively easy to cultivate in acute infections [1]. This is understandable, since the lesion in chronic infections is loaded with activated defence mechanisms. The very appearance of chlamydiae in cells crushed in the isolation procedure, which used to protect them, makes them a vulnerable target for neutralisation. *C. pneumoniae* is generally difficult to isolate even in acute disease conditions, and thus a negative isolation proves nothing in suspected chronic infections. Recently, the form of *Chlamydia* associated with chronic infection has also been reported to occur in vivo in a non-cultivable form, with poor expression of the major outer membrane protein [2].

Serology

The first evidence that *C. pneumoniae* might cause chronic conditions was provided by serology. Studies on antibody prevalences in industrialised countries have shown that, in the general population, antibodies against *C. pneumoniae* are by far the most common and high titred ones among the different chlamydial species [3]. In micro-immunofluorescence, the *C. pneumoniae* titre levels are often comparable to the *C. trachomatis* titres occurring in infertile women with chronic PID, or in both sexes in LGV [4]. These titre levels can be partly explained by a booster effect due to reinfections, but they also suggest infections analogous to chronic deep-sited *C. trachomatis* infections. Serology has been a sentinel test, showing that *C. pneumoniae* infections do not behave like *C. trachomatis* infections in general, and points to the possibility of quite common chronic, generalised infections. As an indicator of chronic infections, however, serology is inadequate. Firstly, it tells nothing of the locality of the possible chronic process. Secondly, *C. pneumoniae* antibodies are so common, especially in the older age classes, that it is difficult to prove an association with a specific disease. Thirdly, epidemics induce temporally high-titred antibodies in control populations, too. Despite these facts, continuously elevated high titred antibodies can be not only a sign of a possible chronic infection, but also a sign of failed defence mechanisms in the battle against an intracellular pathogen. The development of cell-mediated immunity can be more crucial than antibodies. IgA production is seen in the Th2 type of response and seems to be a better marker in chronic chlamydial infections than IgG antibodies [5]. IgA antibodies can be measured from local secretions and are hence helpful in chronic respiratory tract infections [6, 7].

Micro-immunofluorescence

Micro-immunofluorescence (micro-IF) has provided the first evidence of the possible association of *C. pneumoniae,* not only with acute [8], but also with various chronic inflammatory processes [9]. If read with expertise and patience, the results can differentiate between the specific reactions and various interfering noises from antibodies cross-reacting to other chlamydial or bacterial species [10]. The lack of experienced readers is the weak point of the test. Moreover, the reading conditions must be strictly adjusted; the patients and the controls, matched for locality, time, age, sex and social class, must be titrated in simultaneous titrations and the results be read blindfolded by the same reader. In a subjective test like micro-IF, no exact numerical values can be given: they depend not only on the reader, but also on the microscope and reagents used. Unfortunately, there is currently no standardised quality control system for checking the performance of chlamydial micro-IF in different laboratories. Before that can be done, one should approach the results published from various laboratories with some caution.

Unspecific Serological Tests

Unspecific test systems, such as particle-, LPS-EIA- and inclusion-based serological test, being broad-reactive and sensitive to the common antigens presented in the course of chronic infections, may paradoxically be more sensitive in monitoring chronic chlamydial infections.

Immunoblotting

Immunoblotting offers a possibility to measure specific responses to various chlamydial antigens [11–14]. The actual specificity of the reactions is doubtful, since chlamydial proteins possess common epitopes, which are exposed and reactive after PAGE electrophoresis. However, these studies should be continued further, in order to find the specific proteins reactive in chronic chlamydial infections [14]. These, or synthetic peptides derived from them, could then be used in EIA to detect the possible patients with persistent infection.

Immune Complexes

Immune complexes are produced in the battle against the infecting organism and contain principally degradation products of the microbe and antibodies bound to them. After healing, these are removed little by little from circulation. Their consistent presence is a sign of continuous production of new complexes inside the body, i.e. continuous production of microbial antigens and thus a persistent infection. These kinds of complexes are typical of chronic infections and well documented in many viral and bacterial chronic diseases. Two kinds of immune complexes have been reported in suspected chronic chlamydial infections, those containing chlamydial LPS and respective antibodies [15], naturally the majority of IgM type, and those containing antibodies against chlamydial proteins [16].

Immune complexes are not easy to measure. LPS-EIA is tricky to handle [15], and precipitation of complexed antibodies is easily interfered with by co-precipitating antibodies simulating true immune complexes. Moreover, the presence of specific immune complexes does not indicate the exact localisation of the chronic process, i.e. whether it is situated in the lungs or in the venous or arterial side of the circulation. However, a simplified test for specific immune complexes could possibly show which individuals are liable to be harbouring *Chlamydia* in their lungs or vessels and effect of treatment.

Antigen Detection

Antigen detection from circulating immune complexes does not seem to be as sensitive as antibody detection, but it has not yet been studied sufficiently. Both protein and LPS antigens have been found in blood [16], [Tiirala et al., to be published]. Whether these can be detected in excretions in chronic lung infections is unknown. In chronic vascular *C. pneumoniae* infections, the major obstacle is the availability of representative samples from the lesions. Immunocytochemistry has been rewarding in biopsies and autopsies, and arterial operations yield satisfying samples, especially from excised aortic abdominal aneurysms and removed valves. Unspecific staining can be confusing and requires good expertise. LPS staining seems to be most sensitive, but possible movements and deposition of LPS and cross-reactions to *Bartonella* must be kept in mind. The protein antigens sought for should also include chlamydial hsp60 [17]. Immunocytochemistry can provide invaluable data on the pathogenesis of a chronic infection.

Nucleic Acid Detection

The promise of exact diagnosis of chronic *C. pneumoniae* infections seems to lie in nucleic acid amplification methods. The problems to be solved include: (1) how to obtain an adequate sample, (2) how to process it to extract reactive nucleic acids in a proper condition, (3) how to get rid of the interfering components in a biological sample, and (4) how to exclude the contamination of the extremely sensitive test system. One should bear in mind that a method which is fully satisfactory when applied to cell culture samples, is not adequate for tissue samples with minimal amounts of *C. pneumoniae* and ample interfering substances, although a massive amount of human DNA gives a positive signal. PCR has already yielded compelling evidence of the presence of the agent in lesions [18]. In situ hybridisation can, moreover, tell us about the exact localisation of chronic *C. pneumoniae* infections. Sputum [19] and circulating, purified white blood cells [20] constitute easily obtainable material and are a promising possibility in future diagnostics, both at the baseline and following the progression of the disease.

Electron Microscopy

Electron microscopy can be used to identify *C. pneumoniae* particles in lesions, since their morphology can be differentiated from the other vesicles present in the specimen [21]. The sensitivity is low and technique itself is demanding, however. Immune electron microscopic studies are so far lacking.

Diseases Associated with Chronic *Chlamydia pneumoniae* Infection

Chronic Bronchitis

Chronic bronchitis is the disease which immediately comes to mind when we consider possible chronic *C. pneumoniae* infections. It would, however, be difficult to prove this on the basis of comparative antibody studies only, since patients are usually elderly male smokers, who always tend to have high antibody prevalences [22, 23]. Blasi et al. [24, 25] found, in exacerbations of chronic bronchitis, serological evidence to suggest that *C. pneumoniae* was participating in the process. Von Hertzen et al. [26] were unable to find differences in serum IgG antibodies between patients and controls, but the difference in serum IgA prevalences was significant. Moreover, local sputum IgA antibodies against *C. pneumoniae*, lacking for majority of pneumonia patients sputa, were common finding in sputa of chronic bronchitis patients, and *C. pneumoniae* nucleic acids were demonstrated in PCR [19, 26]. *C. pneumoniae* can be added to the bacteria associated with the pathogenesis of chronic bronchitis.

Asthma

C. pneumoniae was associated with asthma by Hahn et al. [27], who found the prevalence of adult onset asthma to be seven times more common after lower respiratory tract infection caused by *C. pneumoniae* than with other causes. Prolonged macrolide treatment was effective in the cases where treatment had been started early in the disease [28]. Childhood asthma has also been associated with *C. pneumoniae*, in which cases macrolide treatment has been effective [29]. IgA and IgE [29] antibodies in serum, secretory IgA and PCR seem to be the best diagnostic methods. The specific IgA content in nasopharynx has been reported to be in relation to the severity of childhood asthma [7]. A persistent *C. pneumoniae* infection may participate in the asthmatic inflammation in lungs and act as a cofactor in asthmatic episodes. This possibility should be studied in detail, since the prevalence of asthma is globally increasing, even in areas without aerial pollution. The first large-scale intervention trial was completed in 1998.

Sarcoidosis

Sarcoidosis is a chronic inflammatory process of unknown origin, with giant cell and granuloma formation, eventually resulting in scarring, and leading to tissue destruction. Persistently elevated *C. pneumoniae* antibody titres were noted in sarcoidosis [30] and these were later studied in detail [14]. Sarcoidosis has been associated with acute episodes of *C. pneumoniae* infection [30, 31]. *C. pneumoniae* is able to persist and replicate within alveolar macrophages [32], and the macrophage products angiotensin converting enzyme (ACE) and lysozyme (LZM), used to monitor the activity of sarcoidosis, correlated positively with *C. pneumoniae* micro-IF titres [30]. However, many antibodies are elevated in sarcoidosis, and an attempt to demonstrate the agent in the affected tissue was unsuccessful [33]. In contrast, PCR was positive in two-thirds of samples in sarcoid lesions of skin among 20 granulomatic lesions [34].

Cancer in the Lungs

Chlamydial infections are associated with malignant tumours, just as *H. pylori* is associated with gastric cancer. *C. trachomatis* is associated with invasive squamous cell carcinoma of the cervix [Koskela et al., to be published], LGV with rectal cancer and *C. pneumoniae* with squamous cell carcinoma of the lungs [35]. The extent to which chronic chlamydial infections promote and contribute to carcinogenesis remains to be studied.

Other Chronic Respiratory Tract Diseases

There are several Swedish reports on *C. pneumoniae* in chronic pharyngitis [36, 37]. The possible association between *C. pneumoniae* and other chronic conditions of the upper respiratory tract has not been studied in depth. Negative and positive reports have been published concerning chronic secretory otitis media [38, 39]. No studies on chronic sinusitis have yet been published.

Immunological Complications

Erythema Nodosum

The occurrence of erythema nodosum, an immunological vasculitis, was noted in the first published epidemic of *C. pneumoniae* [8, 40]. Erythema nodosum has been associated with chlamydial infections since 1965 [41], and some reports of this disease in connection with *C. pneumoniae* infections have been published [42, 43]. Since *C. pneumoniae* infection is a common disease, a search for *C. pneumoniae* is indicated in every erythema nodosum case.

Reactive Arthritis

Recent reports seem to indicate that *C. pneumoniae* is found in reactive arthritis, which tends to appear after respiratory tract infections [44–47], but it is far less common than *C. trachomatis* [2]. Different target cells could be behind this difference. Prolonged antibiotic treatment is effective against *C. trachomatis*-induced reactive arthritis [48], and treatment studies are indicated in *C. pneumoniae*-associated reactive arthritis.

Chronic Fatigue Syndrome

Prolonged convalescence is a typical sequel in chlamydial pneumonias and chronic infection may lead to continuous cytokine production, which, in turn, may affect the patient's physical and mental status. In the Helsinki Heart Study an inverse correlation was noted to *C. pneumoniae* antibodies and/or immune complexes when compared to spare-time physical activity [Leinonen et al., to be published]. In one study on *C. pneumoniae* no correlation with simple IgG antibodies in chronic fatigue syndrome patients was found [49].

Non-Hodgkin Lymphomas

Anttila et al. [50] reported that circulating immune complexes containing chlamydial antigens are found in a significant proportion of patients with non-Hodgkin lymphomas compared with matched healthy blood donors. Whether this is a reflection of the altered immune status of these patients or whether chronic disseminated chlamydial infections may lead to a connection similar to that between *H. pylori* and mucosa-associated lymphoid tissue (MALT) lymphoma remains to be studied.

Chronic Cardiovascular Diseases

Vasculitis Syndromes

In the early 1940s, South American researchers found out that some patients with Buerger's disease were hypersensitive to *Chlamydia* [51–53]. The part played by *C. pneumoniae* in vasculitides has been studied inadequately, since the agent is capable of disseminating in peripheral vessels [54]. Only two publications have appeared on *C. pneumoniae* in vasculitis [55, 56]. These studies should be continued.

Cardiomyopathy

Sutton et al. [57] described a 3-year epidemic of cardiomyopathy in Illinois, with the exceptional feature of elevated chlamydial CF antibodies. The epidemic was not compatible with psittacosis/ornithosis, but its course rather resembled a *C. pneumoniae* epidemic. It is unknown if a "cardiotropic" strain [58] of *C. pneumoniae* or an unknown human chlamydial strain was responsible for the incident. *C. pneumoniae* has been found to associate with subacute myocarditis in Swedish elite orienteers [59].

Arteriosclerosis

Chlamydiae have been associated with arteriosclerosis for about 50 years [60]. In the 1930s psittacosis was known to involve embolic complications and cardiac inflammations, and chlamydiae are now well established as a cause of different carditides [61]. In the 1940s South American researchers found that the intradermal Frei test, measuring hypersensitivity to chlamydial species, was often positive in arteriosclerosis without history of LGV [51–53]. Two excellent reviews on the possible mechanisms involved in infections and arteriosclerosis have appeared recently [62, 63].

Seroepidemiological Studies

The association of *Chlamydia* with atherosclerosis was rediscovered nearly 50 years later, when seroconversion against an epitope of chlamydial LPS was demonstrated during acute myocardial infarction (AMI) [9]. Further studies indicated that patients with AMI and ones with chronic coronary heart disease (CCHD) had stable elevated IgG and IgA antibody titres against *C. pneumoniae* in the micro-IF test. This led to the suggestion that the majority of CCHD cases are associated with chronic *C. pneumoniae* infection, and AMI reflects an exacerbation [9]. Seroconversions were later found to be a sign of a sudden imbalance in relative amounts of chlamydial LPS and antibodies against it [15]. Immune complexes were found in about 70% of the patients with CCHD and their protein-antibody nature pointed to the presence of *C. pneumoniae* in vessel wall [16]. Seroepidemiological association was soon confirmed in Seattle [64]. More than 20 seroepidemiological studies have now been published and, with a few exceptions, they have verified the association (Table 2).

Presence of Chlamydia pneumoniae in Arteriosclerotic Lesions

In vitro, *C. pneumoniae* is able to thrive in vessel wall cells [86]. The presence of the agent in vivo in arteriosclerotic plaques in the coronaries was first demonstrated by Shor et al. [21] by electron microscopy and immunohistochemistry. The presence of *C. pneumoniae* in arteriosclerotic lesions has been verified in over 20 studies by immunocytochemistry, PCR reaction [18], and electron microscopy. Although isolation is difficult, *C. pneumoniae* has been cultivated from lesions [87, 88]. Chlamydial hsp60 is found in plaques [17], and T-cells directed against *C. pneumoniae* can be extracted from atherosclerotic lesions [89], showing that an active battle against *C. pneumoniae* is taking place there. The presence of *C. pneumoniae* in arterial lesions is not limited to coronaries; carotid arteries [70, 82, 90–93], abdominal aortic aneurysms [93, 94], peripheral arteries [54] and aortic stenotic valves [95] show the same phenomenon. The presence of *C. pneumoniae* in healthy areas has mostly been rare, but some studies using PCR have demonstrated it in healthy parts of arteries and in veins [93, 96].

Not all patients with *C. pneumoniae* in their arteriosclerotic lesions present antibodies [12], and vice versa, *C. pneumoniae* particles are not found in all plaques. In immunocytochemical staining LPS and protein antibodies do not give

Table 2. Seroepidemiological studies on the association of *C. pneumoniae* antibodies/immune complexes with coronary heart disease

Study	N° of cases/controls	Disease	Degree of adjustment	Odds ratio (95% confidence interval)
Prospective studies				
Miettinen [65]	28/535	AMI or CHD death	++	2.44 (0.98–6.08)
Saikku [66]	102/102	AMI or CHD death	++	2.6 (1.3–5.2)
Ossewaarde [67]	54/108	AMI and/or angina pectoris	++	2.76 (1.31–5.81)
Davidson [68]	21/35	TWAR organism in coronary arteries at autopsy	+	9.4 (2.6–33.8)
Population controls				
Patel [69]	83/305	Angina or ECG	++++	3.06 (1.33–7.01)
Melnick [70]	326/326	Carotid stenosis	+++	2.0 (1.19–3.35)
Thom [71]	133/62	Coronary stenosis	+++	3.5 (1.7–7.0)
Dahlén [72]	60/60	Coronary stenosis	++	3.9 (1.2–12.7)
Saikku [9]	70/41	AMI or angina	++	3.8 (1.5–9.6)
Leinonen [15]	44/44	Myocardial infarct	++	10.3 (3.4–31)
Linnanmäki [16]	46/46	Coronary stenosis	+	3.9 (1.4–10.6)
Haidl [73]	38/68	CHD by ECG	+	1.5 (0.7–3.5)
Blasi [74]	61/61	AMI	+	3.2 (1.5–6.8)
Thomas [75]	83/93	Ischaemic heart disease or MI	+	5.43 (2.71–10.94)
Mazzoli [76]	29/24	AMI	++	4.1 (1.2–13.9)
Perdikaris [77]	87/50	AMI or CCHD	+	2.8 (1.4–5.9)
Diedrichs [78]	131/63	CHD	+	3.8 (1.7–8.4)
Kark [79]	251/324	AMI	+++	0.74 (0.47–1.17)
Other controls				
Mendall [80]	103/67	AMI or coronary stenosis	++++	7.4 (1.7–33)
Weiss [81]	65/28	Coronary stenosis	–	0.2 (0.1–1.1)
Wimmer [82]	58/52	Ischaemic stroke or TIA	++	2.2 (1.09–4.41)
Thom [64]	461/95	Coronary stenosis	+	1.6 (1.0–2.7)
Aceti [83]	37/60	Myocardial infarct	+	5.2 (1.9–14.2)
Cook [84]	408/1297	AMI or unstable angina	+	2.3 (1.6–3.3)
Gieffers [85]	400/400	Clinical signs of CHD	+	1.8 (1.3–2.4)

identical patterns. This discrepancy may be due to several reasons. Antibodies can be bound to immune complexes in the circulation or in the lesion, where they can be extracted [94]. The development of immune tolerance can lower the antibody content under the detectable limit. *C. pneumoniae* in plaques typically has a patchy appearance [92], which makes it easy to miss the positive area. A "hit-and-run" reaction may also start the process. The finding of *C. pneumoniae* in apparently healthy areas does not exclude its pathogenic role. The agent may be dormant, and in PCR the tissue sample studied is destroyed, which makes it difficult to exclude small lesions, especially under the endothelium. In a study of aortic valves, *C. pneumoniae* was also found in healthy valves, but at old age nearly all valves with *C. pneumoniae* showed damage, while the valves staying healthy were without *C. pneumoniae* [97]. The development of arteriosclerosis takes decades and it is understandable that *C. pneumoniae* can be found in the vessel wall in early adolescence already [96].

The first successful intervention trials [98, 99] and rabbit experiments [100–102] speaking directly in favour of *C. pneumoniae* causing arteriosclerosis, are described in detail elsewhere in this book.

Association of Chlamydia pneumoniae with Risk Factors of Arteriosclerosis

C. pneumoniae infection does not exclude the known risk factors for arteriosclerosis, but has interesting interactions with many of them. It is associated with chronic bronchitis, which is a newly found risk factor for CHD. Chronic vascular infection is influenced by several important risk factors. The incidence of chronic *C. pneumoniae* infections rises steadily with age, possibly due to deterioration of the immunological defence mechanisms in senescence. Gender is another risk factor and males are more susceptible to chronic *C. pneumoniae* infections, perhaps due to their higher iron levels, iron being an indispensable ion for *C. pneumoniae* [103]. Hereditary background is important in CHD, and the HLA system has been associated with *C. pneumoniae* and CHD [72]. Smoking is clearly associated with chronic *C. pneumoniae* infection [22], possibly due to its immunosuppressive effect. In pairs of identical twin discordant for smoking the smoking twin showed diminished cell-mediated immunity and elevated IgA levels suggestive of chronic infection [104]. Physical activity stimulates immunodefence, but high dietary fat makes it possible for fat to precipitate in active *C. pneumoniae* lesions in the vascular wall.

Chronic *C. pneumoniae* infection has been shown to stimulate foam cell formation of macrophages [105], thereby making this lipid deposition possible, and the phase of inflammation may be reflected in the CRP levels [106]. Chronic infection may also contribute to many other established risk factors. *C. pneumoniae* is a potent inducer of cytokines, notably TNF-α and IL-1 [107]. Perhaps due to continuous cytokine production, the lipid profile of serum found in chronic *C. pneumoniae* infections is precisely the same, which is a typical risk factor for CHD: elevated triglyceride and cholesterol levels and a lowered HDL level [108]. Cytokines are possibly behind the obesity seen in chronic *C. pneumoniae* infections

[Leinonen et al., to be published]. Severe essential hypertonia has also been associated with *C. pneumoniae* [109]. The metabolic syndrome (obesity, lipid alterations, elevated glucose, hypertonia) seems to be a risk factor only if it is associated with markers of chronic *C. pneumoniae* infection [Leinonen et al, in press]. Cytokines may also induce fatigue and depression, but their association with chronic *C. pneumoniae* infection is hypothetical at this moment. The development of autoimmunity to hsp60 is quite possible, since chlamydial hsp60 is typical of chronic chlamydial infections and present in plaques [17]. The importance of *C. pneumoniae* infection in atherosclerosis is seen in familiar hypercholesterolaemia, where markers of chronic infection indicate an over fivefold increase in risk for cardiac events in patients [Vuorio et al., to be published]. It is possible that chronic *C. pneumoniae* infection is a confounding factor in many studies on risk factors for atherosclerosis.

What precipitates the actual infarction is unknown. Re-infection [74], other infections such as influenza [110], stress or unknown activators may disturb the balance in the plaque and activate *C. pneumoniae* for abundant multiplication. This could lead to a massive inflammation with adhesin induction and proteolysis. *C. pneumoniae* itself possesses proteolytic enzymes capable of lysing the arterial wall [111]. All this could lead to thrombus formation and/or loosening of the plaque with rupture, leading to infarction.

Future Perspectives

Two chronic disease entities mentioned above, namely cardiovascular diseases and chronic obstructive pulmonary diseases, are, together with pneumonia, among the six big disease killers in the world. The cholesterol hypothesis took nearly a century and 30 years of massive research before it was accepted, and there are still mavericks who point out that statins, which were thought to be the final proof, have many different effects besides the lowering of cholesterol. On the whole, the evidence on chlamydial involvement, although accumulated in only 10 years in a few laboratories, seems impressive at the moment. We have numerous chemotherapeutic drugs effective against the agent. Incidentally, when they appeared on the market, the CHD figures started to decrease. Crucial intervention studies are already going on. But even if their outcome is favourable, the problems are not solved. We do not know whether early treatment with an effective drug will prevent the development of a chronic infection, or in how mild conditions medication would then be indicated. If a chronic condition develops, we do not know how to identify those at risk of developing irreparable damages among the vast majority with only a serological scar from a former *C. pneumoniae* infection. And if a good marker is found, we do not know what therapeutic agent should be used or for how long. There are no narrow-spectrum chlamydiocidic or even chlamydiostatic chemotherapeutic agents, and massive prolonged administration of the current broad-spectrum chlamydia antibiotics could imply disastrous consequences for chemotherapy in a broader sense, with a concomitant upsurge of bacterial resistance. Further studies are therefore urgently needed. An effective vaccine would be an ideal answer, but there is no such vaccine even against *C. trachomatis*, despite 30 years' efforts. Nevertheless problems are solvable through intensive research.

References

1. Schachter J, Moncada J, Dawson CR, Sheppard J, Courtright P, Said ME, Zaki S, Hafez SF, Lorincz A (1988) Nonculture methods for diagnosing chlamydial infection in patients with trachoma: a clue to the pathogenesis of the disease? J Infect Dis 158:1347-1352
2. Gérard HC, Branigan PJ, Schumacher HR, Hudson AP (1998) Synovial *Chlamydia trachomatis* in patients with reactive arthritis/Reiter's syndrome are viable but show aberrant gene expression. J Rheumatol 25:734-742
3. Wang S-P, Grayston JT (1986) Microimmunofluorescence serological studies with the TWAR organism. In: Oriel JD, Ridgway G, Schachter J, Taylor-Robinson D (eds) Chlamydial infections. Cambridge University Press, Cambridge, pp 329-332
4. Wang S-P, Grayston JT (1982) Micro-immunofluorescence antibody responses in *Chlamydia trachomatis* infection, a review. In: Mårdh PA, Holmes KK, Oriel JD, Piot P, Schachter J (eds) Chlamydial infections. Elsevier, Amsterdam, pp 301-316
5. Sarov I, Sarov B, Hanuka N, Glasner M, Kaneti J (1986) The significance of serum specific IgA antibodies in diagnosis of active *Chlamydia trachomatis* infections. In: Oriel D, Ridgway G, Schacter J, Taylor-Robinson D, Ward M (eds) Chlamydial infections. Cambridge University Press, Cambridge, pp 566-569
6. von Hertzen L, Leinonen M, Surcel HM, Karjalainen J, Saikku P (1995) Measurement of sputum antibodies in the diagnosis of acute and chronic respiratory infections associated with *Chlamydia pneumoniae*. Clin Diagn Lab Immunol 2:454-457
7. Cunningham AF, Johnston SL, Julious SA, Lampe FC, Ward ME (1998) Chronic *Chlamydia pneumoniae* infection and asthma exacerbations in children. Eur Respir J 11:345-349
8. Saikku P, Wang S-P, Kleemola M, Brander E, Rusanen E, Grayston JT (1985) An epidemic of mild pneumonia due to an unusual strain of *Chlamydia psittaci*. J Infect Dis 151:832-839
9. Saikku P, Leinonen M, Mattila K, Ekman MR, Nieminen MS, Mäkelä PH, Huttunen J, Valtonen V (1988) Serologic evidence of an association of a novel *Chlamydia*, TWAR, with chronic coronary heart disease and acute myocardial infarction. Lancet ii: 983-985
10. Grayston JT, Golubjatnikov R, Hagiwara T, Hahn DL, Leinonen M, Persson K, Saikku P, Treharne J, Wang S-P (1993) Serologic tests for *Chlamydia pneumoniae*. Pediatr Infect Dis J 11:790-791
11. Campbell LA, Kuo C-C, Wang S-P, Grayston JT (1990) Serological response to *Chlamydia pneumoniae* infection. J Clin Microbiol 28:1261-1264
12. Puolakkainen M, Kuo C-C, Shor A, Wang S-P, Grayston JT, Campbell LA (1993) Serological response to *Chlamydia pneumoniae* in adults with coronary arterial fatty streaks and fibrolipid plaques. J Clin Microbiol 31:2212-2214
13. Puolakkainen M, Campbell LA, Kuo C-C, Leinonen M, Grönhagen-Riska C, Saikku P (1996) Serological response to *Chlamydia pneumoniae* in patients with sarcoidosis. J Infect 33:199-205

14. Maass M, Gieffers J (1997) Cardiovascular disease risk from prior *Chlamydia pnemoniae* infection can be related to certain antigens recognized in the immunoblot profile. J Infect 35:171-176

15. Leinonen M, Linnanmäki E, Mattila K, Nieminen MS, Valtonen V, Leirisalo-Repo M, Saikku P (1990) Circulating immune complexes containing chlamydial lipopolysaccharide in acute myocardial infarction. Microb Pathog 9:67-73

16. Linnanmäki E, Leinonen M, Mattila K, Ekman MR, Nieminen MS, Valtonen V, Saikku P (1993) Presence of *Chlamydia pneumoniae* specific antibodies in circulating immune complexes in coronary heart disease. Circulation 87:1130-1134

17. Kol A, Sukhova GK, Lichtman AH, Libby P (1998) *Chlamydial* heat shock protein 60 localizes in human atheroma and regulates macrophage tumor necrosis factor-a and matrix metalloproteinase expression. Circulation 98:300-307

18. Kuo C-C, Shor A, Campbell LA, Fukushi H, Patton DL, Grayston JT (1993) Demonstration of *Chlamydia pneumoniae* in atherosclerotic lesions of coronary arteries. J Infect Dis 167:841-849

19. von Hertzen L, Alakärppä H, Koskinen R, Liippo K, Surcel H-M, Leinonen M, Saikku P (1997) *Chlamydia pneumoniae* infection in patients with chronic obstructive pulmonary disease. Epidemiol Infect 118:155-164

20. Boman J, Söderberg S, Forsberg J, Birgander LS, Allard A, Persson K, Jidell E, Kumlin U, Juto P, Waldenström A, Wadell G (1998) High prevalence of *Chlamydia pneumoniae* DNA in peripheral blood mononuclear cells in patients with cardiovascular disease and in middle-aged blood donors. J Infect Dis 178:274-277

21. Shor A, Kuo C-C, Patton DL (1992) Detection of *Chlamydia pneumoniae* in coronary arterial fatty streaks and atheromatous plaques. S African Med J 82:158-160

22. Karvonen M, Tuomilehto J, Pitkäniemi J, Naukkarinen A, Saikku P (1994) Importance of smoking for *Chlamydia pneumoniae* infection. Int J Epidemiol 23:1315-1321

23. Verkooyen RP, Vanlent NA, Joulandan SAM, Snijder RJ, Vandenbosch JM, Vanhelden HP, Verbrugh HA (1997) Diagnosis of *Chlamydia pneumoniae* infection in patients with chronic obstructive pulmonary disease by micro-immunofluorescence and ELISA. J Med Microbiol 46:959-964

24. Blasi F, Legnani D, Negretto G, Caratozzolo O, Magliano E, Chiodo F, Pozzoli R, Fasoli A (1992) Incidence and prevalence of *Chlamydia pneumoniae* infection in COAD patients. J Infect 25[Suppl 1]:125-126

25. Blasi F, Legnani D, Lombardo VM, Negretto GG, Magliano E, Pozzoli R, Chiodo F, Fasoli A, Allegra L (1993) *Chlamydia pneumoniae* infection in acute exacerbations of COPD. Eur Respir J 6:19-22

26. von Hertzen L, Isoaho R, Leinonen M, Koskinen R, Laippala P, Töyrylä M, Kivelä SL, Saikku P (1996) *Chlamydia pneumoniae* antibodies in chronic obstructive pulmonary disease. Int J Epidemiol 25:658-664

27. Hahn DL, Dodge RW, Golubjatnikov R (1991) Association of *Chlamydia pneumoniae* (strain TWAR) infection with wheezing, asthmatic bronchitis, and adult-onset asthma. JAMA 266:225-230

28. Hahn DL, Golubjatnikov R (1994) Adult onset asthma and atypical infection: a case series. J Fam Pract 38:589-595

29. Emre U, Sokolovskaya N, Roblin PM, Schachter J, Hammerschlag M (1995) Detection of anti-*Chlamydia pneumoniae* IgE in children with reactive airway disease. J Infect Dis 172:265-267

30. Grönhagen-Riska C, Saikku P, Riska H, Fröseth B, Grayston JT (1988) Antibodies to TWAR - a novel type of *Chlamydia* - in sarcoidosis. In: Grassi C (ed) Sarcoidosis and other granulomatous disorders. Elsevier, Amsterdam, pp 297-301

31. Campbell JF, Barnes RC, Kozarsky PE, Spika JS (1991) Culture-confirmed pneumonia due to *Chlamydia pneumoniae*. J Infect Dis 164:411-413

32. Black CM, Perez R (1990) *Chlamydia pneumoniae* multiplies within human alveolar macrophages. In: Abstracts of the 90th Annual Meeting of the American Society for Microbiology. American Society for Microbiology, Washington, DC, p 80

33. Blasi F, Rizzato G, Gambacorta M, Cosentini R, Raccanelli R, Tarsia P, Arosio C, Savini E, Cantoni C, Fagetti L, Allegra L (1997) Failure to detect the presence of *Chlamydia pneumoniae* in sarcoid pathology specimens. Eur Respir J 10:2609-2611

34. Jackson LA, Campbell LA, Schmidt RA, Kuo C-C, Cappuccio AL, Lee MJ, Grayston JT (1997) Specificity of detection of *Chlamydia pneumoniae* in cardiovascular atheroma - evaluation of the innocent bystander hypothesis. Am J Pathol 150:1785-1790

35. Laurila AL, Anttila T, Läärä E, Bloigu A, Virtamo J, Leinonen M, Albanes D, Saikku P (1997) Serologic evidence of an association of chronic *Chlamydia pneumoniae* infection with lung cancer. Int J Cancer 74:31-34

36. Falck G, Heyman L, Gnarpe J, Gnarpe H (1995) *Chlamydia pneumoniae* and chronic pharyngitis. Scand J Infect Dis 27:179-182

37. Falck G, Gnarpe J, Gnarpe H (1996) Persistent *Chlamydia pneumoniae* infection in a Swedish family. Scand J Infect Dis 28:271-273

38. Goo YA, Hori MK, Voorhies JH Jr, Kuo C-C, Wang S-P, Campbell LA (1995) Failure to detect *Chlamydia pneumoniae* in ear fluids from children with otitis media. Pediatr Infect Dis J 11:100-101

39. Ogawa H, Hashigucci K, Kazuyama Y (1992) Recovery of *C. pneumoniae* in six patients with otitis media with effusion. J Laryngol Otol 106:490-492

40. Kousa M, Saikku P, Kanerva L (1980) Erythema nodosum in chlamydial infections. Acta Dermatovener (Stockholm) 60:319-322

41. Sarner M, Wilson RJ (1965) Erythema nodosum and psittacosis: report of five cases. BMJ 2:1469-1470

42. Erntell M, Ljunggren K, Gadd T, Persson K (1989) Erythema nodosum - a manifestation of *Chlamydia pneumoniae* (strain TWAR) infection. Scand J Infect Dis 21:693-696

43. Sundelöf B, Gnarpe H, Gnarpe J (1993) An unusual manifestation of *Chlamydia pneumoniae* infection: meningitis, hepatitis, iritis and atypical erythema nodosum. Scand J Infect Dis 25:259-261

44. Saario R, Toivanen A (1994) *Chlamydia pneumoniae* as a cause of reactive arthritis. Br J Rheumatol 33:1112 (letter)

45. Braun J, Laitko S, Treharne J, Eggens U, Wu P, Distler A, Sieper J (1994) *C. pneumoniae*: a new causative agent of reactive arthritis and undifferentiated oligoarthritis. Ann Rheum Dis 53:100-105

46. Moling O, Picoretti S, Rielli M, Rimenti G, Vedovelli C, Pristera R, Mian P (1996) *Chlamydia pneumoniae* - reactive arthritis and persistent infection. Br J Rheumatol 35:189-190

47. Braun J, Tuszewski M, Eggens U, Mertz A, Schauer-Petrowskaja C, Döring E, Laitko S, Distler A, Sieper J, Ehlers S (1997) Nested polymerase chain reaction strategy simultaneously targeting DNA sequences of multiple bacterial species in inflammatory joint diseases. I. Screening of synovial fluid samples of patients with spondylarthropathies and other arthritides. J Rheumatol 24:1092-1100

48. Lauhio A, Leirisalo-Repo M, Lähdevirta J, Saikku P, Repo H (1991) Double-blind, placebo-controlled study of three-month lymecycline course in reactive arthritis with special reference to *Chlamydia* arthritis. Arthritis Rheum 34:6-14

49. Komaroff AL, Wang S-P, Lee J, Grayston JT (1992) No association of chronic *Chlamydia pneumoniae* infection with chronic fatigue syndrome. J Infect Dis 165:182 (letter)

50. Anttila TI, Lehtinen T, Leinonen M, Bloigu A, Koskela P, Lehtinen M, Saikku P (1998) Serological evidence of an association between chlamydial infections and malignant lymphomas. Br J Haematol 103:150-156

51. May J (1943) La intradermoreacción de Frei en las arteropatias. Rev Argent Dermatosifil 27:581-582

52. Quiroga, Ambrosetti FE (1943) La reacción de Frei en las endoarteritis obliterantes. Rev Argent Dermatosifil 27:624-625

53. Coutts WE, Davila M (1945) Lymphogranuloma venereum as a possible cause of arterio-sclerosis and other arterial conditions. J Trop Med Hyg 48:46-51

54. Kuo C-C, Coulson AS, Campbell LA, Cappuccio AL, Lawrence RD, Wang S-P, Grayston JT (1997) Detection of *Chlamydia pneumoniae* in atherosclerotic plaques in the walls of arteries of lower extremities from patients undergoing bypass operation for arterial obstruction. J Vasc Surg 26:29-31

55. Väätäinen NJ, Alila MH, Kärkkäinen AT (1993) *Chlamydia pneumoniae* as a trigger of IgA-associated small dermal vessel leukocytoclastic vasculitis (adult Henoch-Schönlein purpura). Eur J Dermatol 7:610

56. Ljungström L, Franzén C, Schlaug M, Elowson S, Viidas U (1997) Reinfection with *Chlamydia pneumoniae* may induce isolated and systemic vasculitis in small and large vessels. Scand J Infect Dis Suppl 104:37-40

57. Sutton GC, Demakis JA, Anderson, Morrisey RA (1971) Serologic evidence of a sporadic outbreak in Illinois of infection by *Chlamydia* (psittacosis-LGV agent) in patients with primary myocardial disease and respiratory disease. Am Heart J 81:597-607

58. Black CM, Johnson JE, Farshy CE, Brown TM, Berdal BP (1991) Antigenic variation among strains of *Chlamydia pneumoniae*. J Clin Microbiol 29:1312-1316

59. Wesslén L, Påhlson C, Lindquist O, Hjelm E, Gnarpe J, Larsson E, Baandrup U, Eriksson L, Fohlman J, Engstrand L, Linglöf T, Nyström-Rosander C, Gnarpe H, Magnius L, Rolf C, Friman G (1992) An increase in sudden unexpected cardiac deaths among young Swedish orienteers during 1979-1992. Eur Heart J 17:902-910

60. Haagen E (1964) Miyagawanellen In: Viruskrankheiten des Menschen, Band I. Dietrich Steinkopff Verlag, Darmstadt, pp 807-1052

61. Odeh M, Oliven A (1992) Chlamydial infections of the heart. Eur J Clin Microbiol Infect Dis 11:885-893

62. Danesh J, Collins R, Peto R (1997) Chronic infections and coronary heart disease: is there a link? Lancet 350:430-436

63. Mattila KJ, Valtonen VV, Nieminen MS, Asikainen S (1998) Role of infection as a risk factor for atherosclerosis, myocardial infarction, and stroke. Clin Infect Dis 26:719-734

64. Thom DH, Wang S-P, Grayston JT, Siscovick DS, Stewart DK, Kronmal RA, Weiss NS (1991) *Chlamydia pneumoniae* strain TWAR antibody and angiographically demonstrated coronary artery disease. Arteriosclerosis Thromb 11:547-551

65. Miettinen H, Lehto S, Saikku P, Haffner SM, Rönnemaa T, Pyörälä K, Laakso M (1996) Association of *Chlamydia pneumoniae* and acute coronary heart disease events in non-insulin dependent diabetic and non-dibetic subjects in Finland. Eur Heart J 17:682-688

66. Saikku P, Leinonen M, Tenkanen L, Ekman MR, Linnanmäki E, Manninen V, Mänttäri M, Frick MH, Huttunen JK (1992) Chronic *Chlamydia pneumoniae* infection as a risk factor for coronary heart disease in the Helsinki Heart Study. Ann Int Med 116:273-278

67. Ossewaarde JM, Feskens EJM, De Vries A, Vallinga CE, Kromhout D (1998) *Chlamydia pneumoniae* is a risk factor for coronary heart disease in symptom-free elderly men, but *Helicobacter pylori* and cytomegalovirus are not. Epidemiol Infect 120:93-99

68. Davidson M, Kuo C-C, Middaugh JP, Campbell LA, Wang S-P, Newman WP, Finlay JC, Grayston JT (1998) Confirmed previous infection with *Chlamydia pneumoniae* (TWAR) and its presence in early coronary atherosclerosis. Circulation 98:628-633
69. Patel P, Mendall MA, Carrington D, Strachan DP, Leatham E, Molineaux N, Levy J, Blakeston C, Seymour Ca, Camm AJ, Northfield TC (1995) Association of *Helicobacter pylori* an *Chlamydia pneumoniae* infections with coronary heart disease and cardio-vascular risk factors. BMJ 311:711-714
70. Melnick SL, Shahar E, Folsom AR, Grayston JT, Sorlie PD, Wang SP, Szklo M (1993) Past infection by *Chlamydia pneumoniae* strain TWAR and asymptomatic carotid athero-sclerosis. Am J Med 95:499-504
71. Thom DH, Grayston JT, Siscovick DS, Wang S-P, Weiss NS, Dailing JR (1992) Associa-tion of prior infection with *Chlamydia pneumoniae* and angiographically demon-strated coronary artery disease. JAMA 268:68-72
72. Dahlén GH, Boman J, Birgander LS, Lindblom B (1995) Lp(a) lipoprotein, IgG, IgA and IgM antibodies to *Chlamydia pneumoniae* and HLA class II genotype in early coro-nary artery disease. Atherosclerosis 114:165-174
73. Haidl S, Juul-Möller S, Israelsson B, Persson K (1992) Ischemic heart disease and anti-bodies to *Chlamydia pneumoniae* (TWAR). Proc Eur Soc Chlamydia Res 2:174
74. Blasi F, Cosentini R, Raccanelli R, Massari FM, Arosio C, Tarsia P, Allegra L (1997) A possible association of *Chlamydia pneumoniae* infection and acute myocardial infarc-tion in patients younger than 65 years of age. Chest 112:309-312
75. Thomas GN, Scheel O, Koehler AP, Basset DCJ, Cheng AFB (1997) Respiratory chlamy-dial infections in a Hong Kong teaching hospital and association with coronary heart disease. Scand J Infect Dis Suppl 104:30-33
76. Mazzoli S, Tofani N, Fantini A, Semplici F, Bandini F, Salvi A, Vergassola R (1998) *Chlamydia pneumoniae* antibody response in patients with acute myocardial infarc-tion and their follow-up. Am Heart J 135:15-20
77. Perdikaris G, Mentis A, Makris Th, Pourmaras G, Dafnou A, Xatzizaharias A, Votieas V, Giamarellou H (1997) Serologic response to *Chlamydia pneumoniae* (Cpn) in Greek adults with chronic coronary heart disease (CCHD) and acute myocardial infarction (AMI) (preliminary report). Clin Infect Dis 25:369
78. Diedrichs H, Schneider CA, Scharkus S, Pfister H, Erdmann E (1997) Prävalenz von Chlamydien-Antikörpern bei Patienten mit koronarer Herzerkrankung. Herz Kreis-lauf 29:304-307
79. Kark J, Leinonen M, Paltiel O, Saikku P (1997) *Chlamydia pneumoniae* and acute myocardial infarction in Jerusalem. Int J Epidemiol 26:730-738
80. Mendall MA, Carrington D, Strachan D, Patel P, Molineaux N, Levi J, Toosey T, Camm AJ, Northfield TC (1995) *Chlamydia pneumoniae*: risk factors for seropositivity and association with coronary heart disease. J Infect 30:121-128
81. Weiss SM, Roblin PM, Gaydos CA, Cummings P, Patton DL, Schulhoff N, Shani E, Frankel R, Penney K, Quinn TC, Hammerschlag MR, Schacter J (1996) Failure to detect *Chlamydia pneumoniae* in coronary atheromas of patients undergoing atherectomy J Infect Dis 173:957-962
82. Wimmer M, Sandmann-Strupp R, Saikku P, Haberl RL (1996) Association of chlamy-dial infection with cerebrovascular diseases. Stroke 27:207-210
83. Aceti A, Mazzacurati G, Amendolea MA, Fennica A, Zechini B, Trappolini M, Puletti M (1996) *H pylori* and *C. pneumoniae* infections may account for most acute coronary syndromes. BMJ 313:428-429 (letter)
84. Cook PJ, Honeybourne D, Lip GYH, Beevers DG, Wise R (1995) Chlamydia pneumoni-ae and acute arterial thrombotic disease. Circulation 92:3148 (letter)

85. Gieffers J, Maass M (1995) Serological response to *Chlamydia pneumoniae* in coronary heart disease. In: Abstracts of the 7th ECCMID, Vienna, no 495, p 95

86. Godzik KL, O'Brien ER, Wang SK, Kuo C-C (1995) In vitro susceptibility of human vascular wall cells to infection with *Chlamydia pneumoniae*. J Clin Microbiol 33:2411-2414

87. Ramirez JA, (1997) *Chlamydia pneumoniae*/atherosclerosis Study Group Isolation of *Chlamydia pneumoniae* from the coronary artery of a patient with coronary atherosclerosis. Ann Intern Med 125:97-98

88. Maass M, Bartels C, Engel PM, Mamat U, Sievers HH (1998) Endovascular presence of viable *Chlamydia pneumoniae* is a common phenomenon in coronary artery disease. J Am Coll Cardiol 31:827-832

89. Mosorin M, Surcel HM, Laurila A, Saikku P, Juvonen T (1998) *Chlamydia pneumoniae* reactive T lymphocytes in atherosclerotic plaque of carotid artery. In: Stephens RS et al (eds) Chlamydial infections. International *Chlamydia* Symposium, San Francisco, pp 423-425

90. Campbell LA, O'Brien ER, Cappuccio AL, Kuo C-C, Wang S-P, Stewart D, Patton DL, Cummings PK, Grayston JT (1995) Detection of *Chlamydia pneumoniae* TWAR in human coronary atherectomy tissues. J Infect Dis 172:585-588

91. Cook PJ, Honeybourne D, Lip GYH, Beevers DG, Wise R, Davies P (1998) *Chlamydia pneumoniae* antibody titers are significantly associated with acute stroke and transient cerebral ischemia - the West Birmingham stroke project. Stroke 29:404-410

92. Yamashita K, Ouchi K, Shirai M, Gondo T, Nakazawa T, Ito H (1998) Distribution of *Chlamydia pneumoniae* infection in the atherosclerotic carotid artery. Stroke 29:773-778

93. Ong G, Thomas BJ, Mansfield AO, Davidson BR, Taylor-Robinson D (1996) Detection and widespread distribution of *Chlamydia pneumoniae* in the vascular system and its possible implications. J Clin Pathol 49:102-106

94. Juvonen J, Laurila A, Alakärppä H, Leinonen M, Surcel HM, Juvonen T, Kairaluoma M, Saikku P (1997) Demonstration of *Chlamydia pneumoniae* in the walls of abdominal aortic aneurysms. J Vasc Surg 25:499-505

95. Juvonen J, Laurila A, Juvonen T, Alakärppä H, Surcel HM, Lounatmaa K, Kuusisto J, Saikku P (1997) Detection of *Chlamydia pneumoniae* in human non-rheumatic stenotic aortic valves. J Am Coll Cardiol 29:1054-1059

96. Taylor-Robinson D, Ong G, Thomas BJ, Rose ML, Yacoub MH (1998) *Chlamydia pneumoniae* in vascular tissues from heart-transplant donors (research letter). Lancet 351:1255

97. Juvonen J, Juvonen T, Laurila A, Kuusisto J, Bodian CA, Alarakkola E, Särkioja T, Kairaluoma MI, Saikku P (1997) Can degenerative tricuspid aoric valve stenosis be caused by a persistent *Chlamydia pneumoniae* infection? A study of 46 cadavers. Ann Intern Med 128:741-744

98. Gupta S, Leatham EW, Carrington D, Mendall MA, Kaski JC, Camm AJ (1995) Elevated *Chlamydia pneumoniae* antibodies, cardiovascular events, and azithromycin in male survivors of myocardial infarction. Circulation 96:404-407

99. Gurfinkel E, Bozovich G, Daroca A, Beck E, Mautner B, Roxis Study Group (1997) Randomised trial of roxithromycin in non-Q-wave coronary syndromes: ROXIS pilot study. Lancet 350:404-407

100. Fong IW, Chiu B, Viira E, Fong MW, Jang D, Mahony J (1997) Rabbit model for *Chlamydia pneumoniae* infection. J Clin Microbiol 35:48-52

101. Laitinen K, Laurila A, Pyhälä L, Leinonen M, Saikku P (1997) *Chlamydia pneumoniae* infection induces inflammatory changes in the aorta of rabbits. Infect Immun 65:4832-4835

102. Muhlestein JB, Anderson JL, Hammond EH, Zhao LP, Trehan S, Schwobe EP, Carlquist JF (1998) Infection with *Chlamydia pneumoniae* accelerates the development of atherosclerosis and treatment with azithromycin prevents it in a rabbit model. Circulation 97:633-636

103. Freidank HM, Billing H (1997) Influence of iron restriction on the growth of *Chlamydia pneumoniae* TWAR and Chlamydia trachomatis. Clin Microbiol Infect 3[Suppl 2]:193

104. von Hertzen L, Surcel HM, Kaprio J, Koskenvuo M, Leinonen M, Saikku P (1998) Effect of smoking on humoral and cell-mediated immune response to *Chlamydia pneumoniae* in twins. J Med Microbiol 47:441-446

105. Kalayoglu MV, Byrne GI (1998) Induction of macrophage foam cell formation by *Chlamydia pneumoniae*. J Infect Dis 177:725-729

106. Mendall MA, Patel P, Ballam L, Strachan D, Northfield TC (1996) C reactive protein and its relation to cardiovascular risk factors: a population based cross sectional study. BMJ 312:1061-1065

107. Kaukoranta-Tolvanen SS, Teppo AM, Laitinen K, Saikku P, Linnavuori K, Leinonen M (1996) Growth of *Chlamydia pneumoniae* in cultured human peripheral blood mononuclear cells and induction of a cytokine response. Microb Pathog 21:215-221

108. Laurila A, Bloigu A, Näyhä S, Hassi J, Leinonen M, Saikku P (1997) Chronic *Chlamydia pneumoniae* infection is associated with a serum lipid profile known to be a risk factor for atherosclerosis. Arterioscler Thromb Vasc Biol 17:2910-2913

109. Cook PJ, Lip GYH, Davies P, Beevers DG, Wise R, Honeybourne D (1998) *Chlamydia pneumoniae* antibodies in severe essential hypertension. Hypertension 31:589-594

110. Meier CR, Jick SS, Derby LE, Vasilakis C, Jick H (1998) Acute respiratory-tract infections and risk of first-time acute myocardial infarction. Lancet 351:1467-1471

111. Valkonen K, Saikku P (1996) Proteinase associated with *Chlamydia pneumoniae*. In: Proceedings of the 3rd Meeting of the European Society for *Chlamydia* Research, Vienna, 11-14 September, 1996. Esculapio, Bologna

Chlamydia pneumoniae: A New Possible Cause of Asthma

D.L. Hahn, L. Allegra

Introduction

Asthma is a chronic respiratory condition of uncertain etiology and often multifactorial that is characterized by chronic bronchial inflammation and airway hyperreactivity that result in episodes of reversible airway obstruction usually manifested as symptoms of cough, shortness of breath and wheeze triggered by a variety of stimuli [1]. Earlier in this century it was generally believed that focal infections were one cause of asthma [2]. Nowadays most experts believe that asthma is exclusively a noninfectious inflammatory lung condition, although a role for viral infections as triggers of asthma exacerbations is widely acknowledged [1]. The current belief in an exclusively noninfectious cause for asthma is based in part on the lack of effectiveness, in producing longlasting asthma remissions, of antibiotic treatment of conventional respiratory pathogens. Recent evidence suggests a causal role for the atypical respiratory pathogen, *Chlamydia pneumoniae*, in the initiation, exacerbation and promotion of asthma [3]. Eradication of this organism from the respiratory tract is difficult and often requires longer than conventional courses of specific antichlamydial antibiotics. It is not likely that antibiotic treatment directed against traditional pyogenic bacteria would eradicate *C. pneumoniae*.

Asthma Epidemiology

Asthma symptoms are present in children and adults worldwide with great variation in prevalence ranging from a few percent in nonindustrialized, rural countries to over 25% in some industrialized nations [4]. Also, asthma prevalence appears to be increasing worldwide [5]. Neither the presence of classic atopy (eczema, allergic rhinoconjunctivitis) [4] nor traditional environmental risk factors (such as air pollution) can explain the wide variations in prevalence between countries or the temporal trends [6]. Many studies have associated antecedent respiratory illnesses (mainly bronchitis and pneumonia) with the development of asthma [7]. Most experts have not considered these associations as evidence that infections can initiate asthma. Instead, interpretations have included: (1) the antecedent "infections" were actually asthma attacks misdiagnosed as infection; or (2) the infections were viral-induced exacerbations of previously unrecognized asthma. Nevertheless, the epidemiologic evidence does not exclude the possibility that viral [8], chlamydial [3] or other atypical infections could explain some of the worldwide cross-sectional and temporal patterns noted for asthma.

Chlamydia pneumoniae Infections

Historical cohort studies on stored sera have demonstrated that up to 70% of seroconversions do not result in documented illness [9]. Thus, most acute infections go unrecognized. *C. pneumoniae* nevertheless accounts for approximately 5% of acute bronchitis and 10% of community-acquired pneumonia [9]. *C. pneumoniae* respiratory infection may also result in pharyngitis, laryngitis, otitis media and sinusitis that often accompany symptoms of lower respiratory tract infection. These illnesses may be persistent and poorly responsive to appropriate antibiotic therapy [10–12]. The association of *C. pneumoniae* with persistent respiratory problems is consistent with the known propensity for *Chlamydia* species to produce chronic infection in target organs and supports the plausibility of the suggestion that asthma could be one manifestation of persistent chlamydial infection in susceptible individuals.

Seroepidemiologic studies agree that *C. pneumoniae* antibody prevalence is low in preschool children, rises steadily to over 50% by early adulthood and continues to increase slowly into old age, suggesting repeat or persistent infection throughout the adult life span [9]. Childhood infection as determined by polymerase chain reaction (PCR) testing can be found in many children who do not develop antibodies until years later, suggesting that infection may occur earlier in life than suggested by the serologic data [13]. A high prevalence of *C. pneumoniae* DNA has been reported in peripheral blood mononuclear cells of heart disease patients (59%) and also in middle-aged blood donors (46%) [14], supporting the presence of persistent systemic infection suggested by the seroepidemiologic data. Such high background rates of infection in the population suggest that it may be difficult to prove that *C. pneumoniae* infection is specifically and causally related to asthma.

Chlamydia pneumoniae in Asthma: Case Reports

In their original 1986 report describing the clinical spectrum of acute TWAR respiratory infection in a university population, Grayston et al. [15] described one culture-positive 35-year-old with persistent symptoms that included wheezing following pneumonia. In 1989, Frydén et al. [16] reported a patient who developed severe chronic asthmatic bronchitis following an acute *C. pneumoniae* infection diagnosed by serology. In 1992 Hammerschlag et al. [10] also reported on a persistently culture-positive health care worker who developed asthmatic bronchitis, and in 1993 Kawane [17] reported a patient with cough-variant asthma, bronchial hyperreactivity, elevated IgE, eosinophilia and high titers of *C. pneumoniae*-specific IgG (1:1024) and IgA (1:32) who responded to macrolide therapy. In 1994 Hahn [18] reported on a 35-year-old man with asthma, eosinophilia, persistent positive cultures and stable IgG titer (1:128) who, after prolonged antibiotic treatment, became culture-negative, had no asthma symptoms or eosinophilia and had normalization of pulmonary function. In 1994 Thom et al. [19] reported on a patient with an acute infection who developed persistent symptoms of new reactive airways disease and Thom [20] also reported a PCR-positive 21-year-old college student with an acute primary infection who developed pneumonia and bronchospasm. Lastly, in 1996 Aldous et al. [21] reported an MIF-positive 4 year-old Tanzanian boy with fever and bronchospasm.

These case reports suggest that acute *C. pneumoniae* infections can initiate new asthma symptoms and that treatment in the acute phase of asthma development can improve or eradicate asthma symptoms, at least in the short-term. These case reports have been supplemented by additional case series of asthma patients with evidence of *C. pneumoniae* infection.

Chlamydia pneumoniae in Asthma: Case Series

Children

In 1991 Korppi et al. [22] studied 188 hospitalized children less than 6 years old with expiratory difficulty and reported 8 who seroconverted as measured by a *Chlamydia* genus-specific enzyme immunoassay (EIA) test but in whom specific tests for *C. trachomatis* were negative. In 1995 Korppi et al. [23] reported additionally that, of 449 children aged 1 month to 8 years with lower respiratory tract infection, 9 of 12 with MIF-positive chlamydial infections (including 2 *C. pneumoniae* infections) had bronchial obstruction. In 1994, Emre et al. [24] reported that 13 (11%) of 118 children aged 5 to 16 years with acute wheezing episodes were culture positive, but only 3 of 13 seroconverted by MIF testing; 9 of 12 culture-positive children had clinical and laboratory improvement in asthma after microbiologic eradication, which was difficult to achieve in some cases. Other observations from that study were one culture-positive child who wheezed for the first time and lack of seroconversion in 6 of 7 persistently culture-positive children. Also in 1994, Cunningham et al. [25] reported on 96 outpatient children with asthma studied by a sensitive nested PCR test; over a 1-year observation period the cumulative rate of PCR positivity was 45 (47%) of 96. Positivity was equally distributed between pharyngeal lavage samples obtained during exacerbations and during asymptomatic periods; however, symptom frequency was associated with detection of *C. pneumoniae*-specific nasal lavage sIgA. The high rates of PCR positivity were confirmed by Johnston [26], who studied children admitted to hospital with wheezing and bronchiolitis and found that respiratory secretions were positive by nested PCR in 18% of patients aged less than 3 months and 58% in those aged over 5 years. In 1995 Prückl et al. [27] reported on 193 children aged 5–16 years with acute or chronic respiratory infections; 3 had PCR-positive gargled-water specimens and also had chronic obstructive bronchitis which had proved resistant to antimicrobial therapy. In 1996 Gnarpe et al. [28] studied 210 children aged 0–15 years with acute respiratory infections and found that 40 (19%) had a positive throat PCR test; 8 PCR-positive children had asthma.

Adults

In 1991, Hahn et al. [29] tested 365 adult outpatients with acute lower respiratory tract illnesses and identified 19 patients with acute *C. pneumoniae* infection diagnosed by serology (19) and culture (1); 9 infected patients wheezed during the acute illness, 4 had exacerbations of previously diagnosed asthma and 4 others had newly diagnosed asthma after illness. In 1994 Hahn and Golubjatnikov [30] reported on two additional patients with acute *C. pneumoniae* infection diagnosed serologically; one patient rapidly developed severe, steroid-dependent asthma and the second had persistent asthma symptoms and chronic obstructive pulmonary disease (COPD). In 1994, Allegra et al. [31] studied 74 adult outpatients with an acute asthma exacerbation and reported that 3 had acute primary and 4 had acute secondary *C. pneumoniae* infections diagnosed serologically; 2 of these 7 had a positive pharyngeal swab for the organism detected by an indirect immunofluorescence test. In 1995 Resta et al. [32] reported on 91 adults with respiratory infections and found serologic evidence of recent infection in 13; 3 had asthmatic bronchitis and 5 had exacerbations of COPD. In 1995 Hahn [33] treated 46 adults with moderate to moderately severe chronic persistent asthma symptoms who were also seroreactive to *C. pneumoniae* (MIF titer ≥ 1:16, median 1:128) and reported that 25 (54%) had major (18) or complete (7) symptom improvement confirmed by pulmonary function testing. In 1996 Hahn [34] also reported on 10 adult outpatients with a first-ever wheezing episode and found that 8 had MIF seroconversions (acute primary infection) and 2 had acute secondary infections; 5 of these 10 developed chronic asthma during follow-up, and another patient was culture-positive later during development of chronic bronchitis. In 1996 Peeling et al. [35] performed detailed serologic testing on 14 asthmatic adults whose sera contained antibodies to the genus-specific chlamydial heat shock protein 60 (CHSP60) antigen. All CHSP60-reactive asthma patients had titers ≥ 1:16 against *C. pneumoniae*-specific IgG and IgA antibodies, and 5 had IgE antibodies detected by immunoblotting against the 60, 62 and/or 70 kDa antigens of *C. pneumoniae*; 13 of 14 CHSP-60 positive patients reported that their asthma began after an acute respiratory infection (the "infectious asthma" syndrome). Lastly, in 1998 Hahn et al. [36] reported treatment results for 3 patients (aged 13, 45 and 65) with severe, steroid-dependent asthma and MIF IgG titers of 1:512; all 3 were able to discontinue oral steroids and remained well-controlled on lesser amounts of inhaled topical therapy (2 adults) or had complete resolution of asthma symptoms (the adolescent).

The case series results provide further evidence that acute *C. pneumoniae* respiratory tract infections can initiate and exacerbate asthma symptoms and that treatment may favorably affect the natural history. However, because of the high background rates of infection in the nonasthmatic population, it is possible that some or all of the infections documented in patients with asthma occurred coincidentally and were not causal. Examination of the results of a growing number of controlled epidemiologic studies could help to determine whether evidence of infection is associated with asthma.

Chlamydia pneumoniae in Asthma: Controlled Studies

In 1991 Hahn et al. [29] reported the first epidemiologic study to find significant associations of *C. pneumoniae* antibody with wheezing during acute respiratory illness and with the subsequent development of asthmatic bronchitis. In that study of 365 adults, the adjusted odds ratio (OR) for an MIF titer of 1:64 or greater and wheezing was 2.1 (1.1–4.2). Comparing 71 exposed cases (titer ≥ 1:64) and 71 unexposed controls (titer < 1:16) with acute respiratory infections, Hahn et al. [29] also reported a highly significant association of antibody with the development of asthmatic bronchitis within 6 months after illness (OR 7.2, 2.2–23.4). In a follow-up study in 1994 Hahn and Golubjatnikov [30] reported a significant association for *C. pneumoniae* seroreactivity (titer ≥ 1:16) and pulmonary function-confirmed adult-onset asthma (100% of asthma cases versus 53% of nonwheezing controls with acute respiratory infections, $P < 0.001$). In 1994 Peters et al. [37] reported on 122 adult patients with acute respiratory illness (ARI) and healthy controls and found that acute MIF antibody was present in 22% of 46 asthma exacerbations compared to 8% of nonasthma ARI ($P < 0.001$) and in 4% of matched controls without ARI ($P < 0.001$). In 1994 Emre et al. [24] studied 188 inner city children aged 5–16 with asthma exacerbations and 41 healthy age- and sex-matched controls and reported that 11% of cases and 5% of controls were culture-positive ($P = NS$). Serologic results were available for 70 cases (including 12 of 13 culture-positive cases) and 24 controls; no MIF antibodies were detected in 58% of culture-positive cases, 55% of culture-negative cases and 46% of controls ($P = NS$). In 1995 Weiss et al. [38] compared 68 adults with bronchospasm and 26 asymptomatic controls and found comparable levels of IgG titers ≥ 1:16 (87% and 92%, respectively, $P = NS$). In 1995 Emre et al. [39] looked for evidence of *C. pneumoniae*-specific IgE by immunoblot in 45 children with and without culture-proven infection and found that 86% of 14 culture-positive asthma cases were positive compared to 9% of culture-positive pneumonia ($P < 0.001$), 18% of culture-negative asthma ($P < 0.001$) and 22% of culture-negative asymptomatic patients ($P < 0.006$). In 1996 Emre et al. [40] reported on 56 patients aged 1–47 years with cystic fibrosis (32 hospitalized cases with an acute exacerbation and 24 clinically stable outpatient controls) and reported that 4 cases and no controls were culture-positive; 3 of 4 culture-positive cases were wheezing. *C. pneumoniae*-specific IgE was detected by immunoblotting in 4 of 4 culture-positive cases, 2 of 18 culture-negative cases and

6 of 20 controls (Chi-square, *P* value = 0.003). In 1996 Hahn et al. [41] performed a case-control study (25 adults with asthma symptoms beginning less than 2 years prior to enrolment and 45 matched controls with normal pulmonary function) and found a significant association of IgA antibody (titer ≥ 1:10) and asthma (72% of cases and 44% of controls, OR 3.7, 1.1–9.0) but comparable prevalence for IgG titers ≥ 1:16 (92% of cases and 84% of controls). Also in 1996, Hahn and McDonald [42] reported that, of 104 adult outpatients with asthma, 68 patients with the infectious asthma syndrome had IgA titers ≥ 1:16 (62%) and IgG titers ≥ 1:16 (93%) significantly more often (*P* < 0.01) than did noninfectious asthma patients (22% and 61%, respectively). In 1996 Björnsson et al. [43] studied 122 subjects with asthma-related symptoms and 75 general population controls and reported that cases with wheezing compared to controls without wheezing had more IgM ≥ 1:16 and/or IgG ≥ 1:512 (OR 6.7, 1.3–35.7). Also, bronchial hyperresponsiveness (BHR) as measured by the methacholine challenge test was associated with IgA titers ≥ 1:32 (cases 22%, controls 8%, OR 3.3, 1.3–8.3). In 1996, Brüggen et al. [44] claimed that 70% of 100 intrinsic adult asthma patients compared to 27% of general population controls had positive *C. pneumoniae* throat antigen detection using a monoclonal antibody immunofluorescence test (*P* < 0.001). In 1998 Cook et al. [45] reported that IgG titers ≥ 1:64 and ≤ 1:256 were associated with severe "brittle" asthma compared to nonasthmatic hospitalised controls (cases 35%, controls 13%, OR 3.99, 3.6–9.9). In 1998 von Hertzen et al. [46] tested consecutive patients with asthma or allergy aged 15 years and older and found that an IgG titer ≥ 1:128 was associated with asthma compared with symptomatic nonasthmatic patients (cases 34%, controls 17%, OR 2.6, 1.4–4.8). They also found that the reported serologic association was stronger for nonatopic asthma (OR 3.3, 1.4–4.7) than for atopic asthma (OR 2.1, 0.7–5.8). Lastly, in 1998 Miyashita et al. [47] reported a series of serologic associations (IgG ≥ 1:16, IgG geometric mean titer (GMT), IgA ≥ 1:16, IgA GMT, IgM ≥ 1:16 or IgG=1:512 or fourfold titer rise) that were all significantly associated with 168 acute exacerbations of asthma compared to 108 matched nonasthmatic controls.

With one exception [38], the seroepidemiologic studies reported significant associations of various aspects of reactive airways disease (wheezing, brochospasm, bronchial hyperreactivity, diagnoses of asthmatic bronchitis or asthma) with various serologic parameters of *C. pneumoniae* infection. The study of Weiss et al. [38] that failed to find any association of bronchospasm and IgG antibodies was characterized by an exceptionally high prevalence of IgG in controls. Another pertinent negative serologic result was reported by von Hertzen et al. [46] who were able to demonstrate significant antibody associations only in females; again, the male control group was notable for having an extremely high antibody prevalence. Cook et al. [45] were unable to demonstrate significant antibody associations in mild asthma. It has been reported that skin test-positive, childhood-onset asthma patients have lesser amounts of antibody [48] and milder disease [7] than adult-onset asthma patients who become symptomatic after an acute respiratory infection (the "infectious asthma" syndrome). An inverse association of skin test positivity and *C. pneumoniae* antibody related to age of onset is depicted in Fig. 1. Emre et al. [24] were able to demonstrate a high-

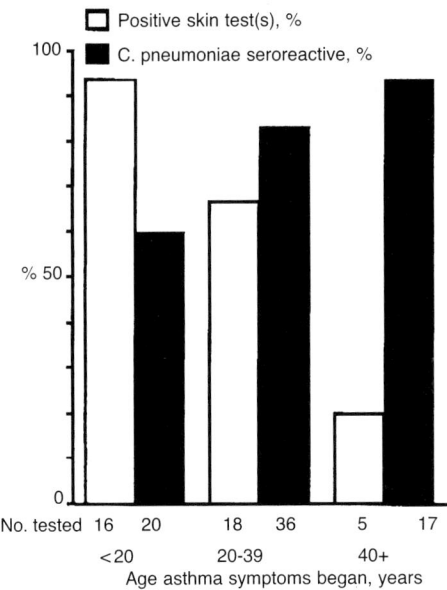

Fig.1. Frequencies of positive skin tests (one or more positive tests against a battery of common aeroallergens) (*open bars*) and *C. pneumoniae* seroreactivity (total Ig titer of 1:16 or greater in the microimmunofluorescence test) (*black bars*) in patients from a primary care outpatient setting. Skin test positivity was significantly related to younger age of reported asthma onset ($P < 0.0001$), and *C. pneumoniae* seroreactivity was significantly related to older age of reported asthma onset ($P < 0.01$)

er prevalence of positive cultures in asthma cases (11%) than controls (5%) but the difference failed achieve statistical significance. Relationships between positive cultures and/or PCR detection in the upper respiratory tract and the presence of deep lung infection in asthma have not been determined.

Associations with fourfold titer rises and/or IgM antibodies can be reliably attributed to acute infections, whereas the association with high stable titers ($\geq 1:512$) in the setting of chronic disease such as asthma is a less certain indicator of acute infection [34, 49]. The majority of the studies reviewed above reported associations of asthma with titer levels deemed "pre-existing" or "chronic." While the associations are specific for *C. pneumoniae* [49], it must be emphasized that these seroepidemiologic studies cannot distinguish between a previous exposure and current persistent infection. Some authors believe that the associations with IgA antibodies of short half-life suggest persistence [41, 47]. The possibility of persistent infection is supported by the clinical observations that treatment appears to be beneficial and that this benefit could be correlated with microbiologic eradication [24, 33]. In a preliminary analysis of screening results in an ongoing international randomized trial of macrolide therapy in adult asthma, proposed and chaired by L. Allegra, P. Black, and F. Blasi, 59% of 459 adult asthma subjects met eligibility criteria for randomization on the basis of an IgG titer ≥ 64 and/or an IgA titer $\geq 1:16$ [50].

One of the major limitations in all the above epidemiological studies in asthma populations is the lack of a true comparison in the general population. With the aim of evaluating the possibility of significant differences between asthmatics and the general population in terms of *C. pneumoniae* seropositivity and chlamydial DNA detection, a large multicenter national epidemiological study is now underway. The PISAC study (Prevalence Italian Study Asthma and *Chlamydia*) is being carried out in Italy and will enrol 450 asthma patients and 1350 subjects randomly selected from electoral rolls. Seroepidemiological prevalence of IgG, IgM, and IgA antibody fractions to *C. pneumoniae* and detection of *C. pneumoniae* DNA in peripheral blood circulating monocytes will be performed in all subjects.

The results of these trials and of others that are being planned will be crucial to answering the question of whether and to what extent persistent and treatable infection is present in asthma.

References

1. Anonimous (1997) Expert Panel Report II. Guidelines for the diagnosis and management of asthma. US Department of Health and Human Services, Public Health Service. National Institutes of Health, National Heart, Lung, and Blood Institute, February
2. Thomas WS (1928) Asthma: its diagnosis and treatment. Hoeber, New York
3. Hahn DL (1996) Intracellular pathogens and their role in asthma: *Chlamydia pneumoniae* in adult patients. Eur Respir Rev 6:224-230
4. The International Study of Asthma and Allergies in Childhood (ISAAC) Steering Committee (1998) Worldwide variation in prevalence of symptoms of asthma, allergic rhinoconjunctivitis, and atopic eczema: ISAAC. Lancet 351:1225-1232
5. Burr ML (1987) Is asthma increasing? J Epidemiol Comm Health 41:185-189
6. Lewis S (1998) ISAAC–a hypothesis generator for asthma? Lancet 351:1220-1221
7. Hahn DL (1995) Infectious asthma: a reemerging clinical entity? J Fam Pract 41:153-157
8. Smith JM (1994) Asthma and atopy as diseases of unknown cause. A viral hypothesis possibly explaining the epidemiologic association of the atopic diseases and various forms of asthma. Ann Allergy 72:156-162
9. Grayston JT (1992) Infections caused by *Chlamydia pneumoniae* strain TWAR. Clin Infect Dis 15:757-763
10. Hammerschlag MR, Chirgwin K, Roblin PM et al (1992) Persistent infection with *Chlamydia pneumoniae* following acute respiratory illness. Clin Infect Dis 14:178-182
11. Falck G, Engstrand I, Gad A et al (1997) Demonstration of *Chlamydia pneumoniae* in patients with chronic pharyngitis. Scand J Infect Dis 29:585-589
12. Falck G, Gnarpe J, Gnarpe H (1997) Persistent *Chlamydia pneumoniae* infection in a Swedish family. Scand J Infect Dis 28:271-273
13. Normann E, Gnarpe J, Gnarpe H et al (1998) *Chlamydia pneumoniae* in children attending day-care-centers in Gävle, Sweden. Pediatr Infect Dis J 17:474-478
14. Boman J, Söderberg S, Forsberg J et al (1998) High prevalence of *Chlamydia pneumoniae* DNA in peripheral blood mononuclear cells in patients with cardiovascular disease and in middle-aged blood donors. J Infect Dis 178:274-277

15. Grayston JT, Kuo C-C, Wang S-P et al (1986) A new *Chlamydia psittaci* strain, TWAR, isolated in acute respiratory tract infections. New Engl J Med 315:161-168

16. Frydén A, Kihlström E, Maller R et al (1989) A clinical and epidemiological study of "ornithosis" caused by *Chlamydia psittaci* and *Chlamydia pneumoniae* (strain TWAR). Scand J Infect Dis 21:681-691

17. Kawane H (1993) *Chlamydia pneumoniae*. Thorax 48:871

18. Hahn DL (1994) Infection as a cause of asthma. Ann Allergy 73:276

19. Thom DH, Grayston JT, Campbell LA et al (1994) Respiratory infection with *Chlamydia pneumoniae* in middle-aged and older adult outpatients. Eur J Clin Microbiol Infect Dis 13:785-792

20. Thom D (1994) Lower respiratory tract infection with *Chlamydia pneumoniae*. Arch Fam Med 3:828-832

21. Aldous MB, West S, Kimaro DN et al (1996) *Chlamydia pneumoniae* (TWAR) infection in Tanzanian children. Trop Doct 26:18-19

22. Korppi M, Leinonen M, Koskela M et al (1991) Bacterial infection in under school age children with expiratory difficulty. Pediatr Pulmonol 10:254-259

23. Korppi M, Leinonen M, Saikku P (1995) Chlamydial infection and reactive airway disease. Arch Pediatr Adolesc Med 149:341-342

24. Emre U, Roblin PM, Gelling M et al (1994) The association of *Chlamydia pneumoniae* infection and reactive airway disease in children. Arch Pediatr Adolesc Med 148:727-732

25. Cunningham A, Johnston S, Julious S et al (1994) The role of *Chlamydia pneumoniae* and other pathogens in acute episodes of asthma in children. In: Orfila J, Byrne GI, Chernesky MA et al (eds) Proceedings of the 8th International Symposium on Human Chlamydial Infections, Chantilly, France. Esculapio, Bologna, pp 480-483

26. Johnston SL (1997) Influence of viral and bacterial respiratory infections on exacerbations and symptom severity in childhood asthma. Pediatr Pulmonol 16:88-89

27. Prückl PM, Aspöck C, Makristathis A et al (1995) Polymerase chain reaction for detection of *Chlamydia pneumoniae* in gargled-water specimens of children. Eur J Clin Microbiol Infect Dis 14:141-144

28. Gnarpe J, Gnarpe H, Normann E et al (1996) *Chlamydia pneumoniae, Mycoplasma pneumoniae* and *Mycoplasma fermentans* PCR in children with acute respiratory tract infections (abstract C-160). In: Abstracts of the 96th General Meeting of the American Society for Microbiology, New Orleans, LA, 19-23 May, 1996, p 29

29. Hahn DL, Dodge R, Golubjatnikov R (1991) Association of *Chlamydia pneumoniae* (strain TWAR) infection with wheezing, asthmatic bronchitis and adult-onset asthma. JAMA 266:225-230

30. Hahn DL, Golubjatnikov R (1994) Asthma and chlamydial infection: a case series. J Fam Pract 38:589-595

31. Allegra L, Blasi F, Centanni S et al (1994) Acute exacerbations of asthma in adults: role of *Chlamydia pneumoniae* infection. Eur Respir J 7:2165-2168

32. Resta O, Monno R, Saracino A et al (1995) *Chlamydia pneumonae* infection in Italian patients. Monaldi Arch Chest Dis 50:173-176

33. Hahn DL (1995) Treatment of *Chlamydia pneumoniae* infection in adult asthma: a before-after trial. J Fam Pract 41:345-351

34. Hahn D (1996) Incident wheezing and prevalent asthma have different serologic patterns of "acute" *Chlamydia pneumoniae* antibodies in adults. In: Proceedings of the 3rd Meeting of the European Society for *Chlamydia* Research, Vienna, Austria. Esculapio, Bologna, p 226

35. Peeling RW, Hahn D, Dillon E (1996) *Chlamydia pneumoniae* infection and adult-onset asthma. In: Proceedings of the 3rd Meeting of the European Society for *Chlamydia* Research, Vienna, Austria. Esculapio, Bologna, p 228 (abstract)

36. Hahn D, Bukstein D, Luskin A et al (1998) Evidence for *Chlamydia pneumoniae* infection in steroid-dependent asthma. Ann Allergy Asthma Immunol 80:45-49

37. Peters BS, Thomas B, Marshall B et al (1994) The role of *Chlamydia pneumoniae* in acute exacerbations of asthma (part 2 of 2). Am J Respir Crit Care Med 149:A341

38. Weiss S, Quist J, Roblin P et al (1995) The relationship between *Chlamydia pneumoniae* and bronchospasm in adults (abstract K39). In: Abstracts of the 35th Interscience Conference on Antimicrobial Agents and Chemotherapy (ICAAC), San Francisco, California. American Society for Microbiology, p 294

39. Emre U, Sokolovskaya N, Roblin P et al (1995) Detection of *Chlamydia pneumoniae*-IgE in children with reactive airway disease. J Infect Dis 172:265-267

40. Emre U, Bernius M, Roblin P et al (1996) *Chlamydia pneumoniae* infection in patients with cystic fibrosis. Clin Infect Dis 22:819-823

41. Hahn DL, Anttila T, Saikku P (1996) Association of *Chlamydia pneumoniae* IgA antibodies with recently symptomatic asthma. Epidemiol Infect 117:513-517

42. Hahn DL, McDonald RA (1996) Association of serum IgA antibody against *Chlamydia pneumoniae* with "infectious" asthma (Abstract C-152). 96th General Meeting of the American Society for Microbiology, New Orleans, LA, 19-23 May, 1996, p 29

43. Björnsson E, Helm E, Janson C et al (1996) Serology of *Chlamydia* in relation to asthma and bronchial hyperresponsiveness. Scand J Infect Dis 28:63-69

44. Brüggen H, Kaspar P, Petro W (1996) Significance of TWAR-antigen immunofluorescence test and serologic *Chlamydia* anti-rLPS antibody test results compared with clinical findings in asthmatic patients. In: Proceedings of the 3rd Meeting of the European Society for *Chlamydia* Research, Vienna, Austria. Esculapio, Bologna, p 227

45. Cook PJ, Davies P, Tunnicliffe W et al (1998) *Chlamydia pneumoniae* and asthma. Thorax 53:254-259

46. von Hertzen L, Töyrlä M, Gimishanov A et al (1998) Asthma, atopy and *Chlamydia pneumoniae* antibodies in adults. In: Stephens RS, Byrne GI, Christiansen G et al (eds) Proceedings of the 9th International Symposium on Human Chlamydial Infection, Napa, CA, ISBN 0-9664383-0-2, pp 171-174

47. Miyashita N, Kubota Y, Nakajima M et al (1998) *Chlamydia pneumoniae* and exacerbations of asthma in adults. Ann Allergy Asthma Immunol 80:405-409

48. Hahn DL, Golubjatnikov R (1994) Age at asthma diagnosis, skin test positivity and *Chlamydia pneumoniae* seroreactivity (part 2 of 2). Am J Respir Crit Care Med 149:A913 (abstract)

49. Grayston JT, Golubjatnikov R, Hagiwara T et al (1993) Serologic tests for *Chlamydia pneumoniae*. Pediatr Infect Dis J 12:790-791

50. Jenkins C, Blasi F, Allegra L, Black P, Hopkins S (1998) *Chlamydia pneumoniae* Asthma Roxithromycin Multinational Study (CARM): seroprevalence results. 4th International Conference on the macrolides, azalides, streptogamins and ketolides, Barcelona, 21-23 January, 1998, p 5

Chlamydia pneumoniae: An Important Pathogen in Chronic Bronchitis

J. Lorenz

The Role of Airway Infections in Chronic Bronchitis

Chronic bronchitis (CB) refers to the presence of chronic cough and recurrent increases in bronchial secretions sufficient to cause expectoration. It is clinically defined by international consensus as production of sputum on most days for a minimum of 3 months a year for at least 2 successive years that cannot be attributed to other pulmonary or cardiac causes [1, 2]. CB can occur with or without airflow limitation. Chronic obstructive pulmonary disease (COPD) is a disorder that is characterized by the presence of airflow obstruction due to CB or pulmonary emphysema [3]. The obstruction is dominant during expiration and is generally at best partially reversible. Reduced expiratory airflow and slow forced emptying of the lung are persistent and typically show progressive deterioration with age. CB is one of the most prevalent chronic diseases in adults, especially in males. In 1978, about 20% of the male working population in Germany fulfilled the diagnostic criteria [4]. In 1970, 10% of German adults over 50 years suffered from CB with chronic airflow obstruction [5]. In western developed countries COPD ranks among the three or four leading causes of death. In 1983 death rates of adults aged 55–65 in Europe and North American countries due to COPD were 17–90/100000 males and 7–30/100000 females [6]. Between 1966 and 1989 the age-adjusted death rates for COPD rose 71% in the USA [7]. Median survival of 62-year-old patients with COPD was 8 years, against 14 years in healthy subjects of the same age [8]. The observed development in morbidity and mortality appears to be related to trends in cigarette smoking in the decades before.

Simple acute bronchitis is not believed to induce long-term effects in the bronchial mucosa in the absence of α1-antitrypsin deficiency or cystic fibrosis. Cigarette smoke is the dominant risk factor in the development of CB and COPD. Other forms of ambient pollutants (e.g., occupational or urban air pollution) are further major precipitants. The hypersecretion of mucus in CB is due to hypertrophy of the submucosal glands and hyperplasia of goblet cells in small airways at the expense of ciliated epithelium, a change referred to as "mucous metaplasia" [9]. It works in concert with squamous metaplasia, ciliary abnormalities and altered mucus rheology. These influences lead to the impairment of mucociliary clearance. Serous acini of the submucosal glands of the large airways that contain humoral antimicrobial factors (e.g., lysozyme and lactoferrin) and antiproteases are reduced at the same time. All these influences together favor bacterial growth and colonization of the bronchial mucosa.

The clinical course of CB is characterized by acute exacerbations. During exacerbations the patients experience worsening of symptoms including increased cough and sputum production, increased sputum purulence, and shortness of breath. These complaints are usually associated with increased bronchial obstruction and pulmonary hyperinflation. Possible causes of exacerbations include environmental pollutants, allergic responses and viral/bacterial infections [10]. Although the etiology of exacerbations may be multifactorial, it was shown that two thirds are bacterial in origin [11]. However, this estimation was based on conventional microbiological culture methods. *Haemophilus influenzae* has been the pathogen most frequently isolated from patients with acute exacerbation of CB. It accounts for about 50% of the isolates, followed by *Streptococcus pneumoniae* and *Moraxella catarrhalis* [10, 12]. Until recently, intracellular pathogens such as *Chlamydia pneumoniae* have been poorly investigated due to the lack of appropriate culture methods or molecular techniques. Pathogens that are isolated during exacerbations can also be found in respiratory secretions in stable disease and are therefore thought to chronically colonize the airways [13]. Chronic bacterial colonization itself is believed to form the source of recurrent purulent exacerbations. Infections may influence the progression of CB in several ways: (a) recurrent acute infectious exacerbations may accelerate the lung damage associated with CB; (b) bacteria may cause acute exacerbations that themselves lead to the progress of pulmonary damage; (c) chronic bacterial colonization may alternatively/additionally attract and activate inflammatory cells and mediators that contribute to progressive tissue damage. The latter mechanism has been adopted from observations in bronchiectasis [14] and has been proposed as the "vicious circle hypothesis" to explain the role of chronic bacterial load [15]. Proteinases, toxic oxidants, and other mediators generated by activated phagocytes are unable to discriminate between microbial pathogens and host cells, and are therefore capable to damage bronchial cells that are essential for the integrity and function of the airways [16, 17].

Several long-term prospective studies have addressed the issue of prognostic implications of recurrent infections on pulmonary function in CB and COPD [18–21]. Three of the four studies came to the conclusion that there is no relation between pulmonary function and the number of airway infections. However, in one study that tried to identify variables associated with the loss of forced expiratory volume (FEV_1), more frequent episodes of infection correlated with a more rapid decline in FEV_1. As a whole, these studies do not deliver clear evidence that bacterial (purulent) infections contribute to the long-term decline in lung function of patients with COPD. Among the variables that affect the abilities of such studies to draw definite conclusions are the heterogeneity of COPD and CB and the definition of an infective episode. It does not appear to be sufficient to take clinical signs and symptoms as the indicator of bronchial bacterial load and intensity of inflammation. Moreover, the literature addressing the interplay between the host's bronchial system and bacteria in CB is restricted to the pathogens most frequently isolated by routine culture methods [10]. An alternative approach to assessing the participation of bacterial infection is to consider the effect of antibiotics. There are no data that evaluate the long-term effects of antibacterial therapy in CB. However, six prospective placebo-controlled trials on the efficacy of antibiotic therapy in acute exacerbations of CB were published between 1965 and 1991. They have been reviewed recently [12]. Earlier studies using relatively small numbers of patients have provided conflicting results, whereas large-scale studies of the late 1980s and the early 1990s demonstrated markedly improved clinical success when antibiotics were included in the treatment of acute exacerbations of CB [22, 23]. In conclusion, the different lines of evidence speak in favor of a significant contribution of airway infections to the progress of CB. Therefore, the presence and number of respiratory infections has – besides lung function data and the absence or presence of comorbidity – been included in a recently proposed system for staging of CB patients [24].

Chlamydia pneumoniae in Acute Airway Infections

On discovery of *C. pneumoniae* it became clear that the TWAR strain is able to cause mucosal respiratory infections besides parenchymal pulmonary infections [25, 26]. Further evidence for this marked "bronchotropism" was delivered by observations of familial outbreaks in which *C. pneumoniae* caused both pneumonia and acute bronchitis in formerly healthy persons [27, 28]. Subsequently, the role of *C. pneumoniae* in various forms of acute respiratory infections was investigated. Its prevalence in common cold was low (Table 1). In two studies from France and Finland the percentage of *C. pneumoniae* infections was 1% in 285 children under 5 years of age [29] and 2% in 200 young adults [30]. *C. pneumoniae* was identified in acute simple bronchitis in 1%–25% of cases (Table 1) [31–34]. One hundred and fourteen Swedish patients aged over 10 years were studied by ENT swab culture and serologically with the microimmunofluorescence test. Eleven patients had a fourfold rise in antibody titres to *C. pneumoniae*, IgM titres of ≥ 1:16, or IgG titres of ≥ 1:1024. A number of additional patients had IgG titres of 1:512, indicating probable acute infection [31]. This study suggested that at least one out of four patients with acute bronchitis is infected by *C. pneumoniae*. However, this remarkably high prevalence could not be confirmed in two additional studies. The Seattle group investigated a total of 743 patients, among them 247 patients with acute bronchitis [32]. The median age of this population was 40 years. With the use of culture, microimmunofluorescence, and polymerase chain reaction (PCR) they found acute *C. pneumoniae* infections in 5%. These were predominantly reinfections as suggested by serological criteria. Control patients were serologically and microbiologically negative. Patients with reinfections were older and had milder disease than patients with primary infections. The bronchitis induced by *C. pneumoniae* was milder in comparison to *Mycoplasma pneumoniae* or viruses. Wheez-

Table 1. Prevalence of *C. pneumoniae* infection in bronchitis

Setting	Methods	Prevalence (%)		Commentary	Country	Reference	
• Acute infection							
CC	C	3/285	(1)	Children <5 ys	France	Aymard	[29]
CC	MIF	4/200	(2)	Young adults	Finland	Mäkelä	[30]
AB	C, MIF	28/114	(25)	Age >10 ys	Sweden	Falck	[31]
AB	C, MIF, PCR	12/247	(5)	Age 40+ 16 ys	USA	Thom	[32]
AB	MIF	1/140	(1)	Age >15 years	Iceland	Jonsson	[33]
LRTI	MIF	5/111	(4)	29 pts had COPD	France	Vernejoux	[34]
AECB	CFT	0/35	(0)		France	Philit	[35]
AECB	C, MIF	2/44	(5)		USA	Beaty	[36]
AECB	IIF, MIF	6/142	(5)		Italy	Blasi	[37]
• Chronic/previous infection							
CB	C, MIF	50/65	(77)	Controls: 73%	USA	Beaty	[36]
AECB	C+IIF, MIF	90/142	(63)	Controls: 46%	Italy	Blasi	[37]
CB	PCR	4/37	(11)		Italy	Blasi	[38]
AECB	MIF	31/36	(89)	Controls: 55%	Finland	Von Hertzen	[39]
CB		36/54	(66)				
CB	MIF, IC, PCR	35/54	(65)	Severe CB: 71%	Finland	Von Hertzen	[40]
CB	MIF, (ELISA)	195/271	(72)	ELISA: 52%	Netherlands	Verkooyen	[41]

CC, common cold; *AB*, acute bronchitis; *LRTI*, lower respiratory tract infections; *AECB*, acute exacerbation of chronic bronchitis; *CB*, chronic bronchitis (stable); *C*, culture; *MIF*, microimmunofluorescence assay; *PCR*, polymerase chain reaction; *CFT*, complement fixation test; *IIF*, indirect immunoflourescence assay; *IC*, circulating immune complexes; *ELISA*, enzyme-linked immunosorbent assay; *COPD*, chronic obstructive pulmonary disease

ing was infrequent and occurred in comparable proportions of cases in viral, mycoplasmal, and chlamydial disease, but cough persisted for 3 weeks in half of the patients infected by *Chlamydia*. Pneumonia caused by *C. pneumoniae* was also remarkably infrequent in the study population, in contrast to a number of other investigations conducted by the same authors. This raises the question of whether the population in this study was representative. In 140 patients from Iceland with acute bronchitis there was only one *C. pneumoniae* infection [33]. The diagnosis was established serologically by microimmunofluorescence. In 111 serologically diagnosed French patients with lower respiratory tract infections, among them 29 COPD patients, 4% were infected by *C. pneumoniae* [34]. In conclusion, the studies available demonstrate that *C. pneumoniae* can induce acute bronchitis, but that its significance varies markedly over time and between geographical areas: the proportion of patients infected with *C. pneumoniae* in Seattle varied between 1.7% and 4.3% from year to year [32]. Future long-term studies will show whether epidemics are among the factors that are responsible for this variation. The prevalence of antibodies against *C. pneumoniae* in healthy adult subjects is over 50% in most western countries. It can be assumed that mild acute respiratory (re)infection is mainly responsible for this phenomenon.

The first study to assess the prevalence of *C. pneumoniae* in acute exacerbations of CB was done by the Seattle group [36]. They investigated a group of 44 hospitalized patients in whom exacerbations of airflow obstruction were due to acute bronchitis without an obvious bacterial pathogen in the sputum using serology and culture from throat swab specimens. *C. pneumoniae* was found in 5% of the patients. The authors argued that endogenous reinfection by *C. pneumoniae* is not a main cause of exacerbations, because there was serologic evidence of previous infection in nearly 80% of cases. Coinfections of *C. pneumoniae* with other bacteria may have been overlooked due to the study design. Blasi and coworkers also used serology and culture (with the help of an indirect fluorescent antibody for identification of *C. pneumoniae*) to analyze a larger group of 142 outpatients with acute purulent exacerbations of COPD [37]. They found IgM titers suggesting new infection in 4% and reinfections (a fourfold increase in IgG and IgG titres ≥ 1:512) in 14% of cases. Swab cultures were negative, possibly for technical reasons. No other intracellular pathogens were found, and there was no difference in clinical presentation from other bacterial causes. The treatment of *C. pneumoniae* infections with appropriate antibiotics was followed by rapid clinical improvement. The two studies suggest that *C. pneumoniae* is responsible for at least 5% of acute exacerbations of CB/COPD. In the future, long-term studies would be especially valuable to assess the precise role of *C. pneumoniae* in exacerbations. The necessity to use state-of-the-art diagnostic tools is underlined by the observation that *C. pneumoniae* is underestimated when inappropriate methods are used [35].

Chlamydia pneumoniae Chronic Infection

Previous or chronic infections due to *C. pneumoniae* are serologically characterized by specific IgG titers of 1:64–1:256 and/or IgA titres of ≥ 1:16 with an increase of less than fourfold between paired samples [42, 43]. It has been suggested that the detection of chlamydial IgG ≥ 1:128 and concomitant IgA ≥ 1:40 is a criterion of chronic infection [43]. Antibodies against *C. pneumoniae* persist for a considerable period of time after acute infection. IgM disappears usually after 4–6 months and IgA within the first year, while IgG persists and may be detected over 3 years in the same patients [31, 44]. Therefore, the observations that elevated IgA levels remain stable in a number of patients with CB, that sero-conversions are rare and circulating immune complexes frequently present, support the hypothesis that infection by *C. pneumoniae* is chronic in at least a part of the patients [45]. This view is further supported by a study from Blasi and coworkers in which *C. pneumoniae* DNA was detected in sputum samples from 4/37 patients with clinically stable COPD using nested polymerase chain detection. Serology was also positive in three of the four DNA-positive patients [38].

Serologic studies showed a very high prevalence of antibodies against *C. pneumoniae* in patients with chronic airway disease (Table 1). Beaty and coworkers found low-level antibodies (IgG 1:16–1:156) in 77% of the patients, but also in 73% of the controls, a surprisingly high proportion [36]. Blasi and cowork-ers observed specific IgG in 63% of COPD patients and in 46% of the controls [37]. This more realistically reflected the seroepidemiology in a healthy adult population. Not only were *C. pneumoniae* antibodies much more prevalent in patients, but also the mean specific IgG titer in patients over 50 years was signif-icantly higher. Von Hertzen and coworkers measured specific IgG and IgA in elderly male chronic bronchitics in stable disease and during acute exacerbation [39]. Some 89% of the exacerbated versus 66% of the stable COPD patients were antibody positive, but only 55% of the 321 age-matched controls. The same group of authors postulated that of a group of 54 COPD patients 65% had chronic *C. pneumoniae* infection based on results of microimmunofluorescence, sputum IgA, specific immune complexes, and PCR [40]. The proportion was even higher (71%) in patients with severe disease. In 271 patients from the Netherlands the presence of specific IgG was 72% with the microimmunofluorescence assay and 53% in a rDNA LPS ELISA [41]. During a surveillance period of median 15 months there were new *C. pneumoniae* infections in 7% of the patients, diagnosed by the use of either one of the two serological methods. The incidence of new infections or reinfections was computed as 2.2 and 5.3/100 person years, respec-tively, in this outpatient group depending on the the diagnostic method.

In total, the diverse studies demonstrate, in good agreement, that antibodies against *C. pneumoniae* are present in about 70% of CB/COPD patients and that the seroprevalence is about 20% higher than in an age-matched healthy popula-tion. Some evidence suggests that this phenomenon represents chronic infection in at least some of the patients. What is the significance of this finding? This ques-tion can only be answered by the use of mechanistic studies that follow the pos-tulates of Robert Koch to demonstrate a link between infection and disease (CB).

The long-term presence of *C. pneumoniae* in the bronchial mucosa of COPD patients may interact with the underlying disease in different ways. Viable bacte-ria have been shown to persist in the airways for many months, even after ade-quate antibiotic therapy [46]. As shown with *C. trachomatis,* these kinds of agents can especially survive in macrophages until they are reactivated by immunosup-pression or coincidental infection with another organism [47–49]. Since coinfec-tions, either viral or bacterial, are frequent in *C. pneumoniae* infections [50], *Chlamydia* may be the initiating pathogen and, after immobilizing the ciliated cells lining the respiratory tract [51], permit the invader, such as *H. influenzae,* to gain access to the lower airways [50]. By this mechanism chronic chlamydial infection may damage the airways by themselves as well as additionally in an indirect fashion. Another possible pathogenic mechanism of *C. pneumoniae* in COPD is its potential to induce bronchospasms. This point is discussed elsewhere in this book.

It has been established that the host immunity following respiratory *C. pneu-moniae* infection is different from that of common bacterial agents. It induces not only immunoglobulins but also a cell-mediated immune response, as demon-strated by the lymphocyte transformation assay [52]. Immunocytochemistry of sputum in *C. pneumoniae*-induced bronchitis indicates intense airway inflammation with increased total and lymphocyte cell counts, later followed by neutrophils and a CD8 (cytotoxic T-cells)-dominated lymphocyte pattern [53]. Bronchoalveolar lavage in *C. pneumoniae*-induced pneumonia is also characterized by lymphocytic inflammation with dominant cytotoxic T-cells in the absence of neutrophilia [54]. Further studies are required to clarify whether the specific interaction between chronic *C. pneumoniae* infection and bronchial host reaction contributes to the progress of CB.

The present data allow the conclusion that the frequent detection of *C. pneumoniae* is a non-random finding in chronic bronchial disease that indicates chronic infection in many cases [50]. The agent is able to induce acute exacerbations of either bronchitis or pneumonia and possibly tissue damage.

References

1. American Thoracic Society (1962) Chronic bronchitis, asthma, and pulmonary emphysema: a statement by the Committee on Diagnostic Standards for Nontuberculous Respiratory Diseases. Am Rev Respir Dis 85:762-768
2. Medical Research Council (1965) Definition and classification of chronic bronchitis for clinical and epidemiological purposes. Lancet 1:775-779
3. American Thoracic Society (1995) Standards for the diagnosis and care of patients with chronic obstructive pulmonary disease. Respir Crit Care Med 152:S78-S121
4. Fruhmann G (1978) Chronische Bronchitis und Berufsfähigkeit. Arbeitsmed Sozialmed Präventivmed 13:215-218
5. Reichel G, Ulmer WT (eds) (1970) Luftverschmutzung und unspezifische Atemwegserkrankungen. Springer, Berlin Heidelberg New York
6. World Health Organisation (1986) Statistics annual of the World Health Organisation, WHO Publications, Geneva
7. Higgins MW, Thom T (1990) Incidence, prevalence, and mortality: intra- and intercountry differences. In: Hensley MJ, Saunders NA (eds) Clinical epidemiology of chronic obstructive pulmonary disease. Dekker, New York, pp 23-43
8. Farzin I, Ulmer WT (1980) Die Lebenserwartung von Patienten mit chronisch obstruktiver Atemwegserkrankung. Prax Pneumol 34:158-168
9. Jeffery PK (1998) Structural and inflammatory changes in COPD: a comparison with asthma. Thorax 53:129-136
10. Murphy TF, Sethi S (1992) Bacterial infection in chronic obstructive pulmonary disease. Am Rev Respir Dis 146:1067-1083
11. Gump DW, Phillips CA, Forsyth BR, McIntosh FK, Lamborn KR, Stouch WH (1976) Role of infection in chronic bronchitis. Am Rev Respir Dis 113:465-473
12. Ball P (1995) Epidemiology and treatment of chronic bronchitis and its exacerbations. Chest 108:S43-S52
13. Monso E, Ruiz J, Rosell A, Manterola J, Fiz J, Morcra J, Ausina V (1995) Bacterial infection in chronic obstructive pulmonary disease: a study of stable and exacerbated outpatients using the protected specimen brush. Am J Respir Crit Care Med 152:1316-1320
14. Cole P (1989) Host-microbe relationships in chronic respiratory infection. Respiration 55:S5-S8
15. Wilson R (1995) Outcome predictors in bronchitis. Chest 108:S53-S57

16. Amitani R, Wilson R, Read R (1991) Effects of human neutrophil elastase and bacterial proteinase enzymes on human respiratory epithelium. Am J Respir Cell Mol Biol 4:26-32

17. Feldman C, Anderson R, Kanthakumar K (1994) Oxidant-mediated ciliary dysfunction in human respiratory epithelium. Free Radic Biol Med 17:1-10

18. Howard P (1970) A long-term follow-up of respiratory symptoms and ventilatory function in a group of working man. Br J Industr Med 27:326-333

19. Bates DV (1973) The fate of the chronic bronchitic: a report of the ten-year follow-up in the Canadian Department of Veteran's Affairs coordinated study of chronic bronchitis. Am Rev Respir Dis 108:1043-1065

20. Fletcher C, Peto R (1977) The natural history of chronic airflow obstruction. BMJ 1:1645-1648

21. Kanner RE, Renzetti AD Jr, Klauber MR, Smith CB, Golden CA (1978) Variables associated with changes in spirometry in patients with chronic obstructive lung disease. Am J Med 67:44-50

22. Anthonisen NR, Manfreda J, Warren CPW, Hershfield ES, Harding GKM, Nelson NA (1987) Antibiotic therapy in acute exacerbations of chronic obstructive pulmonary disease. Ann Intern Med 106:196-204

23. Allegra L, Grassi C, Grossi E et al (1991) Ruolo degli antibiotici nel trattamento delle riacutizzazioni della bronchite. Ital J Chest Dis 45:138-148

24. Grossman RF (1997) Guidelines for the treatment of acute exacerbations of chronic bronchitis. Chest 112:S310-S313

25. Grayston JT, Kuo C-C, Wang S-P, Altman J (1986) A new *Chlamydia psittaci* strain, TWAR, isolated in acute respiratory infections. N Engl J Med 315:161-168

26. Grayston JT, Aldous MB, Easton A, Wang S-P, Kuo C-C, Campbell LA, Altman J (1993) Evidence that *Chlamydia pneumoniae* causes pneumonia and bronchitis. J Infect Dis 168:1231-1235

27. Mordhorst CH, Wang S-P, Grayston JT (1992) Outbreak of *Chlamydia pneumoniae* infection in four farm families. Eur J Clin Microbiol Infect Dis 11:617-620

28. Blasi F, Cosentini R, Denti F, Allegra L (1994) Two family outbreaks of *Chlamydia pneumoniae* infections. Eur Respir J 7:102-104

29. Aymard M, Bebear C, Valette M, Lina B, Layani MP, De Barbeyrac B, Orfila J (1997) Rapport basé sur une enquête microbiologique et sur la literature existante. Etiologie virale des rhinopharyngites et otites aigües de l'enfant. Med Mal Infect 27:456-471

30. Mäkelä MJ, Puhakka T, Ruuskanen O, Leinonen M, Saikku P, Kimpimäki M, Blomqvist S, Hyypiä T, Arstila P (1998) Viruses and bacteria in the etiology of common cold. J Clin Microbiol 36:536-542

31. Falck G, Heyman L, Gnarpe J, Gnarpe H (1994) *Chlamydia pneumoniae* (TWAR): a common agent in acute bronchitis. Scand J Infect Dis 26:179-187

32. Thom DH, Grayston JT, Campbell LA, Kuo C-C, Diwan VK, Wang S-P (1994) Respiratory infection with *Chlamydia pneumoniae* in middle-aged and older outpatients. Eur J Microbiol Infect Dis 13:785-792

33. Jonsson JS, Sigurdsson JA, Kristinsson KG, Guthnodottir M, Magnussen S (1997) Acute bronchitis in adults. How close do we come to its aetiology in general practice? Scand J Prim Health Care 15:156-160

34. Vernejoux JM, Texier-Mougin J, Rio P, Guizard AV, Tunon De Lara JM, Taytard A (1997) Bacterial infectious agents implicated in community-acquired lower airway infections. Rev Pneumol Clin 53:138-143

35. Philit F, Etienne J, Calvet A (1992) Agents infectieux associés aux décompensations des bronchopathies chroniques obstructives et aux attaques d'asthme. Rev Mal Respir 9:191-196

36. Beaty C, Grayston JT, Wang S-P, Kuo C-C, Reto CS, Martin TR (1991) *Chlamydia pneumoniae*, strain TWAR, infection in patients with chronic obstructive pulmonary disease. Am Rev Respir Dis 144:1408-1410

37. Blasi F, Legnani D, Lombardo VM, Negretto GG, Magliano E, Pozzoli R, Chiodo F, Fasoli A, Allegra L (1993) *Chlamydia pneumoniae* infection in acute exacerbations of COPD. Eur Respir J 6:19-22

38. Blasi F, Damato S, De Carli A, Cosentini R, Fagetti L, Raccanelli R, Pagani N, Arosio C, Campi E, Allegra L (1996) Evidence suggesting *Chlamydia pneumoniae* chronic infection in COPD. ICAAC, Poster

39. Von Hertzen L, Isoaho R, Koskinen R, Laippala P, Töyrylä M, Kivelä SL, Saikku P (1996) *Chlamydia pneumoniae* antibodies in chronic obstructive pulmonary disease. Int J Epidemiol 25:658-664

40. Von Hertzen L, Alakärppä H, Koskinen R, Liippo K, Surcel HM, Leinonen M, Saikku P (1997) *Chlamydia pneumoniae* infection in patients with chronic obstructive pulmonary disease. Epidemiol Infect 118:155-164

41. Verkooyen RP, Van Lent NA, Mousavi Joulandan SA, Snijder RJ, Van den Bosch JM, Van Helden HP, Verbrugh HA (1997) Diagnosis of *Chlamydia pneumoniae* infection in patients with chronic obstructive pulmonary disease by micro-immunofluorescence and ELISA. J Med Microbiol 46:959-969

42. Thom H, Grayston JT, Wang S-P, Kuo C-C, Altman J (1990) *Chlamydia pneumoniae* strain TWAR, *Mycoplasma pneumoniae* and viral infections in acute respiratory disease in a University Student Health Clinic population. Am J Epidemiol 132:228-256

43. Hahn DL, Saikku P (1995) Serologic evidence for *Chlamydia pneumoniae* infection in recently symtomatic asthma. Am J Respir Crit Care Med 151[Suppl]:A470

44. Kuo C-C, Jackson LA, Campbell LA, Grayston JT (1995) *Chlamydia pneumoniae* (TWAR). Clin Microbiol Rev 8:451-461

45. Laurila AL, Von Hertzen L, Saikku P (1997) *Chlamydia pneumoniae* and chronic lung diseases. Scand J Infect Dis 104[Suppl]:34-36

46. Hammerschlag MR, Chirgwin K, Roblin PM, Gelling M, Dumornay W, Mandel L, Smith P, Schachter J (1992) Persistent infection with *Chlamydia pneumoniae* following acute respiratory illness. Clin Infect Dis 14:178-182

47. Hanna L, Dawsen CR, Briones O, Thygeson P, Jarvetz E (1968) Latency in human infections with TRIC agents. J Immunol 101:43-50

48. Yang YS, Kuo C-C, Chen WJ (1983) Reactivation of *Chlamydia trachomatis* lung infection in mice by cortisone. Infect Immun 39:655-658

49. Batteiger BE, Fraiz J, Newhall WJ, Katz BP, Jones RB (1989) Association of recurrent chlamydial infection with gonorrhoea. J Infect Dis 159:661-669

50. File TM, Bartlett JG, Casell GH, Gaydos CA, Grayston JT, Hammerschlag MR, Jones RB, Kahn JB, Marrie TJ, Ramirez JA, Saikku P, Schachter J, Schumacher HR, Stamm WE, Stratton CW, Yu VL (1997) The importance of *Chlamydia pneumoniae* as a pathogen. The 1996 Consensus Conference on *Chlamydia pneumoniae* Infections. Infect Dis Clin Pract 6:S28-S31

51. Shemer-Avni Y, Lieberman D (1995) *Chlamydia pneumoniae*-induced ciliostasis in ciliated bronchial epithelial cells. J Infect Dis 171:1274-1278

52. Surcel HM, Syriala H, Leinonen M, Herva E (1993) Cell-mediated immunity to *Chlamydia pneumoniae* measured as lymphocyte blast transformation in vitro. Infect Immun 61:2196-2199

53. Pizzichini MMM, Pizzichini E, Efthemiadis A, Clelland L, Mahony JB, Dolovich J, Hargreave JB (1997) Markers of inflammation in induced sputum in acute bronchitis caused by *Chlamydia pneumoniae*. Thorax 52:929-931

54. Dalhoff K, Maass M (1996) *Chlamydia pneumoniae* pneumonia in hospitalized patients. Clinical characteristics and diagnostic value of polymerase chain reaction detection in BAL. Chest 110:351-356

Chlamydia pneumoniae:
A New Threat for HIV-infected Subjects

R. Cosentini, F. Blasi, L. Fagetti

Introduction

The acquired immunodeficiency syndrome (AIDS), caused by the human immu-nodeficiency virus (HIV), commonly presents infection of the lungs caused by respiratory tract pathogens [1]. The incidence of pulmonary infections in HIV-positive patients is higher than in seronegative subjects [2, 3]. The function-al derangements of cell-mediated immunity, phagocytosis and bacterial killing facilitate bacterial infection in HIV-infected patients [4]. The probability of bac-terial pneumonia progressively increases as the CD4+ cell counts drop during the progression of the disease [5].

Bacterial pneumonia caused by intracellular micro-organisms, including *Chlamydia pneumoniae*, may play a relevant epidemiological role in AIDS patients. However, in contrast to the numerous epidemiological studies carried out in the general population, only limited data are available in the literature regarding *C. pneumoniae* infection in immunocompromised subjects [6–13].

Seroprevalence

The potential role of *C. pneumoniae* as a respiratory pathogen in immunocom-promised patients has been recognised. A seroepidemiological study carried out by Blasi et al. [8] in 1993 showed that *C. pneumoniae* seroprevalence in HIV-1-infected subjects was significantly higher than in healthy subjects for both HIV-1 vertically infected children and HIV-1-infected intravenous drug users. Interest-ingly, in the latter group seroprevalence was also significantly higher than in a group of HIV-1-negative intravenous drug users, suggesting that the risk factor for *C. pneumoniae* infection is immunodeficiency rather than life style (Fig. 1). This was confirmed in a further study by Blasi et al. [10], by evaluating *C. pneu-moniae* seroprevalence in a sample population (100/1200 subjects) of a close com-munity of former injection-drug users. In this study the *C. pneumoniae* sero-prevalence was almost twice as high in the HIV-positive compared to HIV-nega-tive subjects.

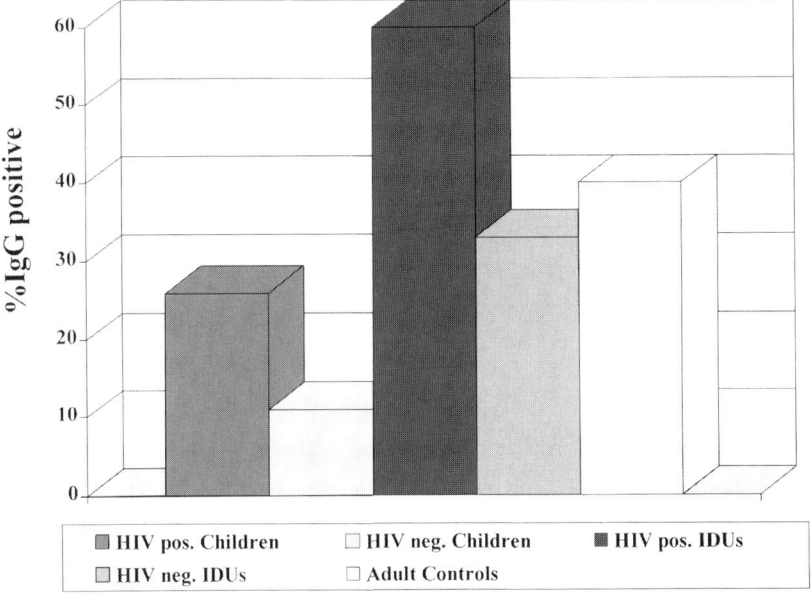

Fig. 1. IgG positivity to *C. pneumoniae* in HIV-positive, HIV-negative, and control subjects. *HIV*, human immunodeficiency virus; *IDUs*, intravenous drug users

However, a recent seroepidemiological study found that *C. pneumoniae* seropositivity was higher in patients with risk factors for HIV infection (particularly injecting drug use and promiscuous heterosexual activity), but the seroprevalence did not significantly differ between HIV-positive and HIV-negative subjects [13].

Incidence of Infection

As far back as 1991 *C. pneumoniae* was isolated by culture in lungs of HIV-infected subjects undergoing fibrebronchoscopy for unexplained pulmonary processes [6] and seroconversion to the agent was demonstrated in an HIV-infected adult patient with pneumonia [7].

Gaydos et al. [9] studied 132 culture-negative bronchoalveolar lavage (BAL) specimens from 108 immunocompromised subjects with radiographically confirmed pulmonary involvement of the disease process. Twelve (11%) of these patients had PCR-EIA-positive specimens. Only two of the 12 infected patients had other microbiological agents implicated in pneumonia. The authors conclude that *C. pneumoniae* should be considered in the evaluation and treatment of pneumonia in immunocompromised patients.

A study carried out on a community of injection-drug users showed that among 210 cases of pneumonia *C. pneumoniae* was the most common pathogen in HIV-negative subjects and third most common pathogen in HIV-positive patients [11]. The authors found that the risk of pneumonia caused by *C. pneumoniae* was three times higher among HIV-positive than HIV-negative subjects. The diagnosis of *C. pneumoniae* was associated with higher CD4 lymphocyte counts than other forms of bacterial infections. This might be due to the fact that diagnosis was reached on the basis of serological testing and that the degree of immunodeficiency alters the predictive value of this type of technique.

Recently, Dalhoff and Maass [12] reported a prospective clinical study on 47 HIV-positive patients, 57 immunocompetent patients with pneumonia and 100 patients with non-infectious bronchopulmonary disorders. In all patients BAL and *C. pneumoniae* culture and DNA detection were performed. The pathogen was frequently detected in the BAL of patients with pneumonia as a sole pathogen. *C. pneumoniae* was detected in 9/57 immunocompetent and in 6/47 immunocompromised patients, whereas no positive results were obtained in the 100 control patients. Coinfections with other organisms were frequent in HIV-positive patients (3/6), but did not occur in the immunocompetent group. Moreover, two of six HIV patients with *Chlamydia* infection had no respiratory symptoms or radiographic abnormalities, and in three, clinical presentation was consistent with the characteristics of the other agents detected. The authors conclude that in the HIV-positive group, the association of *C. pneumoniae* detection and acute pulmonary infection is less clear than in immunocompetent patients, because asymptomatic carriage and isolation of copathogens were found.

Less is known about the role of *C. pneumoniae* in infants and young children. Recent data have shown that this agent is emerging as a common respiratory pathogen also in the paediatric age group [14]. Interestingly, in immunocompetent infants and young children the signs of infection are often localised to the upper respiratory tract [15, 16]. So far, only few studies have addressed the clinical importance of *C. pneumoniae* in immunocompromised children. Blasi et al. [8] have found that HIV-1-infected children seem to be at a higher risk of developing *C. pneumoniae* infection. The same authors recently analysed the rate of antibody seroconversion to *C. pneumoniae* in blood samples of HIV-1-infected and seroreverter children during a 3-year study period [17]. The results of this study showed a high incidence of *C. pneumoniae* infection in HIV-1-infected children. The incidence of *C. pneumoniae* infection appeared to correlate with the degree of immunosuppression and with the viral burden (CD4+ cell count and p24 levels). Conversely, no link was found between the clinical classification of the disease, as assessed by the 1994 CDC guidelines, and seroconversion to *C. pneumoniae*. The incidence of asymptomatic infection was high, suggesting that in immunocompromised children asymptomatic infections are encountered more frequently than symptomatic infections. In HIV-1-infected children anti-*C. pneumoniae* antibody titres generally fell to < 1:16 within 4–6 months of seroconversion. These data confirm the previous report on HIV-1-infected adults [10], suggesting a more immediate drop in antibody titres in HIV-1-infected subjects than in the general population, probably due to impaired antibody synthesis in the immunocompromised host.

Clinical Characteristics

Clinical presentation of *C. pneumoniae* infection in HIV-infected subjects has been described by most authors as similar to that in non-HIV-infected individuals.

Blasi et al. [10] reported an outbreak of *C. pneumoniae* infection in both HIV-infected and non-infected ex-users of injection-drugs. Most of the pneumonia cases recorded in the study occurred in HIV-1-positive patients and the clinical course of pneumonia in these individuals was usually more severe than in non-immunocompromised subjects. It is interesting to note that Boschini et al. [11], in the same community of former injection-drug users, found that the course of *C. pneumoniae* infection was clinically similar in HIV-infected and HIV-non- infected subjects, although the incidence of infection was three times higher in the former than in the latter. A single case of recurrence was observed, and this subject was HIV-infected.

The clinical characteristics of *C. pneumoniae* infection in children appear to differ somewhat from those in adult patients. In a recent report on *C. pneumoniae* infection in HIV-infected children the incidence of asymptomatic infection was high, suggesting that in immunocompromised children asymptomatic infections are encountered more frequently than symptomatic infections [17]. When present, symptoms were generally mild and often disappeared without therapy. Pneumonia was diagnosed in only one case. These observations are in agreement with other studies showing that moderate disease occurs more often in younger children than in older populations [15, 16].

Conclusions

The role of *C. pneumoniae* infection in immunocompromised patients was suggested on the basis of seroepidemiological evidence of a higher prevalence of seropositivity towards this agent in HIV-1-infected subjects than in non-HIV-infected individuals. Seroconversion towards *C. pneumoniae* has been described in HIV-infected adult patients with pneumonia and the agent has also been identified, by both culture and PCR, in BAL fluid of HIV-positive patients with lung infiltrates. A high incidence of *C. pneumoniae* infection has also been described in immunocompromised children, although in this population the infection often appears to be asymptomatic.

However, the most intriguing question is whether this intracellular pathogen could affect the natural history of HIV-1 infection. As yet little is known on whether *C. pneumoniae* interacts with the HIV-1 virus within an infected organism, on the possibility of chronic infection with this organism in immunocompromised hosts, and on the importance of treatment of *C. pneumoniae* infection for the clinical progression of AIDS. Further epidemiological, clinical and laboratory studies are needed to address these interesting topics.

References

1. Fauci AS (1988) The human immunodeficiency virus: infectivity and mechanisms of pathogenesis. Science 239:617-622
2. Polsky B, Gold JWM, Whinbey E et al (1986) Bacterial pneumonia in patients with the acquired immunodeficiency syndrome. Ann Intern Med 104:38-41
3. Witt DJ, Craven DE, McCabe WR (1987) Bacterial infections in adult patients with acquired immunodeficiency syndrome (AIDS) and AIDS-related complex. Am J Med 82:900-906
4. Cohn DL (1991) Bacterial pneumonia in the HIV-infected patient. Infect Dis Clin North Am 5:485-507
5. Noskin GA, Glassroth J (1995) Pulmonary infections in HIV-1 infected patients. In: Semenzato G (ed) AIDS and the lung. European Respiratory Monograph, European Respiratory Society Journal Ltd, Sheffield, pp 255-287
6. Augenbraun MH, Roblin MR, Chirwing K et al (1991) Isolation of *Chlamydia pneumoniae* from lungs of patients infected with the human immunodeficiency virus. J Clin Microbiol 29:401-402
7. Clark R, Mushatt D, Fazal B (1991) Case report: *Chlamydia pneumoniae* pneumonia in HIV-infected man. Eur J Med Sci 302(3):155-156
8. Blasi F, Cosentini R, Clerici Schoeller M et al (1993) *Chlamydia pneumoniae* seroprevalence in immunocompetent and immunocompromised populations in Milan. Thorax 48:1261-1263
9. Gaydos CA, Flower CL, Gill BJ et al (1993) Detection of *Chlamydia pneumoniae* by polymerase chain reaction–enzyme immunoassay in an immunocompromised population. Clin Infect Dis 17:718-723
10. Blasi F, Boschini A, Cosentini R et al (1994) Outbreak of *Chlamydia pneumoniae* infection in an ex injection-drug users community. Chest 105:812-815
11. Boschini A, Smacchia C, Di Fine M et al (1996) Community acquired pneumonia in a cohort of former injection-drug users with and without human immunodeficiency virus infection: incidence, etiologies and clinical aspects. Clin Infect Dis 23:107-113
12. Dalhoff K, Maass M (1996) *Chlamydia pneumoniae* pneumonia in hospitalised patients. Chest 110:351-356
13. Visco Comandini U, Massetti AP, Marchese R et al (1996) *Chlamydia pneumoniae* seroprevalence among HIV-1-infected and uninfected people with known HIV risk factor. AIDS 10:1543-1547
14. Grayston JT (1994) *Chlamydia pneumoniae* (TWAR) infections in children. Pediatr Infect Dis J 13:675-685
15. Falck G, Gnarpe J, Gnarpe H (1997) Prevalence of *Chlamydia pneumoniae* in healthy children and in children with respiratory tract infections. Pediatr Infect Dis J 16:549-554
16. Normann E, Gnarpe J, Gnarpe H, Wettergren B (1998) *Chlamydia pneumoniae* in children with acute respiratory tract infections. Acta Paediatr 87:23-27
17. Cosentini R, Esposito S, Blasi F et al (1998) Incidence of *Chlamydia pneumoniae* infection in vertically HIV-1-infected children. Eur J Clin Microbiol Infect Dis 17:720-723

Chlamydia pneumoniae: Epidemiology of a New Cardiovascular Risk Factor

F. Blasi, R. Cosentini, P. Tarsia

Introduction

In recent decades the understanding of lipid metabolism derangement (hyper-cholesterolaemia and decreased high-density lipoprotein cholesterol) together with tighter control of hypertension, diabetes and smoking habits have led to a substantial decrease in coronary heart disease (CHD) and stroke mortality [1]. Nonetheless, the above risk factors (together with age, gender and family history) are felt to account for approximately 50%–70% of the pathogenesis of cardiovascular diseases [2, 3]. Therefore, scientific attention has recently focused on investigating hypothetical additional risk factors and on a fuller understanding of the development of atherosclerosis, the main pathological process involved in CHD.

Infectious Theory for Atherosclerosis

The inflammatory nature of early atherosclerotic lesions [4, 5], the acute plaque rupture in sites of intense inflammatory infiltration [6], the greater risk of death from cardiovascular disease during and after influenza epidemics or following bacterial infection [7, 8] and the induction of procoagulant activities following infection of endothelial cells or exposure to proinflammatory cytokines [9] all suggest a possible role of infection and inflammation in the pathogenesis of atherosclerosis. The modern "response to injury" model of atherosclerosis recognises that infection may initiate and perpetuate endothelial damage, upon which metabolic, inflammatory, or haemostatic factors may then intervene [4].

The infectious theory for atherosclerosis was first put forward in 1908 by Osler [10]. However, in contrast to Anitschkow's 1913 observations on high-cholesterol diets and atherosclerotic lesions in a rabbit model [11], which were rapidly taken up and gradually expanded, acceptance of Osler's theory was limited during the next two decades [12, 13], and it was generally disregarded until fairly recently.

Viruses and Atherosclerosis

Observations carried out in the late 1970s initially focused attention on viral agents as putative factors in the development of atherosclerosis. Fabricant et al. [14] showed that a herpes-type DNA virus was capable of inducing vascular lesions in chicken closely resembling those of atherosclerosis in humans.

Seroepidemiological studies in humans found a higher prevalence of antibodies to cytomegalovirus (CMV) among patients with atherosclerotic lesions needing vascular surgery than in hyperlipidaemic controls [15]. CMV-specific nucleic acid sequences have been found in advanced stage atherosclerotic plaques by in situ hybridisation (ISH) [16], and by PCR [17]. Viral elements were identified in atheromatous tissue by electron microscopy (EM) [18], and CMV was shown to promote atherosclerosis in a rat model [19]. In addition to involvement in advanced stages of the disease, CMV and herpes simplex virus (HSV) have also been detected in early atherosclerotic lesions of young asymptomatic patients [20]. Earlier studies on HSV had revealed viral mRNA in arterial walls of patients undergoing coronary bypass surgery [21] and demonstrated infection of human endothelial cells [22].

Bacteria and Atherosclerosis

Bacterial involvement in atherosclerosis was first suggested by the finding that coronary artery intimal thickening may be present in pneumonia [23] and other bacterial infections [24]. Dental bacterial infections (caries and periodontal disease) are a source of chronic infection and have been associated with CHD [25].

Helicobacter pylori infection has recently been recognised as the prime cause of peptic ulcers. Features in common between the epidemiology of peptic ulceration and CHD have prompted seroepidemiological studies to test the association between infection with this agent and cardiovascular diseases. Case-control and cross-sectional studies showed that seropositivity to *H. pylori* is a risk factor for CHD [26–28]. It was also suggested that *H. pylori* infection may increase C-reactive protein (CRP) and fibrinogen levels [27], both factors being associated with cardiovascular diseases [29, 30]. However, a recent prospective cross-sectional analysis failed to associate *H. pylori* seropositivity with cardiovascular diseases in a population of 624 elderly subjects [31]. Likewise, in a study on healthy subjects no link was found between *H. pylori* infection and increased concentrations of fibrinogen or other haemostatic factors, which does not support the possibility of infection inducing a tendency towards a procoagulant state [32]. *H. pylori* genomic material was identified in coronary arteries of myocardial infarction cases at autopsy in one series [33] but this finding was not confirmed in aortic aneurysm atherosclerotic plaques [34].

Chlamydia pneumoniae and Atherosclerosis

Convincing evidence has now been put forward that *Chlamydia pneumoniae* is also associated with atherosclerosis and acute cardiovascular events. This evidence rests on seroepidemiological data, identification of genomic material by PCR, immunocytochemistry (ICC), ISH, EM and culture.

Seroepidemiological Evidence (Table 1)

In 1988 Saikku et al. [35] performed a serological study on 40 male patients with acute myocardial infarction (AMI), 30 male patients with chronic CHD and 41 matched controls. Elevated levels of *C. pneumoniae* specific antibodies or immune complexes containing chlamydial lipopolysaccharide (LPS) were observed in 50%–60% of patients with acute myocardial infarction and chronic CHD but in only 7%–12% of controls. Using micro-immunofluorescence, high, stable IgG and IgA titres were observed, with no seroconversion and no IgM antibody response. This suggests a chronic *C. pneumoniae* infection in the AMI and chronic coronary disease groups. Conversely, a significant seroconversion in enzyme immunoassay with LPS antigen was present in AMI patients, but absent in the other two groups. It was therefore suggested that some AMI cases may be associated with acute exacerbation of a chronic *C. pneumoniae* infection. Leinonen et al. [36] showed that immune complexes containing chlamydial LPS were found more commonly in 44 men and women with myocardial infarction than in 44 control subjects.

Saikku's Finnish group then extended their observations to patients participating in the Helsinki Heart Study, a large prospective study on hypercholesterolaemic patients [37]. Sera of 103 patients obtained 3–6 months prior to a cardiac event were matched with those from controls. Raised IgA (but not IgG) titres against *C. pneumoniae* and the presence of immune complexes containing *C. pneumoniae* LPS antigen were associated with an increased risk of developing a cardiac event 6 months later. These associations were independent of age, hypertension and smoking.

Thom et al. studied patients with angiographically demonstrated CHD and compared their *C. pneumoniae* antibody titres with angiographically negative patients [38] and later with normal population control subjects [39]. These studies showed that the risk of CHD was greater among subjects with high antibody titres to *C. pneumoniae* than among subjects with low titres and that the risk was particularly great for coronary artery disease with five or more lesions.

Linnanmäki et al. [40] also evaluated patients with angiographically demonstrated CHD, comparing them with random control subjects in terms of serological evidence of immune complexes containing *C. pneumoniae* LPS. Immune complexes were more common in coronary disease patients than in controls. In this paper an antibody in the protein-specific immune complexes was shown to be specific for *C. pneumoniae* both in the serological testing and by immunoblot.

Table 1. Main findings of seroepidemiological studies on the association between *C. pneumoniae* and atherosclerosis

First author, year of study [reference]	Results
Saikku, 1988 [35]	Significantly higher antibody titres and immune complexes containing *C. pneumoniae* LPS in AMI and CHD patients than in controls
Leinonen, 1990 [36]	Chlamydial LPS-containing immune complexes found more commonly in AMI patients than in controls
Saikku, 1992 [37]	Raised IgA or immune complexes containing *C. pneumoniae* LPS in hypercholesterolaemic patients associated with increased risk of cardiac events
Thom, 1991 [38]	Higher *C. pneumoniae* antibody titres in angiographically demonstrated CHD patients than in angiographically negative subjects
Thom, 1992 [39]	Higher *C. pneumoniae* antibody titres in angiographically demonstrated CHD patients than in normal population control subjects
Linnanmäki, 1993 [40]	Immune complexes containing *C. pneumoniae* LPS more common in angiographically demonstrated CHD than in controls
Melnick, 1993 [41]	Association between antibody titre to *C. pneumoniae* and asymptomatic carotid artery atherosclerosis
Dahlen, 1995 [42]	High *C. pneumoniae* IgG titres associated with early CHD
Mendall, 1995 [43]	*C. pneumoniae* IgG titre > 1:64 independent risk factor for CHD
Miettinen, 1996 [44]	Association between *C. pneumoniae* antibodies and CHD events in nondiabetics, but not in diabetic patients
Carlsson, 1997 [45]	No association between *C. pneumoniae* antibody status and restenosis following PTCA
Laurila, 1997 [46]	High *C. pneumoniae* antibody titres associated with higher triglyceride and lower high-density lipoprotein levels
Blasi, 1997 [47]	*C. pneumoniae* reinfection serological pattern associated with AMI onset
Cook, 1998 [48]	*C. pneumoniae* antibody titres associated with stroke/TIA
Cook, 1998 [49]	Association between *C. pneumoniae* antibody titres and severe essential hypertension

LPS, lipopolysaccharide; *AMI*, acute myocardial infarction; *CHD*, coronary heart disease; *PTCA*, percutaneous transluminal coronary angioplasty; *TIA*, transient ischaemic attack

In 1993 an association between antibody titres to *C. pneumoniae* consistent with past infection and asymptomatic carotid atherosclerosis, as determined by carotid ultrasonography, was found by Melnick et al. [41].

A Swedish study carried out the following year showed that the combination of male sex, certain HLA class II DR genotypes 13a or 17, high lipoprotein (a) levels, and high *C. pneumoniae* IgG antibody titres were strongly associated with angiographically confirmed coronary artery disease [42]. This study indicates that both genetic and infectious factors may be involved in *C. pneumoniae*-associated atherosclerosis.

Mendall et al. [43] conducted a study on *C. pneumoniae* seroprevalence in association with various risk factors in CHD patients and controls attending a general practice health screening clinic in England. *C. pneumoniae* IgG titre > 1:64 was found to be an independent risk factor for CHD.

Most seroepidemiological studies linking *C. pneumoniae* seropositivity and atherosclerosis have been performed on predominantly nondiabetic patients. In view of the fact that diabetic patients are more prone to infection than nondiabetic subjects, Miettinen et al. [44] prospectively evaluated *C. pneumoniae* antibody titres in diabetic and nondiabetic patients to evaluate the effect of this disease on the association between chlamydial infection and atherosclerosis. The risk of serious CHD events was evaluated in the two patient populations. The authors found that elevated baseline *C. pneumoniae* antibody titres were associated with coronary heart events during follow-up in nondiabetic subjects but not in diabetic subjects. The reasons for this finding are not known, but the authors suggested that diabetes is so strong a risk factor that it could mask the effects of weaker risk factors.

Carlsson et al. [45] evaluated the serological pattern of *C. pneumoniae* and CMV antibodies in patients undergoing percutaneous transluminal coronary angioplasty (PTCA). Serology was repeated 6 months after PTCA during a follow-up angiography to test for restenosis. The authors found that *C. pneumoniae* or CMV seropositivity do not appear to be risk factors in the development of restenosis.

It is known that acute infections may interfere with lipid metabolism by increasing triglyceride levels and decreasing high-density lipoprotein cholesterol concentrations. A recent Finnish study investigated the association between *C. pneumoniae* antibodies and serum lipid profile in a population of healthy subjects [46]. High *C. pneumoniae* antibody titres were found to be associated with higher triglyceride and lower high-density lipoprotein levels.

Blasi et al. investigated the possible association between *C. pneumoniae* infection and the onset of myocardial infarction [47]. Further demonstration of the possible role of *C. pneumoniae* chronic infection in the development of CHD was obtained in this study, and the results suggested that an acute infection superimposed on a chronic or latent infection may trigger the onset of myocardial infarction.

Davidson et al. [50] performed a retrospective investigation on premortem serum specimens and autopsy tissues from 60 indigenous Alaska natives. The authors found serological evidence that *C. pneumoniae* infection frequently precedes both the earliest and more advanced lesions of coronary atherosclerosis harbouring this intracellular pathogen.

An association between chlamydial infection and cerebrovascular disease was first suggested by Wimmer et al. [51]. Cook et al. recently confirmed these findings by demonstrating an association between antibody titres to *C. pneumoniae* and acute stroke and transient cerebral ischaemia [48], and severe essential hypertension [49].

During this decade, investigators have linked the increase of serum proteins, such as fibrinogen and CRP, with CHD [29, 30], and these inflammatory mediators may be considered important prognostic indicators of angina. Patel et al. [27] have shown that seropositivity to both *C. pneumoniae* and *H. pylori* is associated with raised fibrinogen levels, which may provide a link between chronic infection and CHD. The association was further confirmed by Toss et al. [52], who found that persistent high *C. pneumoniae* IgA antibody titres are associated with increased fibrinogen levels in patients with unstable CHD. In a recent study Anderson et al. [53] evaluated CRP levels in patients with stable CHD and previous myocardial infarction. The patients were also tested for antibody titre determinations to *C. pneumoniae*, *H. pylori* and CMV. Subjects seropositive to both *C. pneumoniae* and *H. pylori* had an increased prevalence of CHD and myocardial infarction and tended to have higher CRP levels.

Taken together, the above seroepidemiological data seem to indicate an association between *C. pneumoniae* and atherosclerosis. However, these serological studies have been criticised for occasional borderline statistical significance, lack of standardisation of the technique employed for antibody detection and inadequacy of control groups, which are mostly not representative samples of the general population (blood donors, angiographically negative patients etc.). It may be that high *C. pneumoniae* antibody titres simply reflect antigenic cross-reactivity rather than active or past infection. Moreover, occasional reports of a negative association between chlamydial infection and atherosclerosis have appeared [54, 55]. A study by Hahn and Golubjatnikov [56] suggested that cigarette smoking, a risk factor present in most CHD patients, apparently increases the likelihood of *C. pneumoniae* infection. Thus, smoking may act as a confounder of the *C. pneumoniae*–coronary artery disease association. Although the authors suggested that controlling for smoking may have eliminated the association reported in earlier works, confounding risk factors (including smoking) were discounted by statistical methods in later epidemiological studies.

The overall impression, however, is that some degree of association between cardiovascular diseases and high *C. pneumoniae* antibody titres (or immune complexes) has been found repeatedly with different techniques in different laboratories. The studies apply to many different aspects of cardiovascular disease (pre- and post-myocardial infarction, severe hypertension, asymptomatic carotid atherosclerosis, stroke, and TIAs). In the words of Grayston et al., "The sum of the studies is more powerful than any of the parts"[57].

Direct Identification in Atherosclerotic Plaques

So as to accumulate more convincing evidence of the involvement of *C. pneumoniae* infection in atherogenesis, numerous authors have attempted to demonstrate the presence of this organism, or any of its components, in atheromatous tissues (Table 2).

Table 2. Studies on direct identification of *C. pneumoniae* in atheromatous tissues

First author, year of study [reference]	Anatomical site	Method of detection	Proportion of positive specimens
Shor, 1992 [58]	Coronary artery	EM, ICC	5/7
Kuo, 1993 [59]	Coronary artery	EM, ICC, PCR	20/36
Campbell, 1995 [60]	Coronary artery	EM, ICC, PCR	20/38
Kuo, 1995 [61]	Coronary artery	ICC, PCR	8/51
Muhlestein, 1996 [62]	Coronary artery	IMF	66/90
Weiss, 1996 [54]	Coronary artery	EM, PCR	1/58
Ramirez, 1996 [63]	Coronary artery	Culture, EM, ICC,ISH, PCR	7/12
Maass, 1998 [64]	Coronary artery	Culture, PCR	21/70
Kuo, 1993 [65]	Aorta	ICC	7/21
Blasi, 1996 [34]	Aorta	PCR	26/51
Juvonen, 1997 [66]	Aorta	EM, ICC, PCR	12/12
Grayston, 1995 [67]	Carotid artery	ICC, PCR	37/61
Chiu, 1997 [68]	Carotid artery	ICC, IMF	54/76
Yamashita, 1998 [69]	Carotid artery	ICC	11/20
Jackson, 1996 [70]	Carotid artery	Culture, EM, ICC	1/1
Boman, 1998 [71]	Peripheral blood cells	PCR	60/101

EM, electron microscopy; *ICC*, immunocytochemistry; *PCR*, polymerase chain reaction; *ISH*, in situ hybridisation; *IMF*, immunofluorescence

Coronary Artery

The first report in this field was published by Shor et al. in 1992 [58]. The authors observed *C. pneumoniae* elementary bodies (pear-shaped organisms) in coronary artery fatty streaks and atheromatous plaques in ten South African autopsy cases. In seven of these cases there was sufficient material to perform immunoperoxidase staining to detect *C. pneumoniae* species-specific monoclonal antibodies. The immunocytochemical positivity in five of seven cases suggested that the structures observed on electron microscopy were indeed *C. pneumoniae*.

Later work by Kuo et al., also performed on South African autopsy specimens, expanded the number of diagnostic techniques employed for identification of this micro-organism in coronary atherosclerotic lesions [59]. In this study a PCR was employed for the amplification of a *C. pneumoniae*-specific DNA sequence, in addition to culture, serology, EM and ICC. Overall, roughly half of the specimens tested were positive by at least one of the techniques. Culture was the only diagnostic technique to give uniformly negative results in all samples tested. A 1995 study by Campbell et al. [60] employed EM, PCR and ICC to detect *C. pneumoniae* in coronary atherectomy tissues. In addition to demonstration of the agent, this study showed a trend toward a more common occurrence of *C. pneumoniae* in restenosis (following angioplasty) lesions than in native lesions.

The same group [61] failed to detect *C. pneumoniae* in nonatherosclerotic areas of arteries in young subjects (age 15–34 years), suggesting that *C. pneumoniae* is more likely to be associated with atherosclerotic plaques than with healthy tissue.

This finding was later confirmed by Muhlestein et al. [62] in a prospective study on the different incidence of *C. pneumoniae* within coronary arteries of patients with atherosclerosis compared to other forms of cardiovascular disease. The authors found an extremely high rate of infection in patients with symptomatic atherosclerosis compared to a very low rate in patients with normal coronary arteries or coronary artery disease from chronic transplant rejection. This indicates that *C. pneumoniae* is specifically present in atherosclerotic lesions and not in arteries diseased by processes other than atherosclerosis. In contrast, Weiss et al. [54] were able to detect *C. pneumoniae* by culture, EM or PCR in only one of 50 specimens of coronary atheromas.

In 1996 Ramirez et al. [63] were the first to successfully culture *C. pneumoniae* from atherosclerotic plaques of a patient undergoing heart transplantation for CHD. In addition, the microrganism was identified by PCR, ICC, EM and ISH. This study provides direct evidence that viable *C. pneumoniae* is present within atheromatous tissue. A recent study by Maass et al. [64], using culture and PCR, confirmed that a significant proportion of atherosclerotic coronary arteries harbour viable *C. pneumoniae*.

Aorta

Following the identification of *C. pneumoniae* in coronary arteries, other arterial districts were investigated for the presence of bacterial elements. Kuo et al. [65] first documented *C. pneumoniae* in aortic lesions by ICC. The organism was found in both macrophages and smooth-muscle cells.

In a later study, Blasi et al. [34] found *C. pneumoniae*-specific DNA in a significant number of aortic aneurysm atherosclerotic plaques. In the same study the authors failed to identify *H. pylori* in the aortic specimens, ruling out the possibility of direct involvement of the latter pathogen in atherosclerosis. Juvonen et al. [66] confirmed the presence of *C. pneumoniae* components in macrophages located in abdominal aorta aneurysms and in smooth muscle cells beneath the plaques. Identification was obtained by PCR, EM and ICC. The organism was not found in healthy arterial tissue specimens.

Carotid Artery

The presence of *C. pneumoniae* in carotid artery specimens was first explored by Grayston et al. [67] in 1995. Immunocytochemical staining and PCR were performed on five patients undergoing carotid artery surgery and on formalin-fixed tissues from previous carotid endarterectomies. *C. pneumoniae* was frequently present in the atherosclerotic plaques. These results were confirmed by Chiu et al., who found immunocytochemical evidence of the presence of CMV, HSV, and *C. pneumoniae* in carotid endarterectomy specimens [68]. Interestingly, in 77.6% of the diseased arteries at least one micro-organism was detectable and 23.7% of the vessels had two micro-organisms. *C. pneumoniae* was the most commonly detected agent (71% of cases). A further finding was that atherosclerotic plaques with thrombosis were more likely to harbour micro-organisms, suggesting that the presence of infectious agents may predispose to a greater risk of thrombosis. A further immunohistochemical study documented *C. pneumoniae* infection in endothelial cells, macrophages and smooth muscle cells (within and underlying atherosclerotic plaques) in carotid endarterectomy specimens [69].

In 1997 Jackson et al. [70] reported cultural isolation of *C. pneumoniae* from a prospectively obtained carotid endarterectomy specimen. The organism appeared identical to other *C. pneumoniae* isolates by EM morphology, reactivity to species-specific monoclonal antibodies and hybridisation analysis.

In a recent study Boman et al. [71] evaluated the utility of PCR detection of *C. pneumoniae*-specific DNA in peripheral blood mononuclear cells. They found that carriage of circulating *C. pneumoniae*-specific DNA is common both in patients with CHD and in middle-aged blood donors. This technique may be useful in identifying *C. pneumoniae* carriers and as a means of monitoring response to treatment.

Conclusions

Analysing the above studies, it may be inferred that *C. pneumoniae* has been identified in roughly 50% of atheromatous lesions and in only 5% of control samples of arterial tissue. *C. pneumoniae* has been shown to infect and replicate within smooth muscle cells, endothelial cells and macrophages, all of which participate in the development of atherosclerosis as postulated by the "response to injury" theory [2]. This is, however, insufficient to demonstrate a causal relationship between presence of the bacterium and onset or progression of atherosclerosis. It has been suggested that *C. pneumoniae* may act as an "innocent bystander" within atherosclerotic plaques. Macrophages may ingest the micro-organism in the respiratory tract before migrating towards atheromatous lesions. In this situation *C. pneumoniae* may simply thrive within the macrophages without causing harmful effects, thus rendering the association between its presence and atherosclerotic lesions purely coincidental.

Unequivocal demonstration of an aetiological role of *C. pneumoniae* infection in atherosclerosis requires, in accordance to Koch's postulates, induction of atheromatous lesions in animal models following inoculation of the micro-organism and a reduction in cardiovascular events following eradication of the agent with antibiotic treatment. A full and updated description of animal models and intervention trials in *C. pneumoniae*-induced atherosclerosis are reported elsewhere in this book.

References

1. Braunwald E (1997) Shattuck Lecture–Cardiovascular medicine at the turn of the millenium: triumphs, concerns, and opportunities. N Engl J Med 337:1360-1369
2. Solberg LA, Enger SC, Hjermann I et al (1980) Risk factors for coronary and cerebral atherosclerosis in the Oslo study. In: Giotto AM, Smith LC, Allen B (eds) Atherosclerosis. Springer, Berlin Heidelberg New York, pp 57-62
3. Beneditt EP, Gown AM (1980) Atheroma: the arterial wall and the environment. Int Rev Exp Pathol 21:55-118
4. Ross R (1993) The pathogenesis of atherosclerosis: a perspective for the 1990s. Nature 362:801-809
5. Entman ML, Ballantyne CM (1993) Inflammation in acute coronary syndromes. Circulation 88:800-803
6. van der Wal AC, Becker AE, van del Loos CM et al (1994) Site of intimal rupture or erosion of thrombosed coronary atherosclerotic plaques is characterized by an inflammatory process irrespective of the dominant plaque morphology. Circulation 89:36-44
7. Tillett HE, Smith JW, Gooch CD (1983) Excess deaths attributed to influenza in England and Wales: age at death and certified cause. Int J Epidemiol 12:344-352
8. Valtonen V, Kuikka A, Syrjanen J (1993) Thrombo-embolic complications in bacteriaemic infections. Eur Heart J 14:20-23
9. Friedman HM (1989) Infection of endothelial cells by common human viruses. Rev Infect Dis 11:5700-5704
10. Osler W (1908) Diseases of the arteries. In: Osler W (ed) Modern medicine: its practice and theory. Lea & Febiger, Philadelphia, pp 429-447
11. Anitschkow N (1913) Über die Wandänderungen der Kaninchenaorta bei experimenteller Cholesterinsteatose. Beitr Pathol Anat Allg Pathol 56:379-404
12. Frothingham C (1911) The relation between acute infectious diseases and arterial lesions. Arch Intern Med 8:153-162
13. Ophülus W (1921) Arteriosclerosis and cardiovascular disease: their relation to infectious diseases. JAMA 76:700-701
14. Fabricant CG, Fabricant J, Litrenta MM et al (1978) Virus-induced atherosclerosis. J Exp Med 148:335-340
15. Adam E, Melnick JL, Probstfield JL et al (1987) High levels of cytomegalovirus antibody in patients requiring vascular surgery for atherosclerosis. Lancet 2:291-293
16. Petrie BL, Melnick JL, Adam E et al (1987) Nucleic acid sequence of cytomegalovirus in cells cultured from human arterial tissue. J Infect Dis 155:158-159
17. Hendricks MGR, Salimens MMM, Vauboven CPA et al (1990) High prevalence of latently present cytomegalovirus in arterial walls of patients suffering from grade III atherosclerosis. Am J Pathol 136:23-28

18. Gyorkey F, Melnick JL, Guinn GA et al (1984) Herpesviridae in the endothelial and smooth muscle cells of the proximal aorta of atherosclerosis patients. Exp Mol Pathol 40:328-339
19. Span AHM, Grauls G, Bosman F et al (1992) Cytomegalovirus infection induces vascular injury in the rat. Atherosclerosis 92:41-52
20. Yamashiroya HM, Ghosh L, Yang R et al (1988) Herpesviridae in the coronary arteries and aorta of young trauma victims. Am J Pathol 130:71-79
21. Benditt EP, Barrett T, McDougall JK (1983) Viruses in the etiology of atherosclerosis. Proc Natl Acad Sci USA 80:6386-6389
22. Friedman HM, Macarak EJ, MacGregor RR et al (1981) Virus infection of endothelial cells. J Infect Dis 143:266-273
23. Minkowski WL (1947) The coronary arteries of infants. Am J Med Sci 214:623-629
24. Pesonen E, Siitonen O (1981) Acute myocardial infarction precipitated by infectious disease. Am Heart J 101:512-513
25. Mattila KJ, Valle MS, Nieminen MS et al (1993) Dental infections and coronary atherosclerosis. Atherosclerosis 103:205-211
26. Mendall M, Gogin P, Levy J et al (1994) Relation of *Helicobacter pylori* infection and coronary heart disease. Br Heart J 71:437-439
27. Patel P, Mendall MA, Carrington D et al (1995) Association of *Helicobacter pylori* and *Chlamydia pneumoniae* infections with coronary heart disease and cardiovascular risk factors. BMJ 31:711-714
28. Murray LJ, Bamford KB, O'Reilly DPJ et al (1995) *Helicobacter pylori* infection: relation with cardiovascular risk factors, ischemic heart disease, and social class. Br Heart J 74:497-501
29. Liuzzo G, Luigi M, Biasucci L et al (1994) The prognostic value of C-reactive protein and serum amyloid A protein in severe unstable angina. N Engl J Med 331:417-424
30. Yarnell JWG, Baker JA, Sweetman PM et al (1991) Fibrinogen, viscosity and white blood cell count are major risk factors for ischemic heart disease. Circulation 83:836-844
31. Strandberg TE, Tilvis RS, Vuoristo M et al (1997) Prospective study of *Helicobacter pylori* seropositivity and cardiovascular diseases in a general elderly population. BMJ 314:1317-1318
32. Parente F, Maconi G, Imbesi V et al (1997) *Helicobacter pylori* infection and coagulation in healthy people. BMJ 314:1318-1319
33. Cunningham A, Ward M, Matthews R et al (1996) *Helicobacter pylori* and *Chlamydia pneumoniae* in tissues of myocardial infarction cases. 1st European Congress of Chemotherapy, Glasgow, abstract W149
34. Blasi F, Denti F, Erba M et al (1996) Detection of *Chlamydia pneumoniae* and not of *Helicobacter pylori* in atherosclerotic plaques of aortic aneurysms. J Clin Microbiol 34:2766-2769
35. Saikku P, Leinonen M, Mattila K et al (1988) Serological evidence of an association of a novel Chlamydia, TWAR, with chronic coronary heart disease and acute myocardial infarction. Lancet ii:983-986
36. Leinonen M, Linnanmäki E, Mattila K et al (1990) Circulating immune complexes containing chlamydial lipopolysaccharide in acute myocardial infarction. Microb Pathog 9:67-73
37. Saikku P, Leinonen M, Tenkanen L et al (1992) Chronic *Chlamydia pneumoniae* infection as a risk factor for coronary heart disease in the Helsinki Heart Study. Ann Intern Med 116:273-278

38. Thom DH, Wang SP, Grayston JT et al (1991) *Chlamydia pneumoniae* strain TWAR antibody and angiographically demonstrated coronary artery disease. Arterioscler Thromb 11:547-551

39. Thom DH, Grayston JT, Siscovick DS et al (1992) Association of prior infection with *Chlamydia pneumoniae* and angiographically demonstrated coronary artery disease. JAMA 268:68-72

40. Linnanmäki E, Leinonen M, Mattila K et al (1993) *Chlamydia pneumoniae*-specific circulating immune complexes in patients with chronic coronary artery disease. Circulation 87:1130-1134

41. Melnick SL, Sharar E, Folsom AR et al (1993) Past infection by *Chlamydia pneumoniae* strain TWAR and asymptomatic carotid atherosclerosis. Am J Med 95:499-504

42. Dahlen GH, Boman J, Birgander LS, Lindblom B (1995) Lp(a) lipoprotein, IgG, IgA, and IgM antibodies to *Chlamydia pneumoniae* and HLA class II genotype in early coronary artery disease. Atherosclerosis 114:165-174

43. Mendall MA, Carrington D, Strachan D et al (1995) *Chlamydia pneumoniae*: risk factors for seropositivity and association with coronary heart disease. J Infect 30:121-128

44. Miettinen H, Lehto S, Saikku P et al (1996) Association of *Chlamydia pneumoniae* and acute coronary heart disease events in non-insulin dependent diabetics and non-diabetic subjects in Finland. Eur Heart J 17:682-688

45. Carlsson J, Miketic S, Muller KH et al (1997) Previous cytomegalovirus or *Chlamydia pneumoniae* infection and risk of restenosis after percutaneous transluminal coronary angioplasty. Lancet 350:1225 (letter)

46. Laurila A, Bloigu A, Näyhä S et al (1997) *Chlamydia pneumoniae* antibodies and serum lipids in Finnish men: cross sectional study. BMJ 314:1456-1457

47. Blasi F, Cosentini R, Raccanelli R et al (1997) A possible association of *Chlamydia pneumoniae* infection and acute myocardial infarction in patients younger than 65 years of age. Chest 112:309-312

48. Cook PJ, Honeybourne D, Lip GYH et al (1998) *Chlamydia pneumoniae* antibody titres are significantly associated with acute stroke and transient cerebral ischemia. Stroke 29:404-410

49. Cook PJ, Lip GYH, Davies P et al (1998) *Chlamydia pneumoniae* antibodies in severe essential hypertension. Hypertension 31:589-594

50. Davidson M, Kuo C-C, Middaugh GP et al (1998) Confirmed previous infection with *Chlamydia pneumoniae* (TWAR) and its presence in early coronary atherosclerosis. Circulation 98:628-633

51. Wimmer MLJ, Sandmannstrupp R, Saikku P et al (1996) Association of chlamydial infection with cerebrovascular disease. Stroke 27:2207-2210

52. Toss H, Gnarpe J, Gnarpe H et al (1998) Increased fibrinogen levels are associated with persistent *Chlamydia pneumoniae* infection in unstable coronary artery disease. Eur Heart J 19:570-577

53. Anderson JL, Carlquist JF, Muhlestein JB et al (1998) Evaluation of C-reactive protein, an inflammatory marker, and infectious serology as risk factors for coronary artery disease and myocardial infarction. J Am Coll Cardiol 32:35-41

54. Weiss SM, Roblin PM, Gaydos CA et al (1996) Failure to detect *Chlamydia pneumoniae* in coronary atheromas of patients undergoing atherectomy. J Infect Dis 173:957-962

55. Kark JD, Leinonen M, Paltiel O et al (1997) *Chlamydia pneumoniae* and acute myocardial infarction in Jerusalem. Int J Epidemiol 26:730-738

56. Hahn DL, Golubjatnikov R (1992) Smoking is a potential confounder of the *Chlamydia pneumoniae* - coronary artery disease association. Arterioscler Thromb 12:945-947

57. Grayston JT, Kuo C-C, Campbell A, Beneditt EP (1993) *Chlamydia pneumoniae*, strain TWAR and atherosclerosis. Eur Heart J 14:66-71
58. Shor A, Kuo C-C, Patton DL (1992) Detection of *Chlamydia pneumoniae* in coronary arterial fatty streaks and atheromatous plaques. S Afr Med J 82:161-163
59. Kuo C-C, Shor A, Campbell LA et al (1993) Demonstration of *Chlamydia pneumoniae* in atherosclerotic lesions of coronary arteries. J Infect Dis 167:841-849
60. Campbell LA, O'Brien ER, Cappuccio AL et al (1995) Detection of *Chlamydia pneumoniae* TWAR in human coronary atherectomy tissues. J Infect Dis 172:585-588
61. Kuo C-C, Grayston JT, Campbell LA et al (1995) *Chlamydia pneumoniae* (TWAR) in coronary arteries of young adults (15–34 years old). Proc Natl Acad Sci USA 92:6911-6914
62. Muhlestein JB, Hammond EH, Carlquist JF et al (1996) Increased incidence of *Chlamydia* species within the coronary arteries of patients with symptomatic atherosclerotic versus other forms of cardiovascular disease. J Am Coll Cardiol 27:1555-1561
63. Ramirez JA, Ahkee S, Summersgill JT et al (1996) Isolation of *Chlamydia pneumoniae* from the coronary artery of a patient with coronary atherosclerosis. Ann Intern Med 125:979-982
64. Maass M, Bartels C, Engel PM et al (1998) Endovascular presence of viable *Chlamydia pneumoniae* is a common phenomenon in coronary artery disease. J Am Coll Cardiol 31:827-832
65. Kuo C-C, Gown AM, Benditt EP et al (1993) Detection of *Chlamydia pneumoniae* in aortic lesions of atherosclerosis by immunocytochemical stain. Arterioscler Thromb 13:1501-1504
66. Juvonen J, Juvonen T, Laurila A et al (1997) Demonstration of *Chlamydia pneumoniae* in the walls of abdominal aorta aneurysms. J Vasc Surg 25:499-505
67. Grayston JT, Kuo C-C, Coulson AS et al (1995) *Chlamydia pneumoniae* (TWAR) in atherosclerosis of the carotid artery. Circulation 92:3397-3400
68. Chiu B, Viira E, Tucker W, Fong IW (1997) *Chlamydia pneumoniae*, cytomegalovirus, and herpes simplex virus in atherosclerosis of the carotid artery. Circulation 96:2144-2148
69. Yamashita K, Ouchi K, Shirai M et al (1998) Distribution of *Chlamydia pneumoniae* infection in the atherosclerotic carotid artery. Stroke 29:773-778
70. Jackson LA, Campbell LA, Kuo C-C et al (1997) Isolation of *Chlamydia pneumoniae* from a carotid endoarterectomy specimen. J Infect Dis 176:292-295
71. Boman J, Söderberg S, Forsberg J et al (1998) High prevalence of *Chlamydia pneumoniae* DNA in peripheral blood mononuclear cells in patients with cardiovascular disease and in middle-aged blood donors. J Infect Dis 178:274-277

Chlamydia pneumoniae and Atherosclerosis: Mechanisms of Vascular Damage

J.C. Kaski, D.A. Smith

Introduction

In 1908 Sir William Osler first proposed a causative role of infection in the pathogenesis of atherosclerosis [1]. The view that infectious processes may contribute to cardiovascular diseases did not gain wide support, as autopsy and epidemiological studies shifted the attention towards other mechanisms, some of which have now become established risk factors. In recent years, however, it has become apparent that recognised risk factors for coronary heart disease (CHD) do not fully explain the diversity of this disease, or why risk factor modifications have not reduced its incidence as much as has been predicted. Recent observations have prompted research into other potential and hitherto unrecognised influences in the causation of atherogenesis. Amongst these, chronic infection by Gram-negative bacteria and herpesviridae have been shown to have a major role. Current evidence indicates that chronic *Chlamydia pneumoniae* infection may play a causal role in atherogenesis.

Chlamydia pneumoniae and Coronary Heart Disease

The characteristics of *C. pneumoniae* have been described elsewhere in this book. To summarise, *C. pneumoniae* is an obligate, intracellular pathogen which has been found to cause subclinical respiratory infections or "flu-like" symptoms, with serious sequelae being rare [2]. IgG antibodies to *C. pneumoniae* are uncommon among children but increase in early adulthood until the prevalence reaches approximately 70% in men and 50% in women [3].

Seroepidemiological Evidence

Saikku et al. [4] provided the first serological evidence of an association of *C. pneumoniae* with CHD in 1988. Patients with recent myocardial infarction (MI) had significantly elevated IgG and IgA antibodies titres against *C. pneumoniae* compared with controls. Blood samples collected prospectively in the course of the Helsinki Heart Study [5] suggested a relationship between anti-chlamydial IgA or immune complexes containing lipopolysaccharide from *Chlamydia* and the development of acute cardiac events. The association between elevated antibody titres against *C. pneumoniae* and atherosclerosis has since been confirmed by other studies [6–12]. A recent meta-analysis of 18 published seroepidemiological studies, involving over 2700 patients [13], indicated that a raised *C. pneumoniae* antibody titre is associated with a two- to fourfold increased prevalence of CHD. The prevalence of positive serological evidence is approximately 25% higher in men than in women [14], consistent with the higher prevalence of atherosclerosis in men.

Investigations in our institution have shown an association between seropositivity to *C. pneumoniae* and prevalent CHD in a community cross-sectional survey [9], corroborating the findings of other investigators. It was also shown that elevated levels of serum cardiovascular risk factors (fibrinogen, factor VIIa, leucocyte count and C-reactive protein) were associated with an elevated anti-*C. pneumoniae* antibody titre, suggesting that deleterious effects of infection in atherosclerosis may be mediated by activation of inflammatory and procoagulant processes [12]. This finding was supported by observations in an extension of the FRISC trial, in which persistent *C. pneumoniae* infection was found to be independently associated with increased fibrinogen levels [15]. In two other studies [16, 17], a significant proportion of patients admitted with acute MI or unstable angina had serological evidence of chronic or previous *C. pneumoniae* infection. Recently, Davidson et al. [18] found evidence of *C. pneumoniae* in coronary arteries obtained at autopsy and a serological diagnosis of infection in the same individuals 5–14 years earlier, suggesting that *C. pneumoniae* has a role in the pathogenesis of atherosclerosis.

The various serological studies published to date have limitations, particularly with regard to the controls used, the borderline statistical significances sometimes found, and the arbitrary titre cut-off levels selected to indicate seropositivity.

Pathological Evidence

Clearer evidence for an association between *C. pneumoniae* and atherosclerosis has come from direct examination of atherosclerotic tissue. *C. pneumoniae* DNA and elementary bodies have been demonstrated in atheromatous plaques using the polymerase chain reaction (PCR), electron microscopy and immunohistochemical techniques, with the organism found to be located in macrophages [19–22]. In one study *C. pneumoniae* was only in sites of tissue damage and not in normal tissue adjacent to the atherosclerotic lesions, or in normal coronary arteries from control patients [19]. Recent studies have detected *C. pneumoniae* in atherectomy specimens from patients with angina and in atheromatous arteries of patients with other vascular diseases [23]. Muhlestein et al. [24] recently reported immunofluorescence positivity for *C. pneumoniae* in 79% of 90 coronary atherectomy specimens, compared to only 4% of 24 controls. In this study, the presence of *C. pneumoniae* was not related to conventional risk factors, to extent or severity of disease or the clinical status of the patients.

The detection of *C. pneumoniae* in other tissues, including liver, spleen and peritoneal macrophages, in mice [25] has raised the question of whether the organism is disseminated to and persists in multiple tissues in addition to cardiovascular tissue in humans – the so-called innocent bystander hypothesis. When the organism is detected in other tissues, it is usually also detected in cardiovascular tissue from the same patient [26], suggesting that *C. pneumoniae* may be disseminated to other structures but is preferentially localised to cardiovascular tissue.

Monocytes/macrophages probably play an important role in perpetuating chronic *C. pneumoniae* infection and may be responsible for the dissemination of the organism. In vitro *C. pneumoniae* cell replication has been demonstrated by Gaydos et al. [27], although it has not been established whether such growth occurs in vivo. *C. pneumoniae* has recently been isolated and grown from human coronary atherosclerotic tissue in several studies [28–30], thus providing direct evidence of viable bacteria in the coronary circulation.

To investigate the possibility of a direct causal relationship between *C. pneumoniae* and atherogenesis, investigators have attempted to create animal models of atherosclerosis. Moazed et al. [31] examined the relation of infection with *C. pneumoniae* in two different mice models. Apolipoprotein (apo) E-deficient transgenic mice, which spontaneously develop atherosclerosis, and C57BL/6J mice, which only develop atherosclerosis on an atherogenic diet, were evaluated. After intranasal inoculation in these animals, *C. pneumoniae* was persistently demonstrated within aortic atherosclerotic lesions of the apoE-deficient mice using immunocytochemistry (ICC) and PCR, but only transiently in the C57BL/6J mice. Fong et al. [32] reported on a small study of rabbits nasally infected with *C. pneumoniae*. Two of 11 animals demonstrated early and intermediate histological lesions of atherosclerosis. This was corroborated by Laitinen et al. [33], who induced inflammatory changes in the aortas of six of nine rabbits nasally infected with *C. pneumoniae*, and recently Muhlestein et al. [34], who similarly nasally inoculated 30 New Zealand White rabbits and fed them a modestly cholesterol enhanced diet. These animals were then randomised to receive a course of azithromycin or no treatment. Intranasal *C. pneumoniae* infection accelerated intimal thickening, but importantly, treatment with azithromycin prevented accelerated intimal thickening, thus strengthening the aetiological link between *C. pneumoniae* and atherosclerosis.

Atherogenesis and Acute Coronary Syndromes: The Role of Inflammation

In recent years, it has become clear that inflammation plays a vital role in both atherogenesis and the development of acute coronary syndromes. Atheromatous plaque disruption with subsequent thrombus formation is the most common mechanism underlying acute coronary syndromes and rapid disease progression

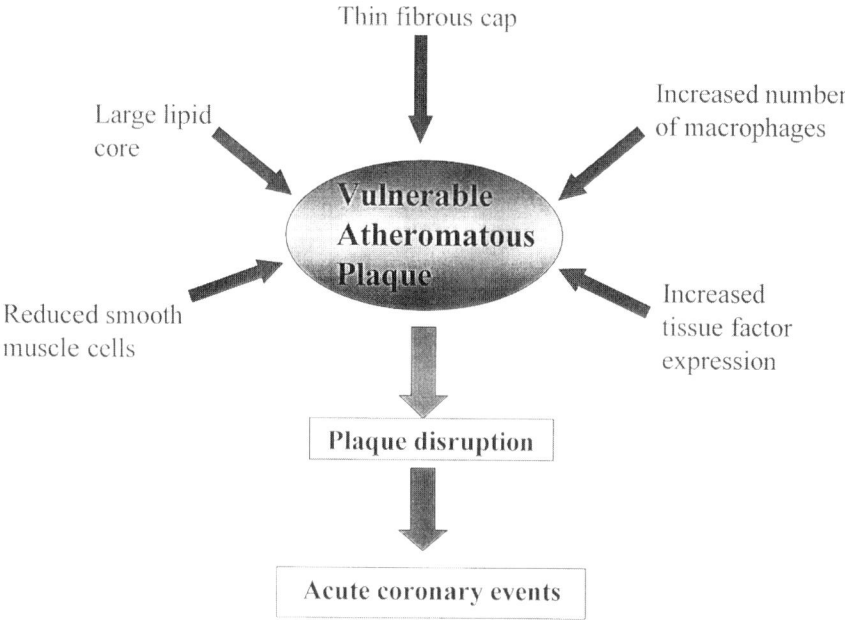

Fig. 1. Factors responsible for plaque vulnerability

[35, 36]. Recent studies have shown that atherosclerotic plaque rupture and "plaque vulnerability" are a function of: an increased number of macrophages within the plaque, the local expression of tissue factor, the presence of a lipid core occupying a large proportion of plaque volume and a thin fibrous cap [37-39] (Fig. 1). When all these factors coincide, the plaque is highly vulnerable [40].

In plaque rupture, the fibrous cap of an atheromatous plaque tears, exposing the highly thrombogenic lipid core to blood in the lumen of the artery. The mechanical strength of the plaque cap is therefore a vital component of plaque stability and depends on the amount and organisation of collagen and other connective tissue proteins [41]. Smooth muscle cells exist in lacunae in the plaque cap, where they produce and maintain the connective tissue matrix on which cap integrity depends. The cap tissue is dynamic, with production of connective tissue matrix proteins by smooth muscle cells being balanced by degradation of the matrix [42] (Fig. 2). Both sides of this equation are detrimentally altered by inflammatory processes within the plaque, with enhancement of connective tissue catabolism being a very important mechanism [41].

Compared to patients with chronic stable angina, patients with acute coronary syndromes have coronary plaques with more extensive macrophage-rich areas [38]. Activated macrophages within plaques produce a range of proteases that lead to proteolytic destruction of connective tissue matrix [43, 44]. By this mechanism, macrophages may be responsible for the "active" phenomenon of plaque

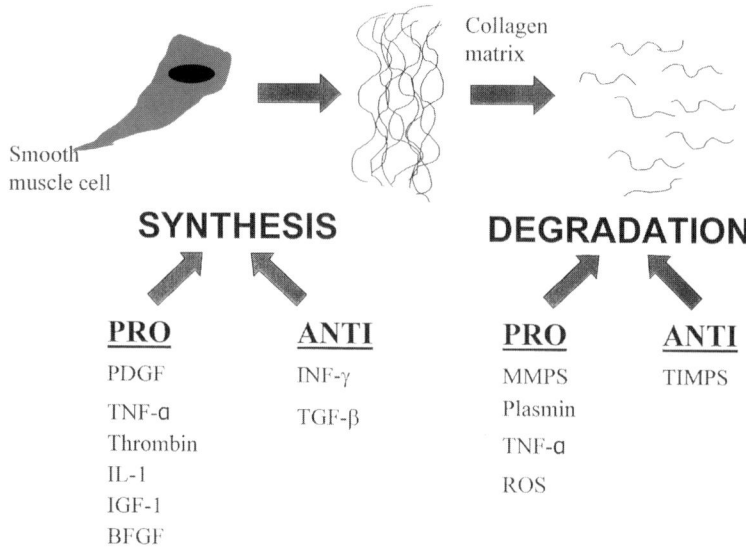

Fig. 2. A schematic illustration of the dynamic state of the fibrous plaque cap. *PDGF,* platelet-derived growth factor; *TNF-α,* tumor necrosis factor-α; *IL-1,* interleukin-1; *IGF-1,* insulin-like growth factor-1; *BFGF,* basic fibroblast growth factor; *INF-γ,* interferon-γ; *TGF-β,* trasforming growth factor-β; *MMPS,* metalloproteinases; *ROS,* reactive oxigen species; *TIMPS,* tissue inhibitors of metalloproteinases

disruption [45, 46]. Vulnerable plaques also have activated T-cells that produce interferon-γ, which affects extracellular matrix collagen production and activates the macrophages [47]. Several stimuli may trigger coronary inflammatory processes, and chronic infection, by different agents, has been implicated. Of all the pathogens implicated to date, *C. pneumoniae* appears to be the most likely to play a role in atherosclerosis.

There are several direct and indirect mechanisms by which infections might initiate or perpetuate atherosclerosis (Fig. 3). Endotoxin secreted by bacteria triggers vascular damage in rabbit [48] and pig [49] models of atherosclerosis and has been shown to bind to lipoproteins in the circulation, some of which are then avidly taken up by macrophages. Infection and activation of macrophages or smooth muscle cells may lead to production of cytokines, major histocompatibility complex upregulation, and synthesis of acute phase proteins such as fibrinogen and C-reactive protein – processes which may perpetuate the inflammatory response [50]. Infections may also directly affect cholesterol metabolism and lipid oxidation [51], creating a more atherogenic lipid profile.

Infection may lead to both a local and a generalised hypercoagulable state, via increased tissue factor expression, following activation and increased levels of monocytes [52] (Fig. 4). As mentioned earlier in this chapter, a recent report by Toss et al. [15] has shown that in unstable patients who took part in the FRISC

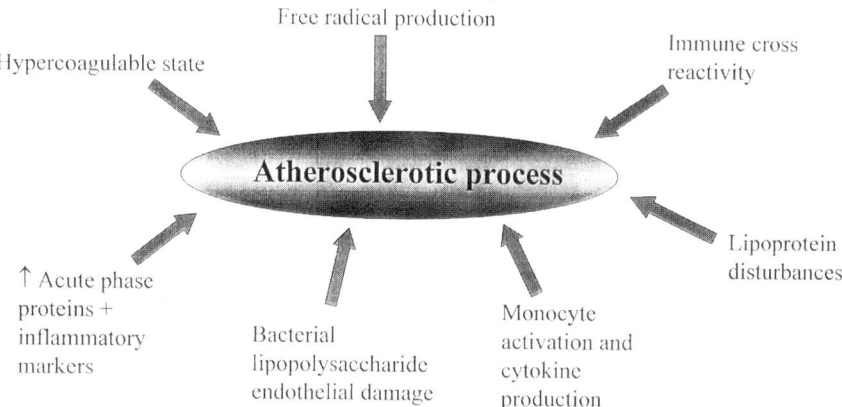

Fig. 3. Possible mechanisms by which infections may contribute to the development of atherosclerosis and acute plaque disruption

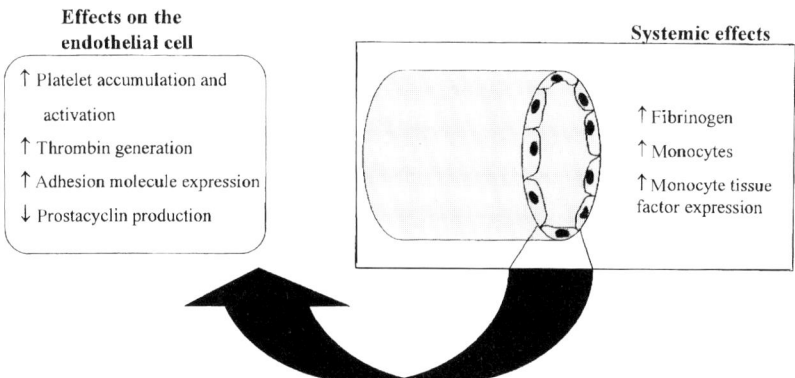

Fig. 4. Mechanisms by which infections can cause a local and generalised hypercoagulable state

study, increased *C. pneumoniae* IgA antibody titres ($\geq 1/64$) were independently associated with increased fibrinogen levels. This finding corroborated earlier work carried out at our institution, which showed that elevated levels of serum cardiovascular risk factors (fibrinogen, factor VIIa, leucocyte count and C-reactive protein) were associated with an elevated *C. pneumoniae* titre [12]. This may therefore increase the risk of local or distal thrombosis. Infection of endothelial cells may also alter thrombin generation on the cell surface, increase platelet accumulation, induce leucocyte adhesion molecule expression or reduce prostacyclin secretion [53].

Mechanisms of Vascular Disease in *Chlamydia pneumoniae* Infection

How *C. pneumoniae* enters atheromatous plaques and whether it has a direct causal role in the pathogenesis of atherosclerosis is speculative. Following pulmonary infection, *C. pneumoniae* may spread systemically, carried within monocytes and macrophages, which may adhere to sites of endothelial damage. The consequences of *C. pneumoniae* uptake by macrophages and the mechanisms of damage at the site of the coronary artery are not known. The organism may simply reside in the macrophage without causing any harmful effects, and any association between *C. pneumoniae* residing in coronary tissue and consequent damage may be purely coincidental [54].

Alternatively, chronic macrophage infection may contribute to local inflammation and development of atheromatous plaques, as suggested by the animal models of infection-induced atherosclerosis described earlier [32–34]. It has been suggested that this process may be analogous to the pathogenesis of trachoma, where the closely related *C. trachomatis* causes blindness as a result of necrosis that follows conjunctival infiltration by macrophages and lymphocytes [55]. Fibrosis may develop in some individuals many years after the original infection, possibly as a result of hypersensitivity rather than as a direct result of the organism itself. *C. pneumoniae* infection may induce a chronic immune activation (mediated by cytokines such as IL-6, and TNF-α [56]) that contributes to direct chronic endothelial cell damage or stimulates the synthesis of acute phase proteins such as fibrinogen [57] and C-reactive protein [58].

An autoimmune hypothesis has recently been suggested. A 57-kDa chlamydial heat shock protein has been identified that has close homology with mycobacterial heat shock protein (which is linked with atherosclerosis) [59]. Birnie et al. [60] recently found that antibodies to heat shock protein (HSP) 65 correlated with the severity and extent of coronary artery disease even after controlling for confounding factors. They also showed a significant reduction in HSP 65 titres after successful *Helicobacter pylori* eradication therapy. More recently, Kol et al. [61] showed that chlamydial HSP 60 colocalises with human HSP 60 within plaque macrophages and that HSP 60 from both species can induce macrophage production of TNF-α and matrix-degrading metalloproteinases. These findings confirmed and expanded work by Xu et al. which suggested a role for mycobacterium HSP 65 in atherogenesis [62]. These studies thus support the hypothesis whereby *H. pylori* and other micro-organisms may induce an immune response to bacterial HSP 60/62/65 and the antibodies produced cross-react with the human HSP 60 [63], thus initiating or contributing to a local inflammatory and auto-immune process.

Finally, the superoxide radical has been implicated in vascular and endothelial damage and plaque disruption. The direct and indirect attack of reactive oxygen species on polyunsaturated fatty acids, essential constituents of biological membranes, has been shown to result in the formation of a number of lipid breakdown products – a process called lipid peroxidation. Once lipid peroxidation is initiated, the reactive intermediates formed induce permanent cell damage [64]. All three major cell types of the arterial lesion – endothelial cells, smooth muscle cells and macrophages – secrete reactive oxygen species [65, 66]. Intriguingly, *C. pneumoniae* has been shown to replicate in vitro in these cell types [27] and therefore may increase lipid peroxidation, although this potential mechanism remains to be studied.

Conclusion

An infectious basis of atherosclerosis may underlie the variable rates of prevalence of coronary artery disease in different parts of the world and the rapidly changing patterns of morbidity and mortality from coronary artery disease, which cannot be explained by conventional risk factors alone. *C. pneumoniae* is a plausible candidate for the initiation or modulation of atherogenesis. The organism may be acting with or independently of other cardiac risk factors. Large-scale randomised antibiotic intervention trials in patients with CHD are under way, and together with work at the basic science level, we hope for an improved understanding of CHD pathogenesis and the development of new effective management strategies in the near future.

References

1. Osler W (1908) Diseases of the arteries. In: Osler W (ed) Modern medicine: its practice and theory. Lea and Febiger, Philadelphia, pp 429-447
2. Saikku P (1992) The epidemiology and significance of *Chlamydia pneumoniae*. J Infect 39:88-90
3. Grayston JT, Campbell LA, Kuo C-C et al (1990) A new respiratory pathogen: *Chlamydia pneumoniae* strain TWAR. J Infect Dis 161:618-625
4. Saikku P, Mattila K, Nieminen S et al (1988) Serological evidence of an association of a novel *Chlamydia* TWAR, with chronic coronary heart disease and acute myocardial infarction. Lancet 2:983-986
5. Saikku P, Leinonen M, Tenkanen L et al (1992) Chronic *Chlamydia pneumoniae* infection as a risk factor for coronary heart disease in the Helsinki Heart Study. Ann Int Med 116:273-278
6. Thom DH, Grayston JT, Siscovick DS et al (1992) Association of prior infection with *Chlamydia pneumoniae* and angiographically demonstrated coronary artery disease. JAMA 268:68-72
7. Melnick SL, Shahar E, Folsom AR et al (1993) Past infection by *Chlamydia pneumoniae* strain TWAR and asymptomatic carotid atherosclerosis. Atherosclerosis Risk in Communities (ARIC) Study Investigators. Am J Med 95:499-504
8. Thom DH, Wang SP, Grayston JT et al (1991) *Chlamydia* strain TWAR antibody and angiographically demonstrated coronary artery disease. Arterioscler Thromb 11:547-551
9. Mendall MA, Carrington D, Strachan DP et al (1995) *Chlamydia pneumoniae*: risk factors for seropositivity and association with coronary heart disease. J Infect 30:121-128
10. Haidl S, Juul-Moller S, Israelsson B et al (1992) Ischaemic heart disease and antibodies to *Chlamydia pneumoniae* (TWAR). Proc Eur Soc Chlam Res 2:174 (abstract)

11. Cook PJ, Lip GY, Zarifis J et al (1996) Is *Chlamydia pneumoniae* infection associated with acute cardiac ischaemic syndromes? J Am Coll Cardiol 324[Suppl A]:807-812

12. Patel P, Mendall MA, Carrington D et al (1995) Association of *Helicobacter pylori* and *Chlamydia pneumoniae* infections with coronary heart disease and cardiovascular risk factors. BMJ 311:711-714

13. Danesh J, Collins R, Peto R (1997) Chronic infections and coronary heart disease: is there a link? Lancet 350:430-436

14. Campbell LA, O'Brien ER, Cappuccio AL et al (1995) Detection of *Chlamydia pneumoniae* TWAR in human coronary atherectomy tissues. J Infect Dis 172:585-588

15. Toss H, Gnarpe J, Siegbahn A et al (1998) Increased fibrinogen levels are associated with persistent *Chlamydia pneumoniae* infection in unstable coronary artery disease. Eur Heart J 19:570-577

16. Cook PJ, Honeybourne D, Lip GY et al (1995) *Chlamydia pneumoniae* and acute arterial thrombotic disease. Circulation 95:3148-3149

17. Aceti A, Mazzacurati G, Amendolea M et al (1996) Relation of C-reactive protein to cardiovascular risk factors: *Helicobacter pylori* and *Chlamydia pneumoniae* infections may account for most acute coronary syndromes. BMJ 313:428-429

18. Davidson M, Kuo C-C, Middaugh JP et al (1998) Confirmed previous infection with *Chlamydia pneumoniae* (TWAR) and its presence in early coronary atherosclerosis. Circulation 98:628-633

19. Kuo C-C, Shor A, Campbell LA et al (1993) Demonstration of *Chlamydia pneumoniae* in atherosclerotic lesions of coronary arteries. J Infect Dis 167:841-849

20. Kuo C-C, Gown AM, Benditt EP, Grayston JT (1993) Detection of *Chlamydia pneumoniae* in aortic lesions of atherosclerosis by immunocytochemical stain. Arterioscler Thromb 13:1501-1504

21. Kuo C-C, Grayston JT, Campbell LA et al (1995) *Chlamydia pneumoniae* (TWAR) in coronary arteries of young adults (15–34 years old). Proc Natl Acad Sci USA 92:6911-6914

22. Grayston JT, Kuo C-C, Coulson AS et al (1995) *Chlamydia pneumoniae* (TWAR) in atherosclerosis of the carotid artery. Circulation 92:3397-3400

23. Ong G, Thomas BJ, Mansfield AO et al (1996) Detection and widespread distribution of *Chlamydia pneumoniae* in the vascular system and its possible implications. J Clin Pathol 49:102-106

24. Muhlestein JB, Hammond EH, Carlquist JF et al (1996) Increased incidence of *Chlamydia* species within the coronary arteries of patients with symptomatic atherosclerotic versus other forms of cardiovascular disease. J Am Coll Cardiol 27:1555-1561

25. Yang Z, Kuo C-C, Grayston JT (1995) Systemic dissemination of *Chlamydia pneumoniae* following intranasal innoculation in mice. J Infect Dis 171:736-738

26. Jackson LA, Campbell LA, Schmidt R et al (1997) Specificity of detection of *Chlamydia pneumoniae* in cardiovascular atheroma. Am J Pathol 150:1785-1790

27. Gaydos CA, Summersgill JT, Sahney NN et al (1996) Replication of *Chlamydia pneumoniae* in vitro in human macrophages, endothelial cells and aortic artery smooth muscle cells. Infect Immunol 64:1614-1620

28. Ramirez JA (1996) Isolation of *Chlamydia pneumoniae* from the coronary artery of a patient with coronary atherosclerosis. The *Chlamydia pneumoniae* Atherosclerosis Study Group. Ann Int Med 125:979-982

29. Maass M, Bartels C, Engel PM et al (1998) Endovascular presence of viable *Chlamydia pneumoniae* is a common phenomenon in coronary artery disease. J Am Coll Cardiol 31:827-832

30. Jackson LA, Campbell LA, Kuo C-C et al (1998) Isolation of *Chlamydia pneumoniae* from a carotid endarterectomy specimen. J Infect Dis 176:292-295

31. Moazed TC, Kuo C-C, Grayston JT et al (1997) Murine models of *Chlamydia pneumoniae* infection and atherosclerosis. J Infect Dis 175:883-890
32. Fong IW, Chiu B, Viira E et al (1997) Rabbit model for *Chlamydia pneumoniae* infection. J Clin Microbiol 35:48-52
33. Laitinen K, Laurila A, Pyhala L et al (1997) *Chlamydia pneumoniae* infection induces inflammatory changes in the aortas of rabbits. Infect Immun 65:4832-4825
34. Muhlestein JB, Anderson JL, Hammond EH et al (1998) Infection with *Chlamydia pneumoniae* acelerates the development of atherosclerosis and treatment with azithromycin prevents it in a rabbit model. Circulation 97:633-636
35. Chen L, Chester MR, Redwood S, Huang J, Leatham E, Kaski JC (1995) Angiographic stenosis progression and cardiac events in patients with stabilised unstable angina. Circulation 91:2319-2324
36. Fuster V, Badimon L, Cohen M et al (1988) Insights into the pathogenesis of acute ischaemic syndromes. Circulation 77:1213-1220
37. Falk E (1989) Morphological features of unstable atherothrombotic plaques underlying acute coronary syndromes. Am J Cardiol 63:114E-120E
38. Moreno P, Falk E, Palacios I et al (1994) Macrophage infiltration in acute coronary syndromes. Circulation 90:775-780
39. Annex B, Denning S, Channon K et al (1995) Differential expression of tissue factor protein in directional atherectomy specimens from patients with stable and unstable coronary syndromes. Circulation 91:619-622
40. Davies MJ (1996) Stability and instability: two faces of coronary atherosclerosis. Circulation 94:2013-2020
41. Davies MJ (1998) Reactive oxygen species, metalloproteinases and plaque stability. Circulation 97:2382-2383
42. Libby PJ (1995) The molecular bases of the acute coronary syndromes. Circulation 91:2844-2850
43. Liuzzo G, Biasucci LM, Gallimore JR et al (1994) The prognostic value of C-reactive protein and serum amyloid A protein in severe unstable angina. N Engl J Med 331:417-424
44. Dollery CM, McEwan JR, Henney A (1995) Matrix metalloproteinases and cardiovascular disease. Circ Res 77:863-868
45. Henney A, Wakeley P, Davies M et al (1991) Localisation of stromelysin gene expression in atherosclerotic plaques by in-situ hybridization. Proc Natl Acad Sci USA 88(18):8154-8158
46. Galis ZS, Sukhova GK, Lark MW et al (1994) Increased expression of matrix metalloproteinases and matrix degrading activity in vulnerable regions of human atherosclerotic plaques. J Clin Invest 94:2493-2503
47. Sernery GGN, Abbate R, Gori AM et al (1992) Transient intermittent lymphocyte activation is responsible for the instability of angina. Circulation 86:790-797
48. Reidy MA, Bowyer DE (1978) Distortion of endothelial repair. The effect of hypercholesterolaemia on regulation of aortic endothelium following injury by endotoxin. A scanning microscopy study. Atherosclerosis 29:459-466
49. Pesonen E, Kaprio K, Rapola J et al (1981) Endothelial cell damage in piglet coronary artery after administration of *E. coli* endotoxin. A scanning and transmission electron microscopic study. Atherosclerosis 40:65-73
50. Hansson GK (1989) Immune mechanisms in atherosclerosis. Atherosclerosis 9:567-588
51. Hajjar DP, Falcone DJ, Fabricant CG et al (1985) Altered cholesterol ester cycle is associated with lipid accumulation in herpes-infected arterial smooth muscle cells. J Biol Chem 260:6124-6128

52. Leatham EW, Bath PM, Tooze JA et al (1995) Increased monocyte tissue factor expression in coronary disease. Br Heart J 73:10-13

53. Visser MR, Tracey PB, Vercellotti GM et al (1988) Enhancing thrombin generation and platelet binding on herpes simplex virus-infected endothelium. Proc Natl Acad Sci USA 85:8227-8230

54. Gupta S, Camm AJ (1997) *Chlamydia pneumoniae* and coronary heart disease: coincidence, association, or causation? BMJ 314:1778-1779

55. Holland MJ, Bailey RL, Hayes LJ et al (1998) Conjuctival scarring in trachoma is associated with depressed cell-mediated immune responses to *Chlamydial* antigens. J Infect Dis 168:1528-1531

56. Kaukoranta-Tolvanen SS, Teppo AM, Laitinen K et al (1996) Growth of *Chlamydia pneumoniae* in cultured human blood mononuclear cells and induction of a cytokine response. Microb Pathog 21:215-221

57. Patel P, Carrington D, Strachan DP et al (1994) Fibrinogen: a link between chronic infection and coronary heart disease. Lancet 343:1634-1635

58. Mendall MA, Patel P, Ballam L et al (1996) C-reactive protein and its relation to cardiovascular risk factors: a population based cross sectional study. BMJ 312:1061-1065

59. Morrison RP, Belland RJ, Lyng K, Caldwell HD (1989) Chlamydial disease pathogenesis. The 57-kD chlamydial hypersensitivity antigen is a stress response protein. J Exp Med 170:1271-1283

60. Birnie DH, Holme ER, McKay IC et al (1998) Association between antibodies to heat shock protein 65 and coronary atherosclerosis. Eur Heart J 19:387-394

61. Kol A, Sukhova GK, Lichtman AH, Libby P (1998) Chlamydial heat shock protein 60 localises in human atheroma and regulates macrophage tumour necrosis factor-α and matrix metalloproteinase expression. Circulation 98:300-307

62. Xu Q, Dietrich H, Steiner HJ et al (1992) Induction of arteriosclerosis in normocholesterolaemic rabbits by immunisation with heat shock protein 65. Arterioscler Thromb 12:789-799

63. Kaski JC, Cox I (1998) Chronic infection and atherogenesis. Eur Heart J 19:366-367

64. Fujita T, Fujimoto Y (1992) Formation and removal of active oxygen species and lipid peroxides in biological systems. Nippon Yakurigaku Zasshi 99:381-389

65. Steinbrecher UP, Parathasarathy S, Leake DS et al (1984) Modification of low density lipoprotein by endothelial cells involves lipid peroxidation and degradation of low density lipoprotein phospholipids. Proc Natl Acad Sci USA 81:3883-3887

66. Morel DW, DiCorleto PE, Chisholm GM (1984) Endothelial and smooth muscle cells alter low density lipoprotein in vitro by free radical oxidation. Arteriosclerosis 4:357-364

Chlamydia pneumoniae and Atherosclerosis: Animal Models

L.A. Campbell, C.-C. Kuo

Introduction

The cumulative seroepidemiologic studies, direct detection of *Chlamydia pneumoniae* antigen in atherosclerotic lesions throughout the arterial tree, and culturing of the organism from atheromatous tissue provide compelling evidence for an association of *C. pneumoniae* with atherosclerosis [1]. However, these findings do not establish causality, which can only be proven through the use of animal models or intervention studies. This chapter will focus on animal models of *C. pneumoniae* and their use in studying pathogenesis, intervention strategies for eradication of acute and chronic infection, and putative roles of *C. pneumoniae* infection on atherogenesis. The recent establishment of mouse and rabbit models of *C. pneumoniae* infection that also are well-defined experimental models of atherosclerosis has provided the opportunity to address the hypothesis that *C. pneumoniae* infection affects the onset, severity, or progression of atherosclerosis.

Animal Models of Pneumonia

In order for animal models to be useful for studying *C. pneumoniae* pathogenesis, several criteria should be met, including: (1) infection should lead to the development of disease/pathology exhibiting characteristics similar to human disease; (2) an immune response should be mounted; (3) Koch's postulate should be fulfilled. Three animal models, mice, rabbits and non-human primates, have been investigated for their susceptibility to *C. pneumoniae* infection [2–8]. Although persistent/chronic infection is established in all three models, the range of clinical symptoms varies from mild in non-human primates to more severe and prolonged in mice. All of these models develop micro-immunofluorescent antibody against *C. pneumoniae* following infection.

The first animal model investigated for susceptibility to *C. pneumoniae* infection was non-human primates, including baboons, rhesus, and cynomolgus monkeys [6, 7]. In these non-human primates, no symptoms of respiratory disease were noted regardless of whether the organism was inoculated via nasopharyngeal, oropharyngeal, or intratracheal routes.

In contrast, both mice and rabbits develop disease following single or repeated inoculation, which is characterized by a multi-focal interstitial pneumonia and systemic infection. In both models, chlamydial inclusions have been seen in macrophages in the lung, supporting in vitro evidence that *C. pneumoniae* can infect and survive in monocytes/macrophages [4, 5]. Histopathology in the lung is most severe early on and is characterized by a severe inflammatory infiltrate consisting of polymorphonuclear leukocytes (PMNLs) (or, in the rabbit, heterophilic granulocytes) which changes to predominantly mononuclear leukocytes later on in the infection and persists for longer periods [2, 3, 5, 8]. A striking pathological feature in both models is the accumulation of perivascular and peribronchial lymphoid cells [2, 5, 8]. This preceding characteristic is distinct from *C. trachomatis*, in which the formation of such foci is observed in chronic or repeated infection in humans and in monkey models. For *C. pneumoniae* infection, the immunopathology of the lung is more severe and longer lasting in mice than in rabbits. Organisms are readily isolated from the lungs and aorta of mice, but not rabbits. In both mouse and rabbit models, persistence of infection in the absence of culture by detection of antigen or DNA has been demonstrated [5, 8, 9]. Because both of these animals also have diet-induced or spontaneously induced genetic models of atherosclerosis, they provide the opportunity for determination of three facets of the effects of *C. pneumoniae* infection on atherogenesis. Specifically, they can be utilized to investigate: (1) whether acute and/or chronic infection with *C. pneumoniae* induces atherosclerosis in normal arteries in the absence of a high-fat/high-cholesterol diet; (2) whether *C. pneumoniae* infection exacerbates progression of the existing lesion; and (3) what the combined effects of infection and diet on atherogenesis are.

Mouse Models of Pneumonia and Atherosclerosis

Several outbred and inbred strains of mice are susceptible to *C. pneumoniae* infection by intranasal (IN) inoculation and develop pneumonia with characteristics of human disease [2]. Following IN inoculation organisms are readily recovered from the lung for up to 3–6 weeks post inoculation and in bronchoalveolar lavage fluids [2, 3]. In addition to the lung, the organism can be cultured from other anatomical sites, including spleen, aorta, and peripheral blood mononuclear cells (PBMCs) [8, 10, 11]. These findings suggest that *C. pneumoniae* infection causes systemic disease. In humans, *C. pneumoniae* has been detected in atheromas, skin granulomas, lung, spleen, liver, lymph node, and PBMCs [12, 13]. Mouse models have proven useful in studying *C. pneumoniae* pathogenesis and its putative roles in atherogenesis. C57BL/6J and apoE-knockout mice have been used to investigate the mechanism of dissemination of the organism from the primary site of infection in the lungs to the atheromatous plaque. These studies have shown that following upper respiratory tract infection, lung macrophages are infected. Infection disseminates to the aorta and effects the progression of atherogenesis [8, 11, 14]. C57BL/6J mice, the background strain of apoE-knockout mice, develop atherosclerosis only when the animals are fed with a high-fat/high-cholesterol diet. In contrast, apoE-knockout mice develop hypercholesterolemia and atherosclerotic lesions spontaneously in a time- and age-dependent manner on a regular chow diet [15-17]. The lesions have characteristics of human atheroma. Following IN or intraperitoneal inoculation of C57BL/6J mice with *C. pneumoniae*, alveolar and peritoneal macrophages are infected, respectively. Additionally, the organism was found in blood monocytes but not in plasma, demonstrating that cell-associated bacteremia occurred during acute infection [11]. In contrast, if mice were inoculated with organisms inactivated by ultraviolet radiation, rendering them non-viable in the same experimental protocol, the organism was not detected in macrophages or PBMCs. Passive transfer of infected macrophages from mice inoculated intranasally or intraperitoneally with *C. pneumoniae* to naive mice by intraperitoneal inoculation demonstrated dissemination of infection to the lung, thymus, spleen, and/or abdominal lymph nodes. These studies have proven infected macrophages serve as a vehicle for dissemination from the lung to other sites by either hematogenous or lymphatic routes.

ApoE-knockout mice have been used to determine whether infection disseminates to the aorta and establishes infection in atherosclerotic lesions as in human disease. Following single or repeated inoculations, *C. pneumoniae* was detected in the aorta intermittently for up to 20 weeks post infection. The organisms were detected by immunostain in foam cells within the developing atherosclerotic lesion [8]. At times at which the aorta was positive for infection, the proportion of mice positive ranged from 33% to 100%. This is in contrast to C57BL/6J mice fed with a non-atherogenic diet. The organism was found in the aorta in only 0.8% of animals up to 2 weeks post infection following a single inoculation [8]. The tropism of *C. pneumoniae* for atheromatous tissues was further demonstrated by inoculation of apoE-deficient mice at 16 weeks of age, at the time when all mice had developed atheroma, which resulted in 100% of mice infected in the aorta [8]. At this age, atheromas have developed to early to intermediate stages. Thus, lesions are found more frequently and are more advanced than in mice inoculated at 8 weeks of age, in which monocyte adherence, a prelude to development of early lesions, is seen. Similar findings on tropism have been observed in humans with examination of autopsy and granulomatous tissues from different anatomical sites. In these specimens, the organism has been found more frequently in atheromas than in other tissues from the same individual [12]. It was not found in other infectious and non-infectious granulomatous diseases, with the exception of sarcoidosis tissues [12]. Interestingly, an association of sarcoidosis and *C. pneumoniae* has been suggested [18]. The higher frequency of infection of mice with more developed atherosclerotic lesions also mimics findings in human tissues, where the organism is found at a somewhat higher frequency in developed than in early lesions. Moreover, the organism is rarely found in human arterial tissue that appears histopathologically normal [19].

The evidence that *C. pneumoniae* infection might accelerate the progression of atherosclerosis has come from experiments with apoE-deficient mice [14]. Mice were fed a normal chow diet and received three inoculations at 8, 9, and 10 weeks of age. At 16 or 20 weeks of age, mice were killed and the aortic arch removed for analysis of lesion size by computer-assisted morphometry. Atherosclerotic lesion measurements were limited to the inner curvature of the aortic arch, the site most vulnerable to the development of lesions in this animal. Comparison of groups of 20 infected and 20 uninfected mice demonstrated statistically significant increases in lesion size in comparison with uninfected mice. The heart was noted to increase in weight at 16 weeks. Infection did not affect blood cholesterol levels.

Similar findings were also observed with another mouse model using low-density lipoprotein receptor (LDLR)-knockout mice fed with a high-cholesterol diet. LDLR-knockout mice have an increased susceptibility to atherosclerosis on a high-cholesterol diet but not with a normal diet. In this model, IN infection alone did not induce atherosclerotic lesions. However, in the presence of a high cholesterol diet, *C. pneumoniae* infection exacerbated lesion progress as measured by computer-assisted morphometry (G. Zhong, personal communication). Collectively, these two studies demonstrate that in either diet-induced or genetically induced hypercholesterolemic mice, *C. pneumoniae* infection accelerates atherosclerosis.

Rabbit Models of Pneumonia and Atherosclerosis

Two rabbit models are available for studying atherosclerosis. One is the New Zealand White (NZW) rabbit, a high-cholesterol-diet-induced model. The other is the Watanabe heritable hyperlipidemic (WHHL) rabbit, a spontaneous genetic model. These two rabbit models have been investigated for their susceptibility to *C. pneumoniae* infection [5]. Both strains develop a moderate multifocal interstitial pneumonia with bronchiolitis and mild vasculitis following IN or intratracheal inoculation. However, in contrast to mice, following a single inoculation, the organism could only be cultured from the upper respiratory tract for 2–3 days post infection. The organism could not be cultured from the lungs, but was observed in interstitial macrophages at this time by electron microscopy, but not at later time. Interestingly, the inclusions contained only organisms in the early development stage, which are non-infectious. These findings are consistent with the inability to culture the organism from the lung. However, the lung tissue was intermittently positive for DNA or antigen for up to 6 weeks post inoculation.

WHHL rabbits were less susceptible to *C. pneumoniae* infection than NZW rabbits [5]. In NZW rabbits following three inoculations, the organism could be isolated from the nasopharynx and trachea up to 2 weeks after inoculation and detected by PCR in the upper and lower respiratory tract for up to 6 weeks. In contrast, the organism could not be cultured from the upper respiratory tract and was detectable by polymerase chain reaction (PCR) and immunocytochemistry (ICC) for 3 weeks in WHHL rabbits. Consequently, subsequent investigations have been conducted in NZW rabbits on normal or high-cholesterol diets to determine whether *C. pneumoniae* respiratory infection induces or accelerates atherosclerosis.

Two studies have dealt with induction of atherogenesis on a normal diet. In the first study, 1-month-old NZW rabbits received a single nasopharyngeal inoculation with *C. pneumoniae* via catheterization. Subsequently, two of ten rabbits showed some pathologic changes in the aorta. One rabbit had an accumulation of foam cells in the aortic arch, a sign of an early lesion, and focal periaortitis in the abdominal aorta [20]. A second rabbit demonstrated spindle cell proliferation of smooth muscle cells in the aorta. These changes were observed 7 and 14 days post inoculation. Both rabbits had bronchiolitis and pneumonitis. Whether these changes persist and progress to typical atherosclerotic lesions has not been determined.

In the second study, NZW rabbits were inoculated twice intranasally, 3 weeks apart with *C. pneumoniae*. Atherosclerotic-like changes were found in the aortas of six of nine NZW rabbits 2–4 weeks after inoculations [21].

One study has evaluated the combined effects of diet and infection on atherosclerosis. NZW rabbits on a diet supplemented with 0.25% cholesterol were inoculated intranasally three times with *C. pneumoniae* [22]. Histological examinations of tissue sections of thoracic aortas 3 months after the final inoculation revealed pathologic changes pertinent to atherosclerosis and increases in the maximal intimal thickness, percentage of luminal circumference, and plaque area index.

In summary, studies in mouse and rabbit models indicate that *C. pneumoniae* infection can induce inflammatory changes similar to those occurring in atherosclerosis and augment the progression of the atherosclerotic lesions.

Animal Models of Persistent Infections and for Evaluation of Antimicrobial Therapy

Seroepidemiologic studies in humans have suggested that chronic infections are common. However, laboratory diagnosis of chronic or persistent infection is not possible because detection of the organism in the respiratory tract in chronic disease by isolation or PCR is difficult. In the mouse model of pneumonia, lung pathology persists despite the failure to isolate the organism. Infection may persist in some animals following a regular course of antibiotic treatment based on the direct detection of *C. pneumoniae* specific DNA or antigen. *C. pneumoniae* has been detected by PCR and ICC in human and animal tissues, including arteries, when the organism has not been isolated. For example, in apoE-deficient mice infected with *C. pneumoniae*, the organism has been isolated from the lung and aorta for up to 3 weeks post inoculation, but has been detected by PCR at both sites as long as 20 weeks post inoculation [8]. One concern about these findings has been whether the organism detected by PCR in culture-negative mice indicates "remnants of the organism" rather than viable, but unculturable organisms. Two lines of evidence indicate infection is persisting. The first is reactivation of infection. Two studies using different strains of mice have shown that lung infection may be reactivated by immunosuppression [9, 23]. Reactivation was achieved in 46%–60% of mice by giving mice six doses of cortisone after the animals had become negative by culture. Control mice given saline continued to be culture-negative although PCR in some cases continued to be positive. The second line of evidence was the survival of live organisms in macrophages and rapid degradation of chlamydial DNA of dead organisms by macrophages in animal experiments [11]. When mice were inoculated intranasally with live organisms, the organism was detected by culture and PCR in alveolar macrophages up to 7 days post inoculation. However, it has been possible to detect chlamydial DNA by PCR only 5 min post inoculation in mice inoculated with UV-inactivated organism. Therefore, it appears that DNA from dead organisms is rapidly degraded by macrophages in vivo.

These findings provide cautionary notes for interpreting drug efficacy studies in animal models or in humans, in which eradication may be indicated by the inability to culture the organism, while direct detection methods may still be positive. To address this question, both mouse and rabbit models have been shown to be useful for evaluating the effects of antibiotic treatment in eradicating infection from the lungs and in suppressing inflammatory reactions and pathologic changes in the aorta from infection.

In a pneumonia model, mice were treated with doxycycline (10 mg/kg of body weight) for 3 days or a single dose of azithromycin (10 mg/kg of body weight) following a single inoculation of *C. pneumoniae*. Both treatment regimens were shown to be effective in clearing the infection based on negative isolation from the lungs. However, 25%–77% of lungs were still PCR positive for *C. pneumoniae* DNA. In addition, no differences in lung pathology were observed between treated and untreated mice. These findings raise the question of whether the presence of DNA and histopathologic changes in the lungs indicate that organisms persist after treatment as they do in untreated mice [24].

Mice have also been used in the evaluation of the efficacy of various antimicrobial agents. In this study, different antibiotics and treatment regimens were compared including amoxicillin-clavulanate (20 mg/kg or 10 mg/kg, 3 × /day for 7 days), ciprofloxacin (40 mg/kg, 3 × /day for 7 days), ofloxacin (50 mg/kg, 2 × /day for 7 days), doxycycline (10 mg/kg, 2 × /day for 7 days), erythromycin (100 mg/kg, 2 × /day for 7 days), or azithromycin (40 mg/kg on the first day, then 30 mg/kg for 3 days). A single inoculation was given to outbred MF1 mice immunosuppressed with cyclophosphamide. Infection was not eradicated in all mice after any treatment regimen, although decreased lung loads were observed [25].

Mice have also been used to evaluate antimicrobial therapy for persistent infection. ApoE-deficient mice were inoculated intranasally three times to establish persistent infection of the lung and aorta. Four weeks after the final inoculation, mice were treated with either roxithromycin (50 mg/kg) or placebo, daily for 7 days by gastric lavage. Although the antibiotic did not clear *C. pneumoniae* from the lungs or the aorta in all mice, the proportion of animals infected in the aorta was lower in roxithromycin-treated than in placebo-treated animals at 14 weeks post inoculation [26]. These studies would suggest that longer treatment regimens may be required for eradication of chronic *C. pneumoniae* infection of the aorta.

Animal models of *C. pneumoniae* infection and atherosclerosis provide the opportunity to further define an etiologic role by determining whether intervention with antimicrobial agents can alter disease progression induced by infection, and identify the most favorable treatment regimens. In the study by Muhlestein et al. described above, treatment of rabbits with azithromycin for 7 weeks reduced the progression of atherosclerosis by the combined factors of a high-cholesterol diet and *C. pneumoniae* infection [22]. However, the organism was detected by immunofluorescence in the aorta of treated rabbits as frequently as in untreated animals.

In conclusion, an etiologic role of *C. pneumoniae* infection in atherosclerosis has not yet been firmly established. However, studies on induction, progression, and intervention studies in animals suggest such a role. Longer-term studies are required to determine whether atherosclerosis-like inflammatory changes seen shortly after infection in rabbit models persist and further develop to classic atherosclerosis in the absence of hypercholesteremia due to diet or predisposing genetic factors. In both mouse and rabbit, infection appears to exacerbate atherosclerosis in conjunction with high serum cholesterol. Future efforts should be directed towards elucidation of the pathogenic and immunologic mechanisms and cascade of events underlying these observed histopathologic changes following respiratory tract infection.

References

1. Grayston JT, Kuo C-C, Campbell LA, Wang S-P, Jackson L (1997) *Chlamydia pneumoniae* and cardiovascular disease. Cardiologia 42:1145-1151
2. Yang Z-P, Kuo C-C, Grayston JT (1993) A mouse model of *Chlamydia pneumoniae* strain TWAR pneumonitis. Infect Immun 61:2037-2040
3. Kaukoranta-Tolvanen SS, Laurila AL, Saikku P, Leinonen M, Liesirova L, Laitinen K (1993) Experimental infection of *Chlamydia pneumoniae* in mice. Microb Pathog 15:293-302
4. Yang Z-P, Cummings PK, Patton DL, Kuo C-C (1995) Ultrastructural lung pathology of experimental *Chlamydia pneumoniae* pneumonitis in mice. J Infect Dis 171:736-738
5. Moazed TC, Kuo C-C, Grayston JT, Campbell LA (1996) An experimental rabbit model of *Chlamydia pneumoniae* infection. Am J Pathol 148:667-676
6. Bell TA, Kuo C-C, Wang S-P, Grayston JT (1989) Experimental infection of baboons (*Papio cynocephalus anubis*) with *Chlamydia pneumoniae* strain "TWAR." J Infect 29:47-49
7. Holland SM, Taylor HR, Gaydos CA, Kappus EW, Quinn TC (1990) Experimental infection with *Chlamydia pneumoniae* in nonhuman primates. Infect Immun 58:593-597
8. Moazed TC, Kuo C-C, Grayston JT, Campbell LA (1997) Murine models of *Chlamydia pneumoniae* infection and atherosclerosis. J Infect Dis 175:883-890
9. Malinverni R, Kuo C-C, Campbell LA, Grayston JT (1995) Reactivation of *Chlamydia pneumoniae* lung infection in mice by cortisone. J Infect Dis 172:593-594
10. Yang Z-P, Kuo C-C, Grayston JT (1995) Systemic dissemination of *Chlamydia pneumoniae* following intranasal inoculation in mice. J Infect Dis 171:736-738
11. Moazed TC, Kuo C-C, Grayston JT, Campbell LA (1998) Systemic dissemination of *C. pneumoniae* infection via macrophages. J Infect Dis 177:1322-1325

12. Jackson LA, Campbell LA, Schmidt RA, Kuo C-C, Cappuccio AL, Grayston JT (1997) Specificity of detection of *Chlamydia pneumoniae* in cardiovascular and non-cardiovascular tissues: evaluation of the innocent bystander hypothesis. Am J Pathol 150:1785-1790

13. Boman J, Söderberg S, Forsberg J, Birgander LS, Allard A, Persson K, Jidell E, Kumlin U, Juto P, Waldenström A, Wadell G (1998) High prevalence of *Chlamydia pneumoniae* DNA in peripheral blood mononuclear cells in patients with cardiovascular disease in middle-aged blood donors. J Infect Dis 178:274-277

14. Moazed TC, Campbell LA, Rosenfeld ME, Grayston JT, Kuo C-C (1998) *Chlamydia pneumoniae* infection accelerates the progression of atherosclerosis in apoE-deficient mice. In: Stephens RS, Byrne GI, Christiansen G, Clark I, Grayston JT, Hatch T, Ridgeway G, Saikku P, Schachter J, Stamm WE (eds) Chlamydial infections. University of California Printing Services, Berkeley, pp 426-429

15. Piedrahita JA, Zhang SH, Hagaman JR, Oliver PM, Maeda N (1992) Generation of mice carrying a mutant apolipoprotein E gene inactivated by gene targeting in embryonic stem cells. Proc Natl Acad Sci USA 189:4471-4475

16. Reddick RL, Zhang SH, Maeda N (1994) Atherosclerosis in mice lacking Apo E. Evaluation of lesional development and progression. Atheroscler Thromb 14:141-147

17. Nakashima Y, Plump AS, Raines EW, Breslow JL, Ross R (1994) ApoE-deficient mice develop lesions of all phases of atherosclerosis. Atheroscler Thromb 14:133-140

18. Grönhagen-Riska C, Saikku P, Riska H, Froseth B, Grayston JT (1988) Antibodies to TWAR – a novel type of *Chlamydia* – in sarcoidosis. In: Grassi C, Rizzato G, Pozzi E (eds) Sarcoidosis and other granulomatous disorders. Excerpta Medica, Amsterdam, pp 297-301

19. Danesh J, Collins R, Peto R (1997) Chronic infections and coronary heart disease: is there a link? Lancet 350:430-436

20. Fong IW, Chiu B, Viira E, Fong MW, Jang D, Mahony J (1997) Rabbit model for *Chlamydia pneumoniae* infection. J Clin Microbiol 35:48-52

21. Laitinen K, Laurila A, Pyhala L, Leinonen M, Saikku P (1997) *Chlamydia pneumoniae* infection induces inflammatory changes in the aortas of rabbits. Infect Immun 65:4832-4835

22. Muhlestein JB, Anderson JL, Hammond EH, Zhao L, Trehan S, Schwobe EP, Carlquist JF (1998) Infection with *Chlamydia pneumoniae* accelerates the development of atherosclerosis and treatment with azithromycin prevents it in a rabbit model. Circulation 97:633-636

23. Laitinen K, Laurila AL, Leinonen M, Saikku P (1996) Reactivation of *Chlamydia pneumoniae* infection in mice by cortisone treatment. Infect Immun 64:1488-1490

24. Malinverni R, Kuo C-C, Campbell LA, Lee A, Grayston JT (1995) *Chlamydia pneumoniae* (TWAR) pneumonitis: effect of two antibiotic regimens on the course and persistence of infection. Antimicrob Agents Chemother 39:45-49

25. Masson MD, Toseland CDN, Beale AS (1995) Relevance of *Chlamydia pneumoniae* murine pneumonitis model to evaluation of antimicrobial agents. Antimicrob Agents Chemother 39:1959-1964

26. Campbell LA, Moazed TC, Kuo C-C, Grayston JT (1997) Preclinical models for *Chlamydia pneumoniae* and cardiovascular disease-hypercholesterolemic mice. Presented at Hoechst Marion Roussel. Roundtable on new concepts in the role of intracellular pathogens in chronic diseases. Sydney, Australia, July 2, 1997

Open and Controlled Intervention Trials for "Unusual" Anti-*Chlamydia pneumoniae* Indications: Asthma, Atherosclerosis, Myocardial Infarction

Clarithromycin Treatment of *Helicobacter pylori* and *Chlamydia pneumoniae* Infections Decreases Fibrinogen Plasma Level in Patients with Ischemic Heart Disease

L. Allegra, R. Cosentini, P. Tarsia

Recent data suggest that active inflammation and/or infection in the coronary arteries may play a role in ischemic heart disease (IHD) [1, 2]. The infectious theory has been suggested by epidemiological, serological, immunohistochemical and in situ hybridization studies, which indicated a possible etiologic role of some viruses and bacteria in the development of atherosclerotic lesions [3–5]. Among the micro-organisms potentially implicated, *Chlamydia pneumoniae* is the most extensively studied in the literature [6–9].

Helicobacter pylori infection, usually acquired in childhood, has also been recently associated with an increased risk of developing IHD [10–13] However, a recent epidemiological study failed to demonstrate an association between *H. pylori* infection and mortality from IHD [14].

The aim of our study was to evaluate changes in plasma fibrinogen level in IHD patients with seropositivity for *H. pylori* and/or *C. pneumoniae*, randomly assigned to antibiotic treatment and followed for 6 months.

A total of 163 consecutive patients with IHD, all admitted to our department or outpatient clinic, were evaluated. For all patients we obtained clinical history, physical examination and blood samples for the following determinations: white blood cell count, erythrocyte sedimentation rate, α-acid glycoprotein, C-reactive protein (CRP), cholesterol level, fibrinogen level, *H. pylori* IgG titer, *C. pneumoniae* IgG, IgA and IgM titers. *C. pneumoniae* IgG and IgA titers were measured again after 1 month in patients with IgG positivity and IgM negativity, in order to exclude *C. pneumoniae* reinfection; patients with basal IgM-positive testing were also excluded.

The inclusion criteria were as follows:
- age between 40 and 75 years;
- angiographically confirmed IHD, with stenosis > 70% in at least one coronary artery, and/or history of previous myocardial infarction (more than 1 month prior to enrolment);
- seropositivity for *H. pylori* and/or *C. pneumoniae* antibodies;
- absence of: acute inflammatory disease, history of neoplastic disease in the previous 5 years, history of acquired or congenital coagulation disorders;
- absence of *C. pneumoniae* acute infection or reinfections.

Six months after randomization all patients underwent blood sampling for all the determinations listed above.

Eligible patients were randomly allocated to treatment or no treatment. All patients gave written informed consent. Fibrinogen level determinations (main variable) were performed blindly by the laboratory technician. Treatment allocation of *H. pylori*-positive and *H. pylori*-negative, *C. pneumoniae*-positive patients was done according to two separate randomization lists generated by a computer. Treatment of *H. pylori*-positive patients, irrespective of *C. pneumoniae*-positivity, consisted of omeprazole 20 mg orally twice a day for 30 days, clarithromycin 500 mg orally twice a day for 14 days and tinidazole 500 mg orally twice a day for 7 days. Treatment of *H. pylori*-negative, *C. pneumoniae*-positive patients consisted of clarithromycin 500 mg orally twice a day for 14 days. The choice of clarithromycin dosage was due to its efficacy in the treatment of *C. pneumoniae* infection. All patients were seen 1 month after randomization for a clinical evaluation and to assess adherence to treatment. Final observation and blood tests were carried out after 6 months in all patients who completed the treatment.

Ninety-seven patients satisfying the inclusion criteria were randomized to treatment (48 patients) or no treatment (49 patients). Five patients of the treated group and eight of the non-treated group did not complete the study, because of the need for coronary artery bypass grafting (one in the treated group and two in the non-treated group) or because of lack of compliance or withdrawal of consent (four in the treated group and six in the non-treated group). Discriminate analysis of the clinical and laboratory data in the 84 patients who completed the study did not detect any difference in baseline variables between the two treatment groups; thus, the two randomization groups were considered to be homogeneous on admission.

The distribution of treated and non-treated patients on the basis of serological results is shown in Table 1.

Table 1. Serological results in treated and non-treated patients

	H. pylori-negative, *C. pneumoniae*-positive	*H. pylori*- and *C. pneumoniae*-positive	*H. pylori*-positive, *C. pneumoniae*-negative
Treated	6	23	14
Non-treated	7	23	11

The means of basal fibrinogen levels were not significantly different in the groups of patients distributed according to serological pattern (3.50 ± 0.70 g/dl in *H. pylori*- and *C. pneumoniae*-positive patients; 3.67 ± 0.76 in *H. pylori*-negative, *C. pneumoniae*-positive patients; 3.60 ± 0.50 in *H. pylori*-positive, *C. pneumoniae*-negative patients). A significant correlation was observed between basal fibrinogen and smoking ($p < 0.05$) and between basal fibrinogen and basal CRP level ($p < 0.01$).

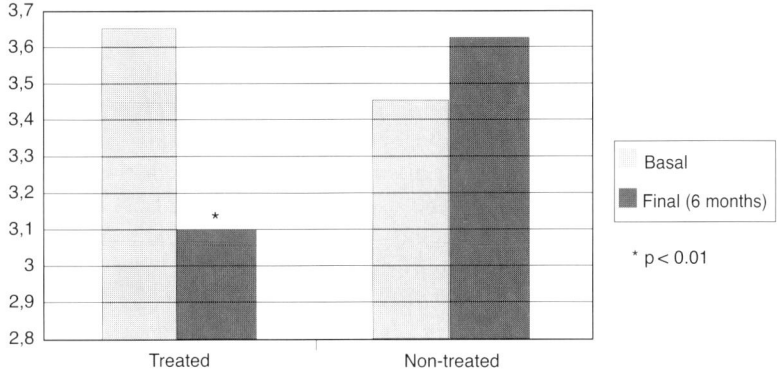

Fig. 1. Fibrinogen levels on admission and at follow-up in treated and non-treated patients

Mean IgG geometric titer in treated patients with single *C. pneumoniae* infection decreased significantly from 725 ± 330 to 225 ± 240 ($p < 0.01$), whereas in the control group mean IgG geometric titer increased after 6 months from 325 ± 470 to 370 ± 480 ($p = \text{NS}$). The difference between mean IgG geometric titer at baseline did not differ significantly between the two groups.

The distribution of fibrinogen and CRP levels on admission and at the 6-month follow-up in treated and non-treated patients is shown in Figs. 1 and 2.

Two recent randomized studies on the treatment of *C. pneumoniae* infection in IHD patients suggested that treatment with macrolides may be effective in decreasing adverse cardiovascular events; the study by Gupta et al. [15] showed that azithromycin treatment of *C. pneumoniae*-positive patients reduced the risk of adverse cardiovascular events during an 18-month follow-up period to values similar to those found in *C. pneumoniae*-negative patients. Gurfinkel et al. [16] found that roxithromycin reduced morbidity and mortality during a 1-month period following non-Q-wave myocardial infarction or unstable angina.

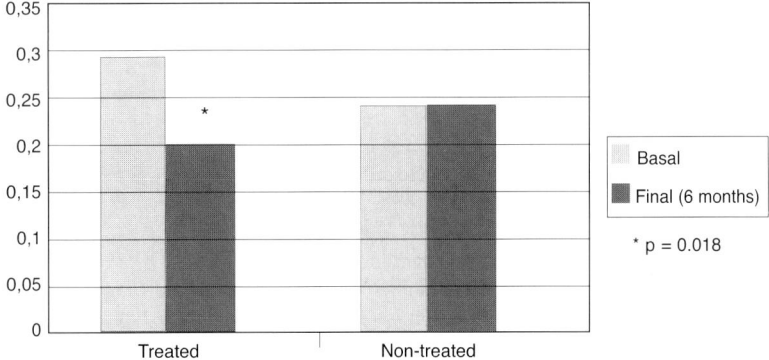

Fig. 2. CRP levels on admission and at follow-up in treated and non-treated patients

We performed a randomized study using a clarithromycin treatment schedule that allowed *H. pylori* eradication displaying antichlamydial activity. The main finding was that treatment significantly reduced fibrinogen levels in IHD patients and this reduction was detectable at 6 months from treatment. The decrease was observed both in the overall study population and in patients with either *C. pneumoniae* or *H. pylori* infection. Interestingly, the greatest reduction (approximately 20%) was found in patients seropositive for both organisms.

This observation suggests that the effect of treatment could be long-lasting and related to its antimicrobial activity, rather than to a possible antinflammatory activity of macrolides [17]. It also supports the link between *C. pneumoniae* or *H. pylori* infections and fibrinogen, further suggested by the significant increase of fibrinogen level in non-treated patients positive for both infections.

In the treated patient groups we observed a reduction in CRP levels which was parallel to the decrease in fibrinogen levels. High CRP concentrations in patients with unstable angina are a strong negative prognostic factor [18]. These data support the hypothesis that *C. pneumoniae* and *H. pylori* infections may contribute to the increase in CRP levels.

Should our data be confirmed in a larger population, in the near future a short, safe and effective course of antibiotic therapy might be suggested as a means of interacting with an "emerging" risk factor, thus obtaining a high epidemiological impact on patients with IHD.

References

1. Nieminen MS, Mattila K, Valtonen V (1993) Infection and inflammation as a risk factor for myocardial infarction. Eur Heart J 14[Suppl K]:12-16
2. Alexander RW (1994) Inflammation and coronary artery disease. N Engl J Med 331:468-469
3. Beneditt EP, Barret T, McDougall JK (1983) Viruses and etiology of atherosclerosis. Proc Natl Acad Sci USA 80:6386-6389
4. Pesonen E, Siitonen O (1981) Acute myocardial infarction precipitated by infectious diseases. Am Heart J 101:512-513
5. Spodick DH, Flessas AP, Johnson MM (1984) Association of acute respiratory symptoms with onset of acute myocardial infarction: prospective investigation of 150 consecutive patients and matched control patients. Am J Cardiol 53:481-482
6. Saikku P (1993) *Chlamydia pneumoniae* as a risk factor in acute myocardial infarction. Eur Heart J 14[Suppl K]:62-65
7. Saikku P, Leinonen M, Mattila K et al (1988) Serological evidence of an association of a novel *Chlamydia*, TWAR, with chronic coronary heart disease and acute myocardial infarction. Lancet ii:983-986
8. Shor A, Kuo C-C, Patton DL (1992) Detection of *Chlamydia pneumoniae* in coronary arterial fatty streaks and atheromatous plaques. S Afr Med J 82:158-161
9. Kuo C-C, Shor A, Campbell LA et al (1993) Demonstration of *Chlamydia pneumoniae* in atherosclerotic lesions of coronary arteries. J Infect Dis 167:845-849
10. Mendall MA, Goggin PM, Molineaux N et al (1994) Relation of *Helicobacter pylori* infection and coronary heart disease. Br Heart J 71:437-439

11. Aceti A, Mazzacurati G, Amendola MA et al (1996) *H. pylori* and *C. pneumoniae* infections may account for most acute coronary syndrome. BMJ 313:428-429

12. Morgando A, Sanseverino P, Perotto C et al (1995) *Helicobacter pylori* seropositivity in myocardial infarction. Lancet 345:1380 (letter)

13. Patel P, Carrington D, Strachan DP et al (1994) Fibrinogen: a link between chronic infection and coronary heart disease. Lancet 343:1634-1635

14. Wald NJ, Law MR, Morris JK et al (1997) *Helicobacter pylori* infection and mortality from ischaemic heart disease: negative result from a large, prospective study. BMJ 315:1199-1201

15. Gupta S, Leatham EW, Carrington D et al (1997) Elevated *Chlamydia pneumoniae* antibodies, cardiovascular events, and azithromycin in male survivors of myocardial infarction. Circulation 96:404-407

16. Gurfinkel E, Bozovich G, Daroca A et al (1997) Randomised trial of roxithromycin in non-Q-wave coronary syndromes: ROXIS pilot study. Lancet 350:404-407

17. Agen C, Danesi R, Blandizzi C et al (1993) Macrolide antibiotics as antiinflammatory agents: roxithromycin in an unexpected role. Agents Actions 38:(1-2)85-90

18. Liuzzo G, Biasucci LM, Gallimore JR et al (1994) The prognostic value of C-reactive protein and serum amyloid A protein in severe unstable angina. N Engl J Med 331:417-424

Antibiotic Treatment in Atherosclerosis and Myocardial Infarction

S. Gupta, J.C. Kaski

Introduction

Evidence is accumulating to suggest that *Chlamydia pneumoniae* may have a role in the development and/or progression of atherosclerotic-related disorders, in particular coronary heart disease (CHD). The evidence for *C. pneumoniae* as a potential causative agent is largely based on the findings of (1) seroepidemiological studies, (2) examination of atheromatous plaque specimens, (3) in vitro experiments and animal models and, recently, (4) preliminary anti-chlamydial antibiotic intervention studies. This chapter aims at focusing on the potential, and intriguing, role of antimicrobial therapy in the secondary prevention of CHD. The findings of the preliminary pilot studies are reviewed, as are the aims and controversies surrounding large-scale, prospective intervention trials, now in progress.

Preliminary Antibiotic Trials in Patients with Coronary Heart Disease

Azithromycin in Male Survivors of Myocardial Infarction: A Pilot Study

Interest in the association between *C. pneumoniae* and CHD began in our institution in 1994. In a cross-sectional population survey in a South London population it was shown that an elevated anti-*C. pneumoniae* antibody titre was associated with prevalent CHD (as defined by Rose questionnaire/electrocardiographic criteria), and that this association persisted even after controlling for established cardiovascular risk factors, such as smoking and social class [1]. In particular, an elevated IgG titre of ≥ 1:64 was associated with a more than sixfold increase in odds ratio for the presence of prevalent CHD. The findings of this first UK-based epidemiological study corroborated the original observations of Finnish [2] and American [3] workers. As an extension to the investigation it was proposed that *C. pneumoniae* may be pathogenetic in athero-thrombosis via the activation of inflammatory and procoagulant markers. This followed the findings of a positive correlation between an elevated anti-*C. pneumoniae* antibody titre and raised levels of C-reactive protein, leucocyte count, fibrinogen and factor VIIa [4]. In addition, one stimulus to the enhanced expression of tissue factor seen on the monocytes of patients with CHD was postulated to be a low-grade chlamydial infection [5].

With the findings of this background research it was next proposed to conduct a pilot intervention study with an anti-chlamydial antibiotic.

In a randomised, placebo-controlled study (funded by the British Heart Foundation) the new-generation macrolide (azalide), azithromycin, was given to a series of male survivors of myocardial infarction (MI) with stable elevated anti-*C. pneumoniae* antibody titres (i.e. stable elevated IgG titre of $\geq 1:64$, taken 3 months apart). The primary aim of this study was to examine for changes in serum and monocyte markers of inflammation and hypercoagulation [6]. An assessment was also made of whether an elevated anti-*C. pneumoniae* antibody titre predicted further cardiovascular events, in 213 consecutive post-MI males stratified according to antibody titres, at a mean 18-month follow-up period [7]. The incidence of future cardiovascular events in those patients with elevated titres (IgG $\geq 1:64$) randomised to azithromycin (single course of 500 mg/day for 3 days, $n = 28$; or a double course, $n = 12$) or placebo ($n = 20$) was also observed.

Azithromycin, a new-generation macrolide, was chosen in view of its efficacy against chlamydial infections and good tolerability. A 3-day course has been shown to be effective treatment against respiratory infections with *C. pneumoniae* [8]. Moreover, the drug achieves strong tissue penetration and, in particular, high macrophage concentration [9], which is highly relevant since this cell is known to harbour *C. pneumoniae*. At the time of study design there was no information available on the effects of broad-spectrum antibiotic therapy in post-MI patients; it was therefore deemed pertinent only to randomise those patients with stable elevated antibody titres (presumed chronic infection) to the trial.

The results of the clinical study are shown in Table 1. There was a fourfold risk of experiencing adverse cardiovascular events among the group with elevated

Table 1. Odds ratios for cardiovascular events in seronegative and seropositive patient groups. (Adapted from [7], with permission)

Group	Total CV events (%)	Unadjusted OR (95% CI)	Adjusted OR (95% CI)
Cp–ve ($n = 59$)	4 (7)		
Cp–I ($n = 74$)	11 (15)	2.4 (0.7-8.0)	2.0 (0.6-6.8)
Cp+ve–NR/P ($n = 40$)	11 (28)	5.2 (1.5-17.8)[*]	4.2 (1.2-15.5)[**]
Cp+ve–A ($n = 40$)	3 (8)	1.1 (0.2-5.3)	0.9 (0.2-4.6)

Comparison of cardiovascular (CV) events are for all groups relative to Cp–ve group [expressed as odds ratio (OR) (95% CI)]. Adjusted OR calculated after controlling for variables: age, diabetes mellitus, smoking status, hypertension, dyslipidaemia and previous coronary revascularisation
Cp–ve, seronegative group of patients; *Cp–I*, group with intermediate antibody titres; *Cp+ve–NR/P*, group with elevated antibody titres either randomised to placebo or not randomised; *Cp+ve–A*, group with elevated antibody titres randomised to azithromycin; *CI*, confidence intervals
[*]$p = 0.008$, [**]$p = 0.03$ relative to Cp–ve group

C. pneumoniae titres compared with the group with negative serology [odds ratio 4.2 (95% CI 1.2–15.5, $p = 0.03$)]. For the high-titre group receiving antibiotic therapy, the adjusted odds ratio was 0.9 (0.2–4.6, $p = $ns), i.e. the same as that in the seronegative group.

Subjects receiving azithromycin had a significant fall in certain levels of serum and monocyte activation markers (monocyte integrins CD11b/CD11c, fibrinogen and leucocyte count, $p < 0.05$) [6]. These findings support the hypothesis that *C. pneumoniae* may be contributory to the progression of atherosclerosis via up-regulation of inflammatory markers.

The study findings suggest that an anti-*C. pneumoniae* antibody titre may be a predictor of further cardiovascular events in male survivors of MI, and that azithromycin may potentially reduce this risk. The results from this pilot study do not help to distinguish between an anti-*C. pneumoniae* effect of azithromycin and a non-antimicrobial (such as anti-inflammatory [10]) effect. In favour of the former, it was intriguing to observe that a greater proportion of patients receiving azithromycin had a fall in their anti-*C. pneumoniae* antibody titres at 6 months, suggesting that the antibiotic may be suppressing infection or accelerating clearance of antibodies. The small size of the study does indicate that a much larger purpose-designed, prospective trial would be necessary to confirm the preliminary findings.

Roxithromycin in Acute Coronary Syndromes

In the "Roxithromycin in Ischaemic Syndromes" (ROXIS) study [11], another pilot randomised intervention trial, the aim was to assess whether the antichlamydial antibiotic, roxithromycin (150 mg twice/day, for 30 days), could decrease the incidence of recurrent ischaemic events in 205 patients presenting with acute coronary syndromes. There was a significant reduction in combined ischaemic events (recurrent ischaemia plus MI plus ischaemic death) at day 31 in the patients randomised to roxithromycin compared with the placebo group (two versus nine events, $p = 0.03$ unadjusted, $p = 0.06$ adjusted). Follow-up results of this study suggest that the benefit derived from therapy may be independent of baseline IgG serology (unpublished). An anti-inflammatory, "plaque-stabilising" effect of macrolide therapy is one postulated mechanism in this clinical setting.

Doxycycline in Patients Undergoing Coronary Artery Bypass Surgery

In a small placebo-controlled study, doxycycline therapy was randomised to a total of 34 non-smoking males with previous coronary artery bypass surgery (CABG) [12]. Following 4 months of chronic therapy (100 mg/daily) no significant differences were noted between the doxycycline-treated and the placebo-treated group in anti-*C. pneumoniae* antibody titres, laboratory-based risk factors for CHD (including lipids, fibrinogen and thrombin fragments) or nitric oxide production (as determined by forearm blood flow responses). The investigators acknowledge that the numbers of patients in the study were too small to assess for clinical effects, that monotherapy alone may not be sufficient to eradicate a chronic chlamydial infection and that antibody serology itself may not be the appropriate surrogate marker to confirm a chronic *C. pneumoniae* infection.

ACADEMIC Study: "Azithromycin in Coronary Artery Disease: Elimination of Myocardial Infection with *Chlamydia*"

The ACADEMIC study is a USA-based, double-blind, randomised study to test whether azithromycin reduces systemic markers of inflammation, antibody titres to *C. pneumoniae* and vascular events in patients with symptomatic CHD (post MI or angiographically demonstrated) [13]. One hundred and fifty patients were randomised to a 3-day acute course of azithromycin (total 1.5 g) followed by a 3-month course of the antibiotic (500 mg weekly), 150 patients to placebo. Preliminary results show a significant stabilisation of certain inflammatory markers [i.e. C-reactive protein, interleukin (IL)-1/IL-6] at 6 months. No difference has been noted in antibody titres or clinical cardiovascular events at 3 months or at 6 months – but again, the study is relatively small. The clinical endpoint (total cardiovascular events) evaluation is awaited at a 2-year follow-up.

Large-scale, Randomised, Antibiotic Trials in Coronary Heart Disease

The interest following the publication of the first two pilot studies of macrolide therapy in the prevention of coronary events has been widespread; in particular the clinical and commercial interest. Although the study of doxycycline in CABG patients and the preliminary findings of the ACADEMIC study have been less optimistic, larger intervention trials are now already underway, with others under design.

WIZARD Study: "Weekly Intervention with Zithromax against Atherosclerotic-Related Disorders"

The WIZARD study, launched in mid-1997, has recruited about 3300 post-MI patients (MI > 6 weeks previously) who have positive anti-*C. pneumoniae* serology ($\geq$ 1:16 IgG). Subjects receive either an acute 3-day course of azithromycin (600 mg/day) followed by a chronic 3-month course of the antibiotic (600 mg, given weekly), or placebo. The primary aim of the study is to assess whether azithromycin reduces total cardiovascular events over a 2.5-year follow-up. The total duration of therapy is arbitrary, albeit based on a logical rationale. An acute course of azithromycin may treat any active *C. pneumoniae* infection, and perhaps stabilise plaque. However, an ongoing chronic course of therapy may be necessary to attempt eradication of a deep-sited infection – where the organism may follow a cyclical pattern of remaining quiescent ("persistent body") and then emerging into an unpredictable active phase – making plaque rupture more susceptible. In the active phase, an adequate local concentration of the drug would be necessary, hence the weekly regimen. The experience of safe, long-term usage of azithromycin is vast, especially in the prophylactic treatment of disseminated

Mycobacterium avium complex disease in HIV-infected patients, who are often given therapy for as long as 2 years [14]. The WIZARD study may not be able to differentiate between any non-antimicrobial action of the antibiotic and antibacterial effects, since only anti-*C. pneumoniae* seropositive patients are included. Provision is made to assess changes in anti-*C. pneumoniae* titres and inflammatory markers during the course of the study. Recruitment of patients is now complete, and endpoints are currently being reviewed.

MARBLE Study: "Might Azithromycin Reduce Bypass-List Events?"

The MARBLE study is a UK-based prospective antibiotic trial. An intrinsic limitation of the British National Health Service system is the realities of waiting lists and times for coronary revascularisation procedures. In an average tertiary cardiothoracic unit some 500–600 patients with severe CHD will be on a typical waiting list for CABG. These patients can expect to wait for up to 12 months for surgery. Such patients often have cardiovascular events while they wait – including readmission with unstable angina, MI and progression in the degree of coronary artery disease [15]. MARBLE aims at randomising such "CABG waiters" to a 3-month course of weekly azithromycin (as in the WIZARD design), or placebo (irrespective of baseline anti-*C. pneumoniae* antibody titre), and to assess whether total cardiovascular events may be reduced during the period waiting for CABG. At time of operation a proportion (20%–25%) of these patients will undergo coronary endarterectomy procedures – and samples of coronary arteries taken at this time will be examined for presence of *C. pneumoniae* and correlations made with serology, inflammatory markers and any effects of antibiotic treatment. The results of the MARBLE study may provide important data on the relationship between antibiotic treatment and effects of infection within coronary arteries. Moreover, this study could have political and socio-economic ramifications for National Health Service CABG waiting lists.

STAMINA Study: "South Thames Antibiotics in Myocardial Infarction and Angina"

A further UK-based study is STAMINA. In this study, patients with acute coronary syndromes ($n = 600$) are being randomised to an azithromycin-based regimen, an amoxycillin-based regimen or placebo. The aim is to treat both *Helicobacter pylori* and *C. pneumoniae* and assess effects on serological markers of infection, inflammatory markers (fibrinogen, C-reactive protein, IL-6) and, secondarily, on clinical cardiovascular events.

Conclusion

Although evidence continues to accumulate suggesting that chronic infection with *C. pneumoniae* contributes to atherogenesis, a direct causal role for *C. pneumoniae* is unproven [16]. A number of questions remain unanswered. The issues of optimal antibiotic therapy, duration of therapy, reinfection rates and role of other infections need further clarification. Furthermore, the question of community-based antibiotic resistance emerging if broad-spectrum antibiotic usage becomes widespread also needs careful risk-benefit analysis [17]. It is postulated (and hoped) that the initial large-scale prospective trials may help to clarify some essential questions. Firstly, whether anti-chlamydial antibiotics, in particular macrolides, may treat a chronic vascular infection with *C. pneumoniae*. Secondly, whether a reduction in cardiovascular events can be achieved. The trials may turn out to demonstrate that these antibiotics possess other beneficial actions, such as anti-inflammatory effects [11]. Finally, it is also possible that the trials may not show a clear-cut benefit in the use of anti-chlamydial therapy in the secondary prevention of CHD. Results from the intervention studies are due early in the next millennium. If the findings are positive, the effects on public health worldwide would be considerable.

References

1. Mendall MA, Carrington D, Strachan D et al (1995) *Chlamydia pneumoniae*: risk factors for seropositivity and association with coronary heart disease. J Infect 30:121-128
2. Saikku P, Mattila K, Nieminen MS et al (1988) Serological evidence of an association of a novel Chlamydia, TWAR, with chronic coronary heart disease and acute myocardial infarction. Lancet 2:983-986
3. Thom DH, Grayston JT, Siscovick DS et al (1992) Association of prior infection with *Chlamydia pneumoniae* and angiographically demonstrated coronary artery disease. JAMA 268:68-72
4. Patel P, Mendall MA, Carrington D et al (1995) Association of *Helicobacter pylori* and *Chlamydia pneumoniae* infections with coronary heart disease and cardiovascular risk factors. BMJ 311:711-714
5. Leatham EWL, Bath PM, Tooze JA et al (1995) Increased monocyte tissue factor expression in coronary disease. Br Heart J 73:10-13
6. Gupta S, Leatham EW, Carrington D et al (1997) The effect of azithromycin in post myocardial infarction patients with elevated *Chlamydia pneumoniae* antibody titres. J Am Coll Cardiol 755:209 (abstract)
7. Gupta S, Leatham EW, Carrington D et al (1997) Elevated *Chlamydia penumoniae* antibodies, cardiovascular events and azithromycin in male survivors of myocardial infarction. Circulation 96:404-407
8. Rizzato G, Montemurro L, Fraioli P et al (1995) Efficacy of a three day course of azithromycin in moderately severe community-acquired pnumonia. Eur Respir J 8:398-402
9. Foulds G, Shepard RM, Johnson RB et al (1990) The pharmacokinetic of azithromycin in human serum and tissue. J Antimicrob Chemother 25[Suppl A]:73-82
10. Black PN (1997) Anti-inflammatory effects of macrolide antibiotics. Eur Respir J 10:971-972
11. Gurfinkel E, Bozovich G, Daroca A et al (1997) Randomised trial of roxithromycin in non-Q-wave coronary syndromes: ROXIS pilot study. Lancet 350:404-407
12. Sinisalo J, Mattila K, Nieminen MS et al (1998) The effect of prolonged doxycycline therapy on *Chlamydia pneumoniae* serological markers, coronary heart disease risk factor and forearm basal nitric oxide production. J Antimicrob Chemother 41:85-92

13. Anderson JL, Muhlestein JB (1998) Azithromycin in coronary artery disease: elimination of myocardial infection with *Chlamydia*. ACADEMIC study. Presented at 47th Scientific Session of American College of Cardiology Meeting, Atlanta, Georgia

14. Havlir DV, Dubé MP, Sattler FR et al (1996) Prophylaxis against disseminated *Mycobacterium avium* complex with weekly azithromycin, daily rifabutin, or both. N Engl J Med 335:392-398

15. Kaski JC, Chester MR, Chen L et al (1995) Rapid angiographic progression of coronary artery disease in patients with angina pectoris. Circulation 92:2058-2065

16. Gupta S, Camm AJ (1997) *Chlamydia pneumoniae* and coronary heart disease: coincidence, association or causation? BMJ 314:1778-1779

17. Gupta S, Kaski JC, Camm AJ (1998) Antibiotic therapy in coronary heart disease: hype versus hope. Br J Cardiol 5:65-66

A Controlled Intervention Study with Antibiotics in Symptomatic Coronary Patients Irrespective of Serology

E. GURFINKEL

Since the first coronary artery bypass surgery in 1967, 30 years have passed with few medical strategies proven effective in the treatment of acute coronary syndromes [1, 2]. In spite of it and many new antithrombotic compounds, a sizable proportion of patients are still developing new ischemic episodes, which may indicate that we have reached a biological barrier where any attempt to increase efficacy leads to the loss of security.

The recent ROXIS trial [3] and its final report [4] support the recent concept that this barrier can be surmounted, raising the possibility that infection and inflammation, which play a key role during the acute phase of symptomatic atherosclerosis, could be treated with a new medical strategy.

The origin of the chronic inflammatory reaction and macrophage activation within atherosclerotic lesions is still unclear, but a multifactorial etiology is likely. The role of other stimuli, such as homocysteine and infection, is still under investigation. Infection, for example, may perpetuate a low-level chronic inflammatory state, either systemically or by direct macrophage infection. *Chlamydia pneumoniae* has been directly identified in macrophages present in atherosclerotic plaques [5].

This evidence suggests that chronic infection may contribute to the chronic inflammatory state of atherosclerosis and be responsible for elevated systemic markers of inflammation. Recently, Birnie et al. [6] showed a correlation between anti-mycobacterial heat shock protein 65 (mhsp65) antibodies and the extent of atherosclerosis. The mhsp65 shares a close homology with human, *Helicobacter pylori*, and *C. pneumoniae* heat shock proteins. Infection might be the origin of a vascular autoimmune reaction.

In addition to this, the human leukocyte antigen (HLA) complex is also implicated in this immune reaction. This system modulates the immune reaction by presenting peptides to effector T-cells. The HLA complex, located in the short arm of chromosome 6, is linked to several chronic diseases by inducing an inadequate or excessive inflammatory response. Atherosclerotic heart disease may prove to be another of these chronic diseases. We also investigated the relationship between unstable angina and the HLA pattern, finding a significant correlation between refractory angina and two HLA alleles: HLA A31 and HLA B4 [7].

All of these were the basis for the ROXIS study [3].

Table 1. Incidence of the composite double and triple endpoints and of component events by intention-to-treat basis

Endpoint	Placebo	ROXIS	p value
	Number %	Number %	
Day 30	(n=100)	(n=102)	
Severe recurrent ischaemia	5 (5)	2 (1.9)	0.277
Myocardial infarction	2 (2)	0 (0)	0.244
Death	2 (2)	0 (0)	0.244
Double endpoint	4 (4)	0 (0)	0.058
Triple endpoint	9 (9)	2 (1.9)	0.032
Day 90	(n=96)	(n=92)	
Severe recurrent ischaemia	6 (6.25)	4 (4.37)	0.747
Myocardial infarction	2 (2.08)	0 (0)	0.497
Death	4 (4.16)	0 (0)	0.122
Double endpoint	6 (6.25)	0 (0)	0.029
Triple endpoint	12 (12.5)	4 (4.37)	0.065
Day 180	(n=96)	(n=92)	
Severe recurrent ischaemia	7 (7.29)	6 (6.52)	0.90
Myocardial infarction	2 (2.08)	0 (0)	0.498
Death	5 (5.2)	2 (2.17)	0.445
Double endpoint	7 (7.29)	2 (2.17)	0.17
Triple endpoint	14 (14.6)	8 (8.69)	0.259

A total of 205 patients with the diagnosis of unstable angina or non-Q-wave myocardial infarction with chest pain within 48 h of presentation were enrolled and immediately randomised in double-blind manner to receive either rox-ithromycin 300 mg per day p.o. or placebo for a minimum of six doses (72 h) to a maximum of 30 days, independently of basal anti-*Chlamydia* antibody titres, as there is no current evidence that IgG titres, as a marker of chronic infection, have any utility in guiding treatment, and knowing that other "*Chlamydia*-like" proteins may activate the immune system and make *Chlamydia* IgG titres less important in clinical decisions. The results are shown in Table 1.

The serological samples in the ROXIS trial revealed that less than 50% of the patients had IgG titres > 1:64 and 72% had titres > 1:32, indicating that a large majority had been exposed to *C. pneumoniae*. In addition, during the ROXIS study we evaluated the inflammatory response through C-reactive protein concentrations in plasma. C-reactive protein levels decreased in both groups after the treatment period, although the decrease was significantly greater in the active treatment arm. A potential anti-inflammatory effect of macrolide antibiotics beyond their bactericidal action [8] remains uncertain and may require different markers of inflammation to evaluate.

Several clinical studies, in various stages of development, will help determine whether infection plays an important role in both the unstable and the quiescent phase of atherosclerosis. If these new studies are consistent with the findings of the ROXIS trial, future therapy for atherosclerotic disease, instead of including even more cardiac drug per patient, may become tailored to a patient's individual risk profile.

References

1. Gurfinkel E, on behalf of the principal contributors (1998) Current treatment and future prospects for the management of acute coronary syndromes. Consensus Recommendation of the 1997 Ushuaia Conference, Tierra del Fuego, Argentina. Clin Drug Invest 15:368-380
2. Gurfinkel E, Fareed J, Antman E, Cohen M, Mautner B (1998) The rationale for the management of acute coronary syndromes with low molecular weight heparins. Am J Cardiol 82:15L-18L
3. Gurfinkel E, Bozovich G, Daroca A, Beck E, Mautner B for the Roxis Study Group (1997) Randomised trial of roxithromycin in non-Q-wave coronary syndromes: Roxis pilot study. Lancet 350:404-407
4. Gurfinkel E, Bozovich G, Livellara G, Beck E, Testa E, Mautner B (1999) Antibiotics for the treatment of non-Q-wave coronary syndromes. The Final Report of the ROXIS Trial. Eur Heart J 15:368-380
5. Grayston JT, Kuo C-C, Coulson AS et al (1995) *Chlamydia pneumoniae* (TWAR) in atherosclerosis of the carotid artery. Circulation 92:3397-3400
6. Birnie DH, Holme ER, McKay IC, Hood S, McColl KE, Hillis WS (1998) Association between antibodies to heat shock protein 65 and coronary atherosclerosis. Possible mechanism of action of *Helicobacter pylori* and other bacterial infections in increasing cardiovascular risk. Eur Heart J 19:387-394
7. Bozovich G, Gurfinkel E, Raimondi E, Padrós K, Mejaíl I, Haas E et al (1997) Major histocompatibility complex and the vulnerable plaque in acute coronary syndromes. Potential modulation of the inflammatory response. Puerto Rico Health Sciences Journal 16:5
8. Kadota JL (1996) Non-antibiotic effects of antibiotics. J Clin Microb Infect [Suppl II]:220-222

Open-Label Before-After Trials of Anti-*Chlamydia pneumoniae* Antibiotics in Asthma

D.L. Hahn

At the time of writing, no randomized, controlled trials of anti-chlamydial antibiotics directed against asthma have been published. Such trials are underway, or are being planned, based upon (1) reported seroepidemiologic associations linking chlamydial infection to asthma (see the chapter, "*Chlamydia pneumoniae*: A New Possible Cause of Asthma") and (2) published case reports [1, 2] and case series [3–5] indicating favorable results of open-label antibiotic administration to patients with asthma who also had culture-confirmed infection, seroreactivity, or both.

Kawane [1] reported the case of a 39-year-old man with cough variant asthma, bronchial hyperreactivity (BHR), eosinophilia, elevated IgE and high serologic titers against *Chlamydia pneumoniae* (IgG 1:1024, IgA 1:32, IgM negative) in whom results were described as successful after treatment with clarithromycin (a macrolide antibiotic) for 2 weeks.

Hahn [2] reported on a patient with symptomatic adult-onset asthma with eosinophilia who was persistently culture-positive for *C. pneumoniae* prior to antibiotic treatment with azithromycin, 1 g, administered orally once weekly for three doses (a single 1-g dose had been approved in the USA for treatment of uncomplicated urogenital *C. trachomatis* infection, and the author reasoned that a longer duration of therapy would be required to eradicate *C. pneumoniae*).

Figure 1 presents details of the serologic and culture findings, pulmonary function results and treatment with prednisone and azithromycin for this patient [2]. Another treated patient for whom culture results were not available is also presented in the figure. Both patients had moderately severe, persistent asthma symptoms that improved temporarily and then relapsed after a 10–14 days' treatment with prednisone (an oral anti-inflammatory agent commonly used in severe asthma). Both patients had temporary improvement in asthma symptoms and pulmonary function after a 5–14 days' treatment with azithromycin (a macrolide antibiotic with in vitro activity against *C. pneumoniae*); both relapsed after finishing the antibiotics, which failed to eradicate *C. pneumoniae* in the culture-positive case. Subsequent administration of azithromycin, 1 g orally once weekly for 3 weeks, achieved microbiologic eradication in the culture-positive patient and long-lasting improvement in asthma symptoms and pulmonary function in both patients.

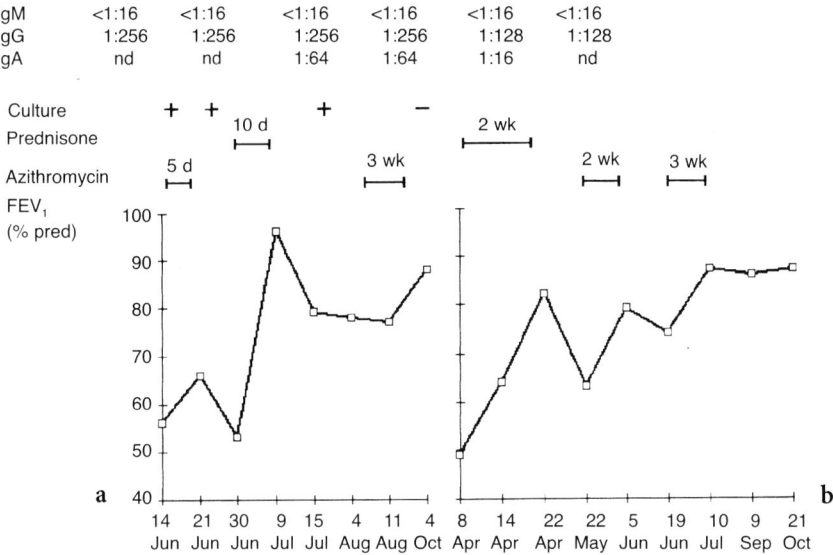

Fig. 1a, b. *Chlamydia pneumoniae* serologic results (specific IgM, IgG, IgA by micro-immunofluorescence assay), culture findings, medication use (oral prednisone, azithromycin) and forced expiratory volume in 1 s (FEV₁) for two patients with adult-onset asthma. **a** 40-years-old African-American male who developed persistent asthma symptoms following a respiratory illness; **b** 36-years-old Caucasian female who developed asthma following an episode of community-acquired pneumonia

On the basis of clinical observations such as those illustrated in Fig. 1, Hahn [3] treated 46 adults with persistent moderate to moderately severe non-steroid-dependent asthma who were also seroreactive to *C. pneumoniae* (total Ig titer ≥1:16, median 1:128). The antibiotics used were doxycycline, 100 mg orally twice daily or azithromycin, 1 g weekly. The treatment duration was 3–9 weeks (median 4 weeks). Follow-up was an average of 6 months post-treatment (range 1.5–36 months). Overall, 25 (54%) of 46 patients had a complete or major improvement in asthma at follow-up that was correlated with improvement in pulmonay function. Complete remission and normalization of pulmonary function was achieved in 7 patients, while 18 had major improvement, defined as a significant clinical improvement with decreased medication use. Improvement was significantly more likely to occur in patients with early disease ($p=0.01$) and before the development of fixed obstruction ($p< 0.01$). The author speculated that this pattern was consistent with chlamydial pathogenesis and called for the performance of randomized, controlled trials before recommending for or against anti-chlamydial treatment in asthma. Hahn et al. [5] subsequently extended the clinical observations of a positive treatment response in seroreactive asthmatics to include patients with severe, steroid-dependent asthma. In the case of patients whose asthma symptoms remained poorly controlled despite administration of systemic steroids, they suggested a careful search for evidence of chlamydial infection. Because accurate diagnostic testing has not yet been established for chronic *C. pneumoniae* infection. They suggested it might even be reasonable in selected cases to prescribe empirical therapy (around 6 weeks with an antibiotic effective against *C. pneumoniae*).

Emre et al. [4] reported on treatment results in 12 culture-positive children with acute wheezing episodes seen at an inner-city emergency department. They reported that 9 of the 12 patients had laboratory and symptom improvement after microbiologic eradication. Antibiotics employed were erythromycin or clarithromycin for 10 days to 2 weeks in most cases. One patient remained culture positive after two 10-day treatment courses with clarithromycin but was later culture negative after 3 weeks of erythromycin. The authors noted that the response to therapy was related to the severity of asthma (the milder the disease, the better the results). They hypothesized that *C. pneumoniae* can produce chronic infection leading to chronic airway inflammation and bronchial hyperresponsiveness in susceptible individuals.

Current asthma therapies are palliative, not curative. For unknown reasons, asthma morbidity and mortality are rising worldwide. Since the underlying cause(s) for asthma are unknown, carefully controlled randomized trials of antibiotics in various asthma patient populations are clearly warranted to determine the appropriate role for antibiotic treatment of asthma in children and adults.

References

1. Kawane H (1993) *Chlamydia pneumoniae*. Thorax 48:871
2. Hahn DL (1994) Infection as a cause of asthma. Ann Allergy 73:276
3. Hahn DL (1995) Treatment of *Chlamydia pneumoniae* infection in adult asthma: a before-after trial. J Fam Pract 141:345-351
4. Emre U, Roblin PM, Gelling M et al (1994) The association of *Chlamydia pneumoniae* infection and reactive airway disease in children. Arch Pediatr Adolesc Med 148:727-732
5. Hahn D, Bukstein D, Luskin A et al (1998) Evidence for *Chlamydia pneumoniae* infection in steroid-dependent asthma. Ann Allergy Asthma Immunol 80:45-49

Treatment of Chronic Infection with *Chlamydia pneumoniae* in Asthma

P. Black

In recent years evidence has emerged that *Chlamydia pneumoniae* may have a role in the pathogenesis of asthma. As a result preliminary studies have been conducted on the use of anti-chlamydial antibiotics in subjects with asthma and serological evidence of infection with *C. pneumoniae*. These studies are discussed below.

David Hahn suggested a role for *C. pneumoniae* in asthma after he and his colleagues conducted a study of 365 subjects who presented with an acute respiratory illness in a primary care setting [1]. Nineteen of the subjects had acute infection with *C. pneumoniae* diagnosed serologically. Nine of these individuals had wheezing as part of their acute presentation, and four of them developed newly diagnosed asthma with this illness. Hahn and his colleagues went on to report a small case control series which demonstrated an association between IgA (but not IgG) antibodies to *C. pneumoniae* and in adults with recent-onset asthma (odds ratio = 3.7, 95% CI 1.2–11.5) [2]. Other workers have also reported an association between *C. pneumoniae* and asthma. Bjornsson and co-workers measured antibodies to *C. pneumoniae* in 197 adults who had been enrolled in the European Community Respiratory Health Survey [3]. Twenty-two per cent of the subjects with bronchial hyperresponsiveness had elevated levels of IgA to *C. pneumoniae*, compared with 8% of subjects without bronchial hyperreponsiveness (odds ratio = 3.3, 95% CI 1.3–8.3). There was no association between the geometric mean titre of IgG antibodies and bronchial hyperresponsiveness. Cook et al. compared titres of antibodies to *C. pneumoniae* in 46 subjects with severe chronic asthma with 1518 subjects admitted to hospital with diagnoses other than asthma or COPD [4]. The subjects with severe asthma were significantly more likely to have IgG antibodies ≥ 1:64 or IgA antibodies ≥ 1:8.

Macrolide antibodies have activity against *C. pneumoniae,* but interest in the steroid-sparing properties of macrolides in patients with asthma predates the first description of *C. pneumoniae* by many years. In 1959 Kaplan and Goldin reported that troleandomycin (TAO), a macrolide antibiotic, was useful in the treatment of "infectious asthma" and led to a reduction in the requirement for medication, including steroids [5]. Itkin and Menzel confirmed these observations in a small controlled trial with 12 subjects. They demonstrated significant improvements in lung function with TAO and suggested that this might be due to inhibition of corticosteroid metabolism [6]. Spector et al. confirmed that the use of TAO allowed a reduction in the dose of methylprednisolone in a larger study with 74 subjects [7]. It was Szefler and his colleagues who showed that TAO did indeed inhibit the metabolism of the methylprednisolone and led to an increase in the half-life of methylprednisolone from 2.46 h to 4.63 h [8]. Although it is clear that the main effect of TAO is to inhibit the metabolism of corticosteroids, there has been an ongoing debate about whether macrolide antibiotics might have other properties wich are useful in the treatment of asthma [9]. Several uncontrolled studies have demonstrated a greater reduction in the dose of methylprednisolone than one would expect solely from the effects of TAO on the metabolism of corticosteroids. An example is the study by Flotte and Loughlin, where the dose of methylprednisolone was reduced from 15.3 mg to 1.4 mg per day in nine children treated with TAO [10]. In addition, three open uncontrolled studies with macrolide antibiotics have been performed in patients with asthma who were not on treatment with oral corticosteroids. Miyatake et al. administered 200 mg of erythromycin three times a day for 10 weeks to 23 subjects with asthma who were not on treatment with oral or inhaled corticosteroids or any other asthma medicines [11]. The provocative concentration of histamine required to produce a 20% fall in the FEV_1 (PC_{20}) increased from 0.13 mg/ml to 0.35 mg/ml. In other words, there was a reduction in bronchial hyperresponsiveness and this was of a similar magnitude to the change one would expect to see with inhaled corticosteroids. Another uncontrolled study showed a threefold decrease in bronchial hyperresponsiveness in children with asthma who were treated with roxithromycin for 8 weeks [12]. None of the subjects were on treatment with oral corticosteroids, and theophylline levels did not change during the study. In a similar uncontrolled study, roxithromycin was also reported to reduce bronchial hyperresponsiveness [13].

With open, uncontrolled studies, however, not all of the improvement may be due to the effect of the study medicine. There may be a placebo effect, and participation in a study may improve compliance with other therapies. Nelson and his colleagues addressed this issue by conducting a double-blind, randomised, placebo-controlled study of TAO in the treatment of steroid-dependent asthma [14]. Seventy-five subjects were enrolled. At the end of 1 year, 57 subjects remained in the study. At this time the mean dose of methylprednisolone was 6.3 mg/day in the subjects on TAO and 10.4 mg/day in the placebo group. In addition, steroid side effects were greater in the TAO group. These findings can be explained by the known steroid-sparing effects of TAO. In another double-blind, placebo-controlled trial of TAO, undertaken in 18 children, the reduction in the dose of methylprednisolone was no greater than one would anticipate from the steroid-sparing effects of TAO [15]. These studies do not suggest that TAO has properties which are useful in the treatment of asthma above and beyond their steroid-sparing effect, but it should be borne in mind that there was no specific selection of subjects with evidence of infection with C. pneumoniae.

After he had identified an association between C. pneumoniae and asthma, Hahn conducted a treatment trial [16]. He enrolled 46 adults with asthma who were seropositive for C. pneumoniae. In this group the mean duration of asthma was 5.5 years. This was an open, uncontrolled study and the subjects were treated with either doxycycline, erythromycin or azithromycin. The duration of treatment varied from 3 weeks to 9 weeks. Eighteen of the subjects had a marked improvement in their symptoms and another seven had a complete remission. Emre et al. addressed the issue of treatment for *C. pneumoniae* in a group of children who presented to the emergency department with wheezing [17]. Samples were obtained for culture and serology from 118 children between the ages of 5 years and 16 years when they came to the emergency department. Of these children, 110 had been previously diagnosed with asthma. *C. pneumoniae* was grown from the nasopharyngeal swab in 13 children. Interestingly, seven of the children with positive cultures did not have antibodies to *C. pneumoniae*. Twelve of the children with positive cultures were treated with either erythromycin or clarithromycin for 10 days to 3 weeks and all became culture negative. Nine of these children had a substantial improvement in the symptoms. This was not just due to the resolution of the acute attack, because many were substantially better than they had been before the acute exacerbation. As has already been discussed, open uncontrolled trials have major limitations. Nonetheless, these two studies provide a strong argument for conducting a randomised, controlled trial of anti-chlamydial antibiotics in subjects with asthma who have evidence of infection with *C. pneumoniae*.

My colleagues and I have recently completed a randomised, placebo-controlled, cross-over trial of roxithromycin in subjects with uncontrolled asthma [18]. This study was not originally designed to look at the effect of treating *C. pneumoniae* infection in patients with asthma. Indeed, our original hypothesis was that roxithromycin had anti-inflammatory effects, but we did perform a post-hoc analysis to look at the effect of *C. pneumoniae* serology on the response to treatment. Subjects were eligible to take part in the study if they were on treatment with ≥400 µg of inhaled steroids and had daily symptoms and an $FEV_1 < 80\%$ of predicted. These subjects were not on treatment with oral corticosteroids. There were two 4-week treatment periods separated by a 4-week washhout period. Subjects received either 150 mg b.i.d. of roxithromycin or matching placebo in the first treatment period and the alternate treatment in the second treatment period. The endpoints were peak expiratory flow rate (PEFR), symptom scores and the use of rescue medication as recorded by the subjects on daily diary cards. There were 19 subjects, with a mean age of 51.8 ± 2.8 years and a mean FEV_1 of $60.3 \pm 3.6\%$ of predicted. Surprisingly the subjects fared better during treatment with placebo than with roxithromycin. During the last 2 weeks of each treatment period the mean morning PEFR was 323 l/min with roxithromycin and 336 l/min with placebo ($p = 0.06$). Daytime symptom scores were 1.9 for roxithromycin and 1.7 for placebo ($p = 0.04$), and the average use of rescue medication during the day was 3.9 puffs for roxithromycin and 3.5 puffs for placebo ($p = 0.02$).

Thirteen of the 19 subjects had antibodies to *C. pneumoniae*. For the post-hoc analysis the subjects were classified into three groups:
1. IgG ≥1:64 and IgA ≥1:16 ($n = 4$)
2. IgG ≥1:64 and IgA <1:16 ($n = 9$)
3. IgG <1:64 and IgA <1:16 ($n = 6$)

In contrast to the other two groups, the subjects with IgA antibodies ≥1:16 fared better during the treatment with roxithromycin. In this group, with positive IgA antibodies, the mean morning PEFR was 273 l/min with roxithromycin and 254 l/min with placebo ($p=0.05$). The other endpoints also favoured roxithromycin although they were not statistically significant.

It is not clear why unselected subjects fared worse with roxithromycin than placebo. It is possible that roxithromycin has unanticipated pro-inflammatory effects. Certainly in mice roxithromycin has been shown to promote release of IL-1 and TNF-α from peritoneal macrophages [19]. The observation of a benefit of treatment with roxithromycin in subjects with IgA antibodies is of interest in view of the epidemiological findings linking IgA antibodies to *C. pneumoniae* with asthma. Great caution should be exercised, however, in interpreting post-hoc analyses involving small numbers of subjects, because the findings may well have arisen by chance. If nothing else, our findings provide a reason for conducting further studies.

Clearly there is a need for a large, randomised, controlled trial to look at the effect of treatment for *C. pneumoniae* in subjects with asthma and high titres of antibodies to *C. pneumoniae*. Such a study is under way at the present time. The CARM study (*Chlamydia pneumoniae*, asthma, roxithromycin, multinational study) is being conducted in Australia, New Zealand, Italy and Argentina. To be eligible subjects have to be between 18 and 60 years old and have a diagnosis of asthma, an FEV_1 between 5% and 90% of predicted and bronchodilator reversibility of ≥15%. The subjects also need to have a high enough symptom score and IgG antibodies to *C. pneumoniae* ≥1:64 and/or IgA antibodies ≥1:16. The subjects are randomised to 6 weeks' treatment with roxithromycin 150 mg b.i.d. or placebo. The subjects are then followed up for 6 months. Prior to, during and after treatment with roxithromycin or placebo the subjects record their PEFR, symptoms and medication use on a daily diary card. Other endpoints are quality of life as measured using the Asthma Quality of Life Questionnaire [20] and changes in the titre of antibody to *C. pneumoniae*. Two hundred and forty subjects have been randomised to treatment, and the study will be completed in 1999.

Cleary it is too early to know whether antibiotic treatment for *C. pneumoniae* will be helpful in the management of asthma. The result of the CARM study is awaited with interest. It is worth remembering, however, that *C. pneumoniae* is an intracellular pathogen and may not be easily eradicated with short courses of antibodies. Hammerschlag et al. described a number of subjects who remained culture positive for *C. pneumoniae* despite treatment with one or more courses of tetracycline or doxycycline of up to 3 weeks' duration [21]. Even when a subject becomes culture negative this does not necessarily mean that the organism has been eradicated – it may persist in the body in a latent form. There are anecdotal reports of subjects whose asthma improved while they were on treatment with anti-chlamydial antibiotics but became worse again after the antibiotic was discontinued [9]. These observations raise important questions about the design and interpretation of future studies to treat chronic infection with *C. pneumoniae*. Will it be enough to suppress infection with *C. pneumoniae,* or do we need to eradicate this organism? If we do need to eradicate it, will treatment with one antibiotic suffice or will combination therapy with two or more antibiotics be necessary? For how long will we need to continue this treatment? Even when the result of the CARM study is available, it may raise as many questions as it answers.

References

1. Hahn DL, Dodge R, Golubjatnikov R (1991) Association of *Chlamydia pneumoniae* (strain TWAR) infection with wheezing, asthmatic bronchitis and adult onset asthma. JAMA 266:225-230
2. Hahn DL, Anttila T, Saikku P (1996) Association of *Chlamydia pneumoniae* IgA antibodies with recently symptomatic asthma. Epidemiol Infect 117:513-517
3. Bjornsson E, Hjelm E, Janson C, Fridell E, Boman G (1996) Serology of *Chlamydia* in relation to asthma and bronchial hyperresponsiveness. Scand J Infect Dis 28:63-69
4. Cook PJ, Davies P, Tunnicliffe W, Ayres JG, Honeybourne D, Wise R (1998) *Chlamydia pneumoniae* and asthma. Thorax 53:254-259
5. Kaplan MA, Goldin M (1959) The use of triacetyloleandomycin in chronic infectious asthma. In: Welch H, Marti-Ibauez F (eds) Antibiotic annual 1958-1959. Interscience, New York, pp 273-276
6. Itkin IH, Menzel ML (1970) The use of macrolide antibiotic substances in the treatment of asthma. J Allergy 45:146-162
7. Spector SL, Katz FH, Farr RS (1974) Troleandomycin: effectiveness in steroid-dependent asthma and bronchitis. J Allergy Clin Immunol 54:367-379
8. Szefler SJ, Rose JQ, Ellis EF, Spector SL, Green AW, Jusko WJ (1980) The effect of troleandomycin on methylprednisolone elimination. J Allergy Clin Immunol 66:447-451
9. Black PN (1996) The use of macrolides in the treatment of asthma. Eur Respir Rev 6:240-243
10. Flotte TR, Loughlin GM (1991) Benefits and complications of troleandomycin in young children with steroid-dependent asthma. Pediatr Pulmonol 10:178-182
11. Miyatake H, Taki F, Taniguchi H, Sizuki R, Takagi K, Satake T (1991) Erythromycin reduces the severity of bronchial hyperesponsiveness in asthma. Chest 99:670-673
12. Shimizu T, Kato M, Mochizuki H, Tokuyama K, Morikawa A, Kuroume T (1994) Roxithromycin reduces the degree of bronchial hyperresponsiveness in children with asthma. Chest 106:458-461
13. Kamoi H, Kurihara N, Fujiwara H, Hirata K, Takeda T (1995) The macrolide antibacterial roxithromycin reduces bronchial hyperresponsiveness and superoxide anion production by polymorphonuclear leukocytes in patients with asthma. J Asthma 32:151-197
14. Nelson HS, Hamilos DL, Corsello PR, Levesque NV, Buchmeier Ad, Bucher BL (1993) A double-blind study of troleandomycin and methylprednisolone in asthmatic subjects who require daily corticosteroids. Am Rev Respir Dis 147:398-404
15. Kamada AK, Hill MR, Ikle DN, Manon Brenner A, Szefler SJ (1993) Efficacy and safety of low-dose troleandomycin therapy in children with severe, steroid-requiring asthma. J Allergy Clin Immunol 91:873-882
16. Hahn DL (1995) Treatment of *Chlamydia pneumoniae* infection in adult asthma: a before-after trial. J Fam Pract 41:345-351
17. Emre U, Roblin PM, Gelling M, Dumornay W, Rao M, Hammerschlag MR, Schacter J (1994) The association of *Chlamydia pneumoniae* infection and reactive airway disease in children. Arch Pediatr Adolesc Med 148:727-732

18. Black PN, Bagg B, Brodie SM, Robinson E, Cooper B (1998) A double-blind, crossover study of roxithromycin in the treatment of asthma. Eur Respir J 12[Suppl 28]:190s (abstract)

19. Kita E, Sawaki M, Mikasa K, Hamada K, Takeuchi S, Maeda K, Narita N (1993) Alterations of host response by a long term treatment of roxithromycin. J Antimicrob Chemother 32:285-294

20. Juniper EF, Johnston PR, Borkhoff CM, Guyatt GH, Boulet LP, Haukioja A (1995) Quality of life in asthma clinical trials: comparison of salmeterol and salbutamol. Am J Respir Crit Care Med 151:66-70

21. Hammerschlag MR, Chirgwin K, Roblin PM, Gelling M, Dumornay W, Mandel L, Smith P, Schachter J (1992) Persistent infection with *Chlamydia pneumoniae* following acute respiratory illness. Clin Infect Dis 14:178-182

Chlamydia pneumoniae Infections in Children

G.L. Biscione, S.L. Johnston

Introduction

There has been considerable recent interest in the role of *Chlamydia pneumoniae* (CP) infection in both adults and children. The major interest with regard to children relates to its role in causing atypical pneumonia, and its possible role in the pathogenesis of bronchial, asthma. The prevalence of childhood asthma and other wheezing disorders has increased over the past few decades in most parts of the world [1]. This illness causes substantial morbidity and mortality in children, and their management is associated with increasing healthcare costs [2]. The etiology of asthma is complex, involving interactions between genetic susceptibility, allergen exposure and external aggravating factors such as air pollution, smoking and respiratory infections. The nature of the relationship between viral and bacterial infections in early childhood and the development of recurrent wheezing is controversial. The relationships between wheezing, coughing and respiratory distress and age, gender, atopy, viral infections, congenital structural abnormalities and baseline lung function (airway mechanics and hyperresponsiveness) are also dynamic and complex [3].

In the past decade the importance of viral upper respiratory tract infections in acute exacerbations of asthma in both adults and children has been highlighted [4–6]. More recently a possible role for atypical bacteria, such as *Mycoplasma* and CP in the pathogenesis of asthma has been proposed. It has been suggested that the CP infection may have crucial importance in both the initiation and exacerbation of bronchial asthma. The data concerning *Mycoplasma pneumoniae* relate to a possible role for infection in the pathogenesis of severe asthma in adults [7], while those for CP are more complex. In this chapter we will discuss CP infection in children.

Chlamydia pneumoniae, Childhood Pneumonia and Childhood Asthma

Studies Using Culture and/or Serology

CP is a recently discovered third species of the genus *Chlamydia* [8]. It has been associated with atypical pneumonia, exacerbations of chronic obstructive airway disease and atherosclerosis [9, 10]. In the past decade attention has been focused on the interaction between CP and bronchial asthma [11]. Although considerable knowledge has been accumulated about CP infections in adults, comparatively little information exists about the role of this pathogen in the etiology of respiratory tract infections in infants and younger children.

When CP infections are symptomatic, atypical pneumonia is the most common clinical syndrome associated with the infection. Cough, sore throat and sinusitis are also common features and have a more gradual onset than is the case with other infectious agents such as viruses, *Legionella pneumophila* or *Mycoplasma* species. However, asymptomatic infection is also one of the characteristics of CP and this has often been documented in childern of 6–12 years of age [12]. Although frequently asymptomatic, CP infection is common in children [13], and several studies have reported the presence of CP in children using culture and/or serology. A multicenter study in the USA on children aged 3–12 years with radiographically confirmed community-acquired pneumonia found evidence of infection with CP, by serology or nasopharyngeal culture, in 28% of patients studied [14]. Interestingly, serological evidence of acute infection was found in only 23% of the patients with CP isolated from nasopharyngeal culture.

Among subjects in Iceland [15], using the micro-immunofluorescence (MIF) test, immunoglobulin G (IgG) seropositivity rates were found to be relatively low in children aged under 10 years (14%) but rose linearly with age, reaching 66% in the 60- to 69-year group. Very similar results were obtained in a study in Slovenia, where MIF IgG antibody was detected in 9% of children under 5 years but the proportion rose with age, reaching 65% in those over 50 years [16].

It is clear, then, that CP antibody detection rates rise with increasing age: they are very low in young children, but the majority of 70-year-old individuals have evidence of a previous infection [17].

Because wheezing is a key symptom during respiratory infections in infancy and childhood and one of the most frequent causes of consultation in pediatric practice, it has been hypothesized that otherwise aymptomatic CP infection may result in the first symptoms of a newly diagnosed asthmatic syndrome or an exacerbation of previously known asthma in children.

Emre et al., in their study on asthmatic children [18], were among the first to highlight the importance of chlamydial infections in exacerbations of asthmatic children. They studied 118 children with acute episodes of wheezing and 41 healthy controls, and found 11% of asthmatic and 5% of control children to be culture positive for CP in nasopharyngeal specimens. The culture-positive wheezy children were given open antibiotic treatment, and 75% showed clinical improvement after eradication of the organism.

Serological and culture-based studies suggest that CP infections are generally quite rare before 3 years of age and occur mainly after 5 years. But it should be emphasized that the prevalence of CP is widely underestimated, with a large proportion of infections being asymptomatic. Furthermore, even symptomatic infections may be underestimated due to the lack of sensitive serological or culture procedures to obtain a specific diagnosis. Tissue culture of respiratory secretions or nasopharyngeal aspirate for isolation of organisms is difficult compared to *C. trachomatis,* and many serological tests rely on complement fixation, which is not species specific. More complicated "specific" tests, such as the MIF test, although widely used and the best avialable current methodology, can cross-react with other *Chlamydia* species [19, 20]. For this reason, recent years have seen the development of more sensitive techniques for detecting chlamydial infections, such as the polymerase chain reaction.

Studies Using the Polymerase Chain Reaction

The development of the PCR has provided an alternative diagnostic method for etiological agents that are difficult to culture or detect by other methods [21]. PCR assays have been developed for detection of rhinoviruses and human coronaviruses, and also for CP [22–24].

Recently, more than 300 children seeking attention for acute respiratory infections were investigated for evidence of CP infection in a study by Normann et al. [25]. Serology was found useful for diagnosis of infection only in children over 5 years of age. Using PCR, prevalences of 8% and 10% of CP were found in male and female children aged less than 2 years; 17% and 19%, respectively, in the age group 2–4 years; and 32% and 21% in the age group 5–16 years. These investigators concluded that younger children were more often found to have a moderate disease, but might have been ill for a long period.

In another study, Jantos et al. [26] examined oropharyngeal specimens to esthablish the prevalence of CP in a large number of infants and children admitted to hospital because of acute lower respiratory tract infection. This was one of the few studies to use cell culture, PCR, enzyme immunoassay and serology for the detection of CP infection. Of 290 patients with a mean age of 3.7 years, only 3 (1%) were found to be infected with CP.

In recent years we have carried out several studies using nested PCR for the major outer membrane protein (MOMP) of CP. We chose PCR rather than serology because we were interested in the presence of this atypical organism rather than in past infection. In the initial study employing this technique, we used a DNA-based PCR to detect simple presence of the organism. We investigated 290 nasal aspirate samples taken from 9- to 11-year-old children with acute asthma exacerbations. The positivity rate was only 1% of specimens, suggesting that in the year and populations studied, CP was not a major pathogen associated with asthma exacerbations [27]. The sensitivity of the PCR used for this study was relatively low, detecting infection with around 10^4 organisms. We therefore used a nested PCR to increase the sensitivity to around 5 organisms. We found much higher identification rates than expected. In a longitudinal analysis 47% of the children were positive at some stage during the year-long study, and in a cross-sectional analysis the prevalence of CP infection was 24%. Interestingly, the detection rate did not differ between asymptomatic children and those with exacerbations (28% and 24% respectively). Several children were positive on more than one occasion, and those that were positive were more likely to be positive when subsequently tested than those who had previously been negative ($p > 0.05$), suggesting chronic infection. Sequence analysis confirmed the identity of the organism and revealed no sequence variations also suggesting chronic infection. Independent PCR for a different part of the genome confirmed the initial results and thus eliminated the possibility of contamination with plasmid DNA [27]. Of further interest was the finding of a similar frequency of children with CP-specific IgA in their nasal secretions (30% of children had raised levels), and a correlation between the presence of CP by PCR and the level of IgA, again suggesting chronic infection. Finally, we found a significant relationship between the level of IgA and the number of asthma exacerbations the children reported during the study ($p < 0.001$), suggesting a relationship between the immune response to CP and asthma severity [27].

Chronic Infection

The above data strongly suggest that chronic colonization of the respiratory tract with CP is likely. Therefore, investigation of the proinflammatory responses induced by chronic infection of the respiratory tract may be of great interest in understanding the pathogenesis of athma associated with CP infection.

In order to confirm our results in a separate population, we subsequently studied 37 infants and 41 children admitted to Southampton General Hospital with acute respiratory illness (wheeze, bronchiolitis, pneumonia or upper respiratory tract symptoms). In this study we used a nested reverse transcription (RT) PCR method to detect CP RNA and thus recognize replicating organisms. The prevalence of CP observed was high in infants and increased with age (from 18% in children under 3 months of age to 58% in children over 5 years of age, p for trend < 0.08). The overall rate of CP positivity for the 78 children was 37% [28]. These data suggest that the prevalence of CP infection in this population of wheezy children is much higher than previously suspected, and further studies comparing normal and wheezy children are clearly required.

Confirming the speculation that CP infection may become chronic especially in the lung, in an American study [29], CP was eradicated from the nasopharynges of 26 (78.8%) of 33 children and adults with community-acquired pneumonia who were treated with azithromycin. The investigators tested 55 isolates of CP obtained from 46 of these patients in vitro against azithromycin. Seven patients remained culture positive after treatment. The minimal inhibitory concentrations (MICs) of azithromycin for isolates from two patients increased fourfold after therapy. However, all patients with persistent infection improved clinically despite the presence of CP.

Immunity to *Chlamydia pneumoniae* in Children

Multiple or repeat infections with CP are common, suggesting that there is little natural immunity to chlamydial infections [30], and the intracellular and indeed intravacuolar life cycle of *Chlamydia* makes immunity complicated. However, there is evidence that acquired immunity develops with repeated exposure to *Chlamydia* infection. IgG, IgM and IgA responses to CP have all been detected. Indeed serological studies have demostrated IgG antobody with increasing prevalence by age: from <5% in children under 5 years of age, through 5%–10% in children 5–10 years of age and 30%–40% in teenagers to 50% in the middle-aged and elderly [31].

In the study by Emre et al. [18], CP was isolated in 13% of the patients and eradication of chlamydial infection resulted in clinical and spirometric improvement of the airway disease. Later, the same investigators [32] demonstrated the presence of anti-CP IgE by immunoblotting in 85.7% of culture-positive patients with wheezing, in contrast to only 9.1% of culture-positive patients with community-acquired pneumonia who were not wheezing. The presence of anti-CP IgE by immunoblotting was not associated with the presence of anti-CP IgG and IgM by immunofluorescence. The results of this study suggested that the production of specific IgE may be an underlying mechanism leading to reactive airway disease in some patients with CP infection.

We have recently demonstrated the ability of CP to infect Hep-2 repiratory epithelial cells in a chemically defined culture minimal medium supplement (HITES) and have examined the effects on pro-inflammatory cytokine release. Messenger RNA levels of interleukin-6 (IL-6) and IL-8 were found to be elevated over the 72-h study period in the infected cells compared with the uninfected controls. It is likely the function of the cytokines released from epithelial cells is to act either alone or in synergy with other pro-inflammatory factors to attract and activate inflammatory cells such as neutrophils. This would provide an important early signaling system for the initiation and development of the mucosal immune response in the early stages of infection [33].

Conclusions

In this chapter we have reviewed evidence that CP is an important cause of community-acquired lower respiratory tract infections in children. Furthermore, CP may well also be involved in the pathogenesis of bronchial asthma at a very early age in life. It may also have a key role in the development of respiratory disease both in acute infections and via chronic colonization.

Most previous epidemiological investigations of CP infection in children have been based on serological studies which have problems with species specifity, and may therefore over- or underestimate the importance of this atypical pathogen. In addition, because not all CP infections evoke detectable systemic antibody responses, serological studies may have underestimated the true prevalence of CP. We should also consider that many of the previous studies were not specifically designed to address the questions they have studied and therefore have clear shortcomings in terms of patient numbers, control populations and detection methods. The development of more advanced techniques of molecular biology such as PCR will enable rapid diagnosis, which may be helpful in determining of the most appropriate chemotherapy.

Younger children represent a dynamic population in which genetic and environmental influences interact in a still poorly understood way. Whether CP can act as an adjuvant in early atopic airway sensitization, or could be involved in the pathogenesis of transient wheezy syndromes, is a fascinating area of speculation. Further research into the role of CP in respiratory disease in children is clearly required.

References

1. Hahn DL (1996) Intracellular pathogens and their role in asthma: *Chlamydia pneumoniae* in adult patients. Eur Respir Rev 6:38,224-230
2. Pedersen S, Silverman M, Martinez F (1998) Early intervention in childhood asthma. Eur Respir J 12:1-2
3. Martinez FD, Wright AL, Taussig LM, Holberg CJ, Halonen M, Morgan WJ (1995) Asthma and wheezing in the first six years of life. The Group Health Medical Associates. N Engl J Med 332:133-138
4. Pattemore PK, Johnston SL, Bardin PG (1992) Viruses as precipitants of asthma symptoms. I. Epidemiology. Clin Exp Allergy 22:325-336
5. Johnston SL, Pattemore PK, Sanderson G, Smith S, Lampe F, Josephs L, Symington P, O'Toole S, Myint SH, Tyrrell DAJ, Holgate ST (1995) Community study of role of viral infections in exacerbations of asthma in 9-11 year old children. 310:1225-1228
6. Nicholson KG, Kent J, Ireland DC (1993) Respiratory viruses and exacerbations of asthma in adults. BMJ 307:982-986
7. Kraft M, Cassell GH, Henson JE, Watson H, Williamson J, Marmion BP, Gaydos CA, Martin RJ (1998) Detection of *Mycoplasma pneumoniae* in the airways of adults with chronic asthma. Am J Respir Crit Care Med 158:998-1001
8. Grayston JT (1989) *Chlamydia pneumoniae*, strain TWAR. Chest 95:664-669
9. Blasi F, Legnani D, Lombardo VM (1993) *Chlamydia pneumoniae* infection in acute exacerbations of COPD. Eur Respir J 6:19-22
10. Saikku P, Leinonen M, Mattila M, Ekman P, Nieminen MS, Makela PH, Huttunen JK, Valtonen V (1988) Serological evidence of an association of a novel *Chlamydia*, TWAR, with coronary heart disease and acute mycardial infarction. Lancet ii:983–986
11. Hahn DL, Dodge RW, Golubjatnikov R (1991) Association of *Chlamydia pneumoniae*, strain TWAR, infection with wheezing, asthmatic bronchitis and adult onset asthma. JAMA 226:225-230
12. Thomas B, Taylor-Robinson D (1996) *Chlamydia pneumoniae* infections. In: Mynt S, Taylor-Robinson D (eds) Viral and other infections of the human respiratory tract. Chapman & Hall, London, pp 341-357
13. Hyman CL, Augenbraun, MH, Roblin PM, Schachter J, Hammerschlag MR (1991) Asymptomatic respiratory tract infection with *Chlamydia pneumoniae* TWAR. J Clin Microbiol 29:2082-2083
14. Block S, Hedrick J, Hammerschlag MR, Cassel GH, Craft JC (1995) *Mycoplasma pneumoniae* and *Chlamydia pneumoniae* in pediatric community-acquired pneumonia: comparative efficacy and safety of clarithromycin vs. erythromycin ethylsuccinate. Pediatr Infect Dis J 14:471-477
15. Einarsson S, Sigurdsson HK, Magnusdottir SD, Eriendsdottir H, Briem H, Gudmundson S (1994) Age specific prevalence of antibodies against *Chlamydia pneumoniae* in Iceland. Scand J Infect Dis 26:393-397

16. Kese D, Hren-vencelj H, Socan M, Beovic B, Cizman M (1994) Prevalence of of antibodies to *Chlamydia pneumoniae* in Slovenia. Eur J Clin Microbiol Infect Dis 13:523-524

17. Saikku P (1994) Diagnosis of acute and chronic *Chlamydia pneumoniae* infections. In: Orfila J, Byrne GI, Chernesky MA et al (eds) Chlamydial infections. Proceedings of the 8th International Symposium on Human Chlamydial Infections, Chantilly, pp 163-72

18. Emre U, Roblin PM, Gelling M Dumornay W, Rao M, Hammerschlag MR, Schachter J (1994) The association of *Chlamydia pneumoniae* infection and reactive airway disease in children. Arch Pediatr Adolesc Med 148:727-732

19. Bourke SJ (1993) Chlamydial respiratory infections. BMJ 306:1219-1220

20. Ozanne G, Lefebvre J (1992) Specificity of the microimmunofluorescence assay for the serodiagnosis of *Chlamydia pneumoniae* infections. Can J Microbiol 38:1185-1189

21. Saiki RK, Scharf S, Faloona F, Mullis KB, Horn GT, Erlich HA, Armheim N (1985) Enzymatic amplification of B-globulin genomic sequences and restriction site analysis for the diagnosis of sickle-cell anemia. Science 230:1350-1354

22. Gaydos CA, Quinn TC, Eiden JJ (1992) Identification of *Chlamydia pneumoniae* by DNA amplification of the 16s RNA gene. Clin Microbiol 30:796-800

23. Campbell LA, Perez Melgosa M, Kuo C-C, Grayston JT (1992) Detection of *Chlamydia pneumoniae* by polymerase chain reaction. J Clin Microbiol 30:434-439

24. Johnston SL, Cunningham A,Ward M (1993) The polymerase chain reaction in the diagnosis of *Chlamydia pneumoniae* infections in clinical samples. Am Rev Respir Dis 147:A573

25. Normann E, Gnarpe J, Gnarpe H, Wettergren B (1998) *Chlamydia pneumoniae* in children with acute respiratory tract infections. Acta Paediatr 87:23-27

26. Jantos CA, Wienpahl B, Schiefer HG, Wagner F, Hegemann JH (1995) Infection with *Chlamydia pneumoniae* in infants and children with acute lower respiratory tract disease. Pediatr Infect Dis J 14:117-122

27. Cunningham AF, Johnston SL, Julious SA, Lampe FC, Ward ME (1998) Chronic *Chlamydia pneumoniae* infection and asthma exacerbations in children. Eur Respir J 11:345-349

28. Biscione GL, Xie P, Johnson A-W BR, Johnston SL (1998) Prevalence of *Chlamydia pneumoniae* in children admitted to hospital with acute respiratory illness using PCR. Am J Respir Crit Care Med 137:A23

29. Roblin PM, Hammerschlag MR (1998) Microbiological efficacy of azithromicin and susceptibilities to azithromicin of isolates of *Chlamydia pneumoniae* from adults and children with community-acquired pneumonia. Antimicrob Agents Chemother 42:194-196

30. Johnston SL (1997) Influence of viral and bacterial respiratory infections on exacerbations and symptom severity in childhood asthma. Pediatr Pulmonol Suppl 16:88-89

31. Ward ME (1997) *Chlamydia* host and host cell interactions. In: McCrae MA, Saunders JR, Smyth CJ, Stow ND (eds) Molecular aspects of host-pathogen interaction. Society for General Microbiology Symposium 55. Cambridge University Press, Cambridge, UK

32. Emre U, Sokolovskaya N, Roblin PM, Schachter J, Hammerschlag MR (1995) Detection of anti-*Chlamydia pneumoniae* IgE in children with reactive airway disease. J Infect Dis 172:265-267

33. Cunningham AF, Johnston SL, Ward ME (1999) Hep-2 epithelial-like cells secrete interleukin-8 in response to infection with *Chlamydia pneumoniae*. FASEB Lett (submitted)

Perspectives and Perceptions on the Clinical Relevance of *Chlamydia pneumoniae* Infection

L. ALLEGRA, F. BLASI, R. COSENTINI

Introduction

Although the identification of *Chlamydia pneumoniae* as a third species of the *Chlamydia* genus may be considered as fairly recent, an impressive wealth of research on this pathogen has been published during the past 10 years. This book has been devised as an attempt to assemble the mass of data at our disposal in an orderly fashion so as to present the reader with a comprehensive and updated review of the very diverse aspects of *C. pneumoniae* infection. This has been made possible by the fact that the chapters are authored either by the "parents" of the discovery of *C. pneumoniae* or by investigators who are currently exploring the most advanced research fields regarding this pathogen.

The microbiological aspects of this third chlamydial species have now been extensively investigated but there are still lines of research that will have to be pursued. The diagnostic methods currently available to document *C. pneumoniae* infection have been expanded, and polymerase chain reaction (PCR) techniques have been successfully and increasingly applied in both acute and chronic infection. In this book the potential usefulness of PCR is fully addressed, and its application in combination with serology seems the most promising diagnostic method for chronic *C. pneumoniae* infection.

The chapters devoted to the epidemiological and clinical aspects of *C. pneumoniae* infection illustrate the worldwide diffusion of this micro-organism and the wide spectrum of both respiratory and extrapulmonary presentations of infection.

However, some lines of research will require particular attention in the future. In this chapter we will highlight those aspects we feel present the greatest interest in terms of social impact and understanding of the basic mechanisms of disease.

Chlamydia pneumoniae Infection in Chronic Bronchitis and Asthma

Chronic obstructive pulmonary disease (COPD) is still a major cause of morbidity and mortality in many countries. Smoking has been identified as the principal risk factor, but only a minority of cases of COPD can be explained by smoking. The role of infections in this disease is still controversial.

The role of *C. pneumoniae* infection in acute exacerbations of COPD has been demostrated by different groups, and approximately 5%–10% of exacerbations appear to be involved. However, more important is the possibility that COPD patients may harbor chronic *C. pneumoniae* infection. In these patients the relevance of chronic infection may be twofold: persistence of the micro-organism in the respiratory tract may facilitate access of different pathogens to the lower airways; longstanding infection might trigger what is traditionally described as the vicious circle of chronic bronchitis. According to this hypothesis infection may both play an etiological role in the development of the disease and act as a worsening factor. Epithelial damage, impairment of defense mechanisms and an increase in the inflammatory and oxidative burden within the airways may all accelerate the functional and anatomical derangements associated with the disease.

Similarly, *C. pneumoniae* infection is now felt to be responsible for approximately 10% of acute exacerbations of asthma. More intriguing is the possibility that persistent *C. pneumoniae* infection participates in asthma inflammation and acts as a co-factor in asthmatic episodes. Large-scale intervention trials are currently under way to test the effect of anti-*C. pneumoniae* antibiotic treatment on the natural course of the disease. Given the overall rise in asthma prevalence worldwide, these studies are of particular importance.

Chlamydia pneumoniae Infection in Atherosclerosis

The accumulated seroepidemiological, electron-microscopic, immunohistochemical, cultural, and molecular biology data have convincingly demonstrated the existence of an association between persistent *C. pneumoniae* infection and atherosclerosis. The challenge has now shifted to unequivocally demonstrating that *C. pneumoniae* plays a causal role in the development or progression of atherosclerosis, rather than simply act as an innocent bystander. Both animal model studies and intervention trials seem to indicate that *C. pneumoniae* infection may indeed be actively involved in the disease, although definitive conclusions will be drawn only after the completion of ongoing large-scale trials. A future line of research will be the definition of subsets of coronary heart disease patients who will benefit most from treatment to eradicate *C. pneumoniae*. For example, unstable angina patients, in whom infection/inflammation may play an active part in plaque instability, are plausible candidates for extensive treatment trials.

Should the role of *C. pneumoniae* infection be confirmed in chronic respiratory and extrapulmonary diseases, eradication of this micro-organism and/or prevention of infection by means of large-scale vaccination may prove to have a major impact on public health worldwide.